Advances in UPPER EXTREMITY SURGERY AND REHABILITATION

Advances in UPPER EXTREMITY SURGERY AND REHABILITATION

Edited by

John A. Boswick, Jr., MD, FACS

Attending Surgeon
Saint Joseph, General Rose, and Veterans Hospitals
Former
Professor of Surgery
and
Chief, Hand Surgical Service
University of Colorado

AN ASPEN PUBLICATION®
Aspen Publishers, Inc.

1986

Rockville, Maryland
Royal Tunbridge Wells

Aspen Publishers, Inc.
1600 Research Boulevard
Rockville, Maryland 20850

Library of Congress Cataloging in Publication Data

Advances in upper extremity surgery and rehabilitation.

Updated and expanded versions of presentations made at the 12th Annual Rocky Mountain International Symposium on Hand Surgery, held in Vail, Colo., in Aug. 1984.
"An Aspen publication."
Includes bibliographies and index.
1. Hand—Surgery—Congresses. 2. Extremities, Upper—Surgery—Congresses. I. Boswick, John A., 1926–
II. Rocky Mountain International Symposium on Hand Surgery (12th : 1984 : Vail, Colo.) [DNLM: 1. Arm—surgery—congresses. 2. Arm Injuries—rehabilitation—congresses. WE 805 A244]
RD559.A27 1986 617'.57 86-3448
ISBN 0-87189-286-3

Printed in the United States of America
1 2 3 4 5

Contents

Preface

In this book experts from around the world present the most recent concepts and techniques in upper extremity surgery and rehabilitation. During the past several years there have been numerous advances in upper extremity surgery, including the treatment of rheumatoid disease, the management of fractures and burn injuries. Studies in the fields of joint motion and the pathomechanics of joint deformities following disease and injury have provided information that has made possible more accurate diagnosis and selective treatment methods. These topics are covered in a complete and concise manner in this volume.

Dr. Damian Ireland gives us, in an easily understood manner, his current thoughts on *Carpal Kinematics* and *Bone Grafting for Scaphoid Nonunion.* A most comprehensive chapter on *The Rheumatoid Wrist,* a subject of vital importance to a hand surgeon, has been contributed by Dr. Lennart Mannerfelt. Chapters on *Injuries of the Wrist* and *Mallet Finger* are clearly and logically presented by Mr. Neville Kay. The chapter on Flaps by Dr. Ravin Thatte is an elaborate and detailed presentation. Mr. Thomas Wadsworth's chapters on *Injuries of the Capitular Epiphysis* and the Pathomechanics of Deformity of the MP joints are from the most recent work in rheumatic diseases and the hand. Dr. Juan Fernandez' outstanding chapter on *Supracondylar Fractures of the Phalanges* is one of the most clearly written articles on this subject. The latest techniques in managing The Burned Hand are discussed by Raymond Warpeha. The chapters on Shoulder Reconstruction by Melvin Post, and Total Wrist Arthroplasty by Robert Volz, reflect most recent advances in these areas.

Advances In Upper Extremity Surgery and Rehabilitation had its start at the 12th Annual Rocky Mountain International Symposium on Hand Surgery held in Vail, Colorado in August 1984. At the Symposium the speakers discussed their latest ideas, practices, and thoughts on potential changes in practice. They have updated and expanded these presentations for inclusion here.

We hope this volume will both interest and assist all those who have the privilege of working with hand patients.

John A. Boswick, Jr., M.D.

Contributors

Juan Angelats, M.D., F.A.C.S.
Assistant Professor of Surgery
Loyola University Stritch School of Medicine
Maywood, Illinois

John A. Boswick, Jr., M.D., F.A.C.S.
former Professor of Surgery and Chief, Hand Surgery Service
University of Colorado Health Sciences Center
Denver, Colorado

Mack L. Clayton, M.D.
Clinical Professor of Surgery (Hand)
University of Colorado Health Sciences Center
Denver, Colorado

Donald C. Ferlic, M.D.
Assistant Clinical Professor of Surgery
University of Colorado Health Sciences Center
Denver, Colorado

David G. Ferguson, M.D.
Consultant in Accident and Emergency Medicine
Royal Hallamshire Hospital
Sheffield, England

Juan M. Fernandez Vazquez, M.D., F.A.C.S.
Assistant Professor of Surgery
Nacional Hospital of Mexico
Mexico City, Mexico

Charles Hamlin, M.D.
Assistant Clinical Professor of Surgery (Hand)
University of Colorado Health Sciences Center
Denver, Colorado

Robert Horner, M.D., F.A.C.S
Assistant Clinical Professor of Orthopedic Surgery
University of Colorado Health Sciences Center
Denver, Colorado

Damian C.R. Ireland, M.D., F.R.A.C.S.
Orthopedic Surgeon
Alfred Hospital, Monash University
Windsor, Victoria, Australia

Neville R.M. Kay, M.D., F.R.C.S.
Consultant Orthopedic Surgeon
Royal Hallamshire Hospital
Sheffield, England

Laurance A. Kirwan, M.D., F.R.C.S.
former Instructor in Surgery
University of Colorado Health Sciences Center
Denver, Colorado

Claude A. Luekens, Jr., M.D.
Assistant Clinical Professor of Surgery
University of Colorado Health Sciences Center
Denver, Colorado

Lennart Mannerfelt, M.D.
Hand Unit Goldenbuhl Hospital
University of Tubingen
Villingen, West Germany

Pat McKenna, O.T.R.
Staff Occupational Therapist
St. Anthony Hospital
Denver, Colorado

Marilyn Meyers, O.T.R
Staff Occupational Therapist
St. Anthony Hospital
Denver, Colorado

Nashaat Naam, M.D.
former Instructor in Surgery
University of Colorado Health Sciences Center
Denver, Colorado

R. Oetker, M.D.
Hand Unit Goldenbuhl Hospital
University of Tubingen
Villingen, West Germany

Uddhav A. Patil, M.S., M.Ch.
Lecturer
Department of Plastic Surgery
Lokmanya Tilak Municipal Medical College
Bombay, India

Melvin Post, M.D., F.A.C.S.
Professor of Surgery
Northwestern University
Chicago, Illinois

Debbie Post, O.T.R
Staff Occupational Therapist
Rose Medical Center
Denver, Colorado

Ravin L. Thatte, M.D.
Honorary Professor and Head Department of Plastic Surgery
Lokmanya Tilak Municipal Medical College
Bombay, India

Robert G. Volz, M.D., F.A.C.S.
Professor of Orthopedic Surgery
University of Arizona Health Sciences Center
Tucson, Arizona

Thomas G. Wadsworth, M.Ch.Orth, F.R.C.S.(Eng), F.A.C.S.
Consultant Orthopaedic Surgeon
St. Bartholomew's, Homerton, and St. Leonard's Hospitals;
Consultant in Hand Surgery
Manor House Hospital;
Honorary Lecturer
Medical College of St. Bartholomew's Hospital
London University
London, England

Raymond L. Warpeha, M.D., F.A.C.S.
Professor of Surgery
Loyola University Stritch School of Medicine
Maywood, Illinois

Richard A. Warren, M.D., F.R.C.S.
Senior Registrar in Accident and Emergency Medicine
Royal Hallamshire Hospital
Sheffield, England

1

Rheumatoid Disease of the Shoulder

Donald C. Ferlic and
Mack L. Clayton

Surgery to the shoulder in patients with rheumatoid arthritis is a relatively infrequent event; in our series of patients who have undergone surgery, only 4% had shoulder surgery.[1] The reasons that shoulder surgery is not commonly necessary are:

- Decreased glenohumeral function can often be compensated by normal scapulothoracic motion.
- Shoulder involvement is usually insidious.
- Patients with multiple involved joints often draw attention to other joints.
- Nonoperative treatment, including physical therapy, an occasional steroid injection, and rest, is often adequate to control pain.

Lower extremity surgery must be considered first in the patient with multiple joint involvement, because this will put less demand on the shoulder for crutch walking and perhaps eliminate the necessity for surgery. The patient who will most likely require shoulder surgery is the one who has multiple upper extremity joint involvement with pain and needs the shoulder to position the hand.

Indications and Contraindications

Patient selection is extremely important when considering major reconstructive shoulder surgery. A considerable amount of physical therapy is necessary to obtain optimal results, and surgery on an unmotivated patient is sure to bring disappointment. Surgery should be considered when pain is not controlled by good medical management and is unresponsive to conservative measures. Surgery has been very successful in relieving pain, but caution should be taken when considering shoulder surgery in the rheumatoid patient for decreased range of motion without pain. A moderate gain in motion in some patients with multiple joint involvement, however, may be enough to increase their functional capacity by allowing them to fulfill the most important function of the shoulder, that is, to permit the patient to reach the top of the head and both ends of the gastrointestinal tract.

Preoperative Evaluation

Our preoperative radiological evaluation includes an anteroposterior (AP) view in internal rotation and axillary and Grashey views in external rotation of the shoulder. The Grashey view is taken with the x-ray tube angled at 35° to the patient's shoulder (Fig 1-1). This opens the glenohumeral joint, making evaluation of the articular surface possible (Fig 1-2). The standard AP view is necessary to evaluate the acromioclavicular joint. The axillary lateral view demonstrates subluxation and loss of glenoid bone stock. Arthrograms may be helpful when a large rotator cuff tear is suspected, to better plan the operative procedure. It is also useful to review the postoperative exercises before surgery so the patient has a good idea of what will follow.

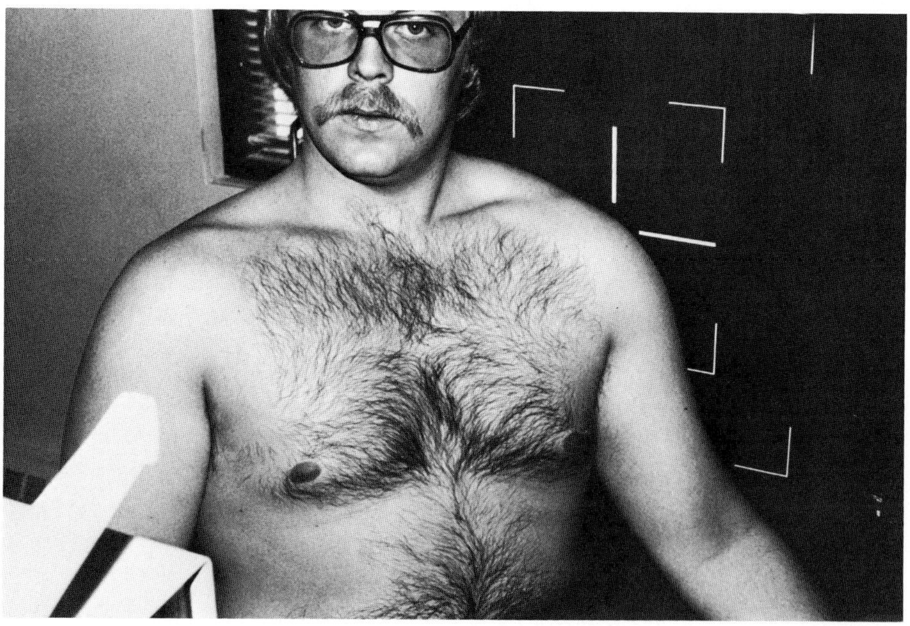

Fig 1-1. Method of taking Grashey view of the shoulder with x-ray beam angled 35° to the shoulder.

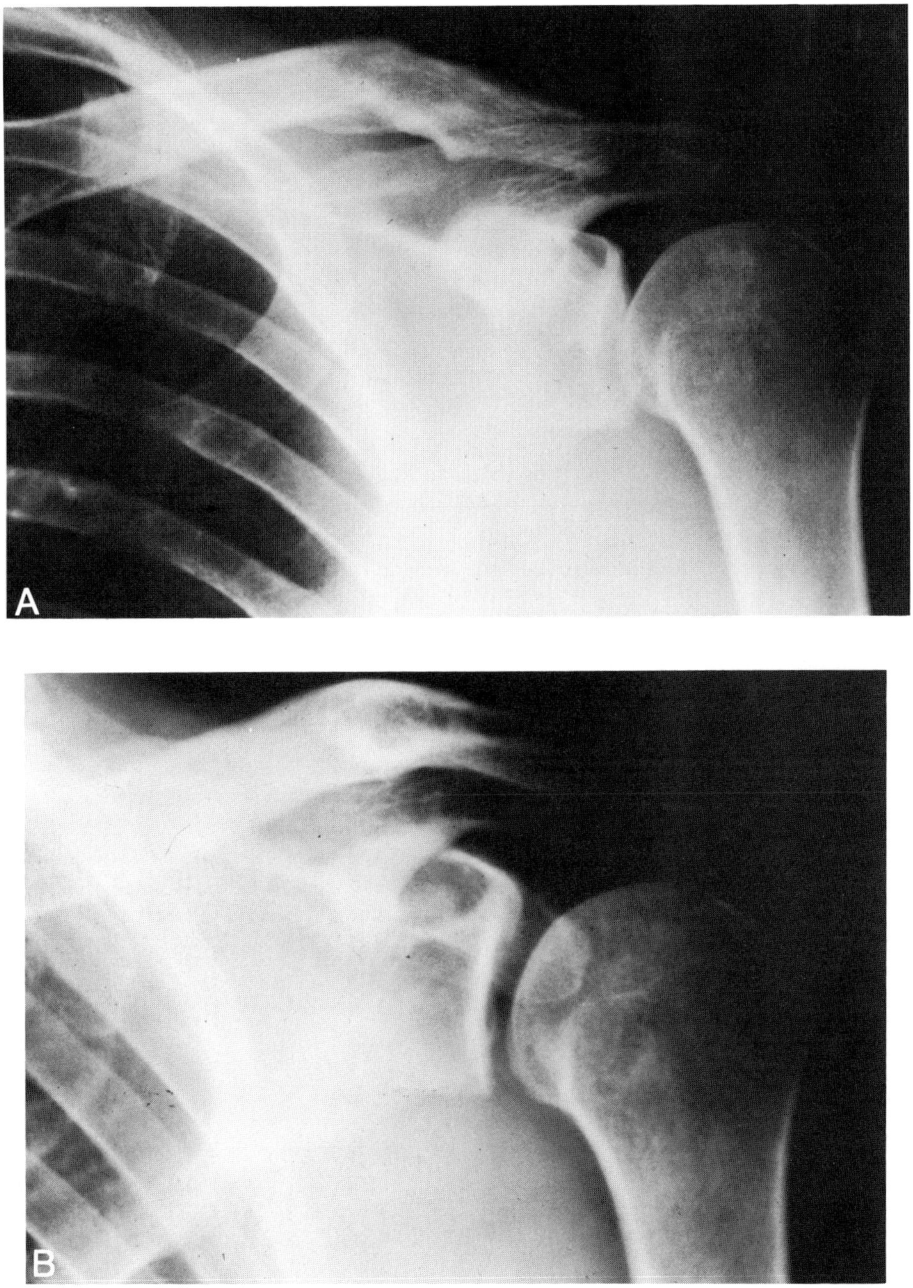

Fig 1-2. *A,* Standard AP view of the shoulder. *B,* Grashey view showing the articular surface of the shoulder joint.

Treatment Options

In the last decade the emphasis of surgery of the rheumatoid shoulder has certainly been on prosthetic arthroplasty, just as it has been for other joints,[2-12] but it is important that other procedures not be forgotten, as they might be useful in earlier stages of the disease before prosthetic arthroplasty is indicated.

Any of the several bursae about the shoulder may become inflamed and swollen. Painful bursitis can be treated with a local steroid injection, but excision may be necessary. The subdeltoid is the most commonly involved bursa and may be large and painful. Resection of the distal end of the clavicle[8,13,14] may be all that is necessary to relieve pain if it can be shown that the pain originates from the acromioclavicular joint. This may sometimes be the site of symptoms, even though there are x-ray changes in the glenohumeral joint. An injection of local anesthetic into the acromioclavicular joint may help make the diagnosis.

Synovectomy in stage II disease may relieve pain and retard the destructive processes.[13,15,16] Synovectomy of the bursa and glenohumeral joint is occasionally successful and may be indicated to relieve pain where there is good motion and preservation of articular cartilage. We have found arthroscopic synovectomy to be a valuable procedure for relieving pain in the patients with rheumatoid synovitis with normal articular surfaces on x-ray (Fig 1-3). Total acromionectomy has been shown to relieve pain in stage III disease with excellent range of motion resulting.[13,17] This procedure should be done rarely because the deltoid power is weakened, shoulder stability is diminished, and crutch walking, which may be necessary in the rheumatoid patient, may be

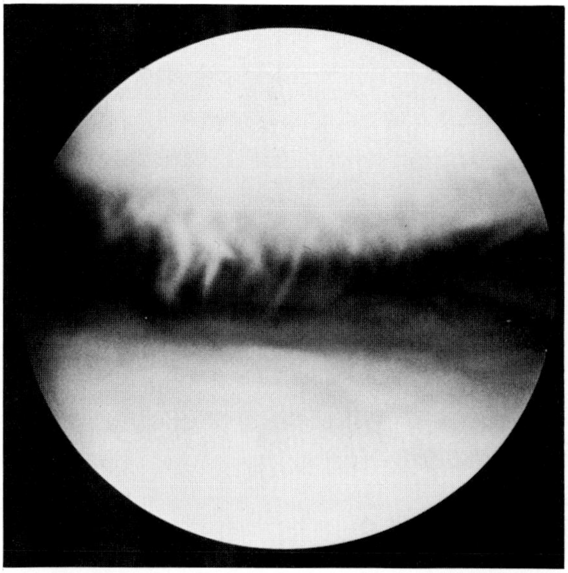

Fig 1-3. Arthroscopic view of a shoulder with degenerative changes in the articular surface of the humerus. The humeral head is on top; the glenoid is on the bottom. The glenoid labrum is visualized in the background to the right.

difficult. Neer and Marberry[18] flatly condemn radical acromionectomy because of persistent pain and weakness of the shoulder. Instead, the anterior acromioplasty, as advocated by Neer,[19] which eliminates the above objections, is used. The bicipital tendon may become inflamed, frayed, or ruptured. The intra-articular portion of this tendon may need to be resected and the remainder of the tendon decompressed from beneath the transverse humeral ligament.

The rotator cuff is a frequent source of symptoms in the rheumatoid shoulder. Simple tendinitis can often be treated with anti-inflammatory medication or an occasional steroid injection, but frequent injections are not used because of increased incidence of tendon rupture and articular cartilage degeneration. Tendinitis and bursitis may give rise to impingement at the coracoacromial arch, and decompression is indicated; this is performed by excision of the coracoacromial ligament and an anterior acromionectomy. Small holes in the rotator cuff may require repair, but large rotator cuff tears may be more difficult in the rheumatoid patient because of attenuation of tissue. Some cases of rotator cuff rupture are irreparable even with extensive mobilization of the supraspinatus, superior transposition of the scapularis, or use of a bicipital tendon patch.

Three other procedures in particular need to be mentioned. The first, osteotomy of the glenoid and humeral neck (double osteotomy) has been shown by Benjamin et al[20] to relieve pain and increase the joint space by x-ray appearance. The second procedure is glenoidectomy. This is not as good as a total shoulder prosthesis, but it has been effective in relieving pain. (Fig 1-4). The third procedure is arthrodesis. We agree with those who feel that there is no place for shoulder fusion in rheumatoid arthritis[13,20] because of the multiple-joint component of the disease. Others[14] believe that if other joints in the extremity are mobile and the disease is quiescent, arthrodesis may be considered. We have seen one such patient in whom arthrodesis was performed but other joints became debilitated later on, and the stiff shoulder, although painless, proved to be a marked hindrance.

Prosthetic replacement is now the mainstay of shoulder surgery for rheumatoid arthritis. All of the preceding procedures are occasionally useful by themselves or in conjunction with replacement surgery. Prosthetic replacement of the shoulder joint has been developed because less radical procedures, such as resectional arthroplasties and arthrodeses, have failed consistently to produce satisfactory results.

There are two types of total shoulder prostheses. One is the nonconstrained type, such as those designed by Neer and Gristina, and the other is the constrained device, such as the Michael Reese prosthesis designed by Post,[12] which may be useful in cases of dislocation, irreparable rotator cuff tears, or paralysis. We feel that the nonconstrained shoulder prosthesis should be used in all but the most unusual cases of rheumatoid arthritis, and our experience has been mostly with the Neer device, starting first with the hemiarthroplasty. A subacromial spacer (Fig 1-5) was then introduced, to be used with an irreparable rotator cuff. This was first made out of chromium-cobalt alloy and was used without

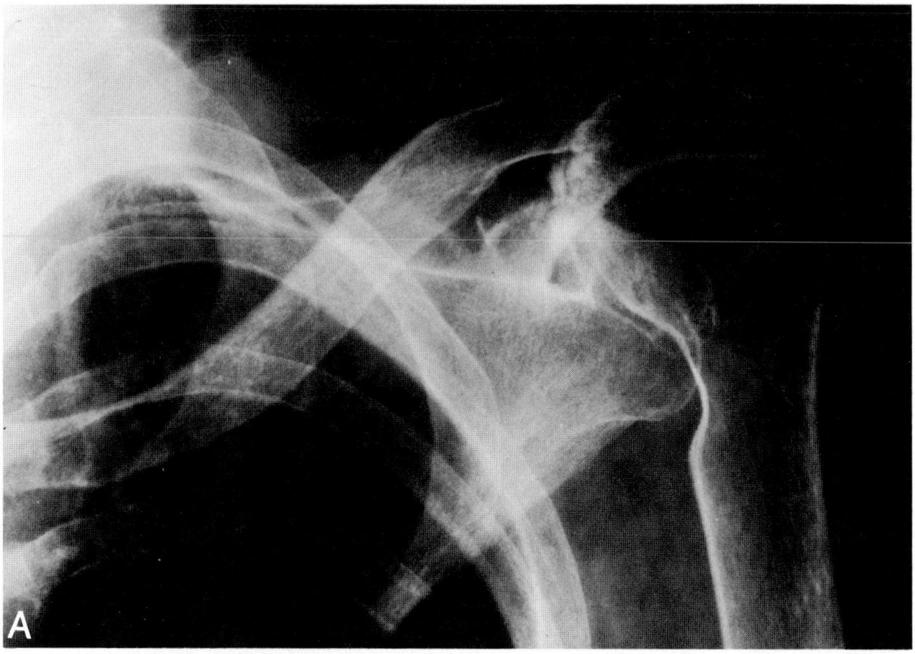

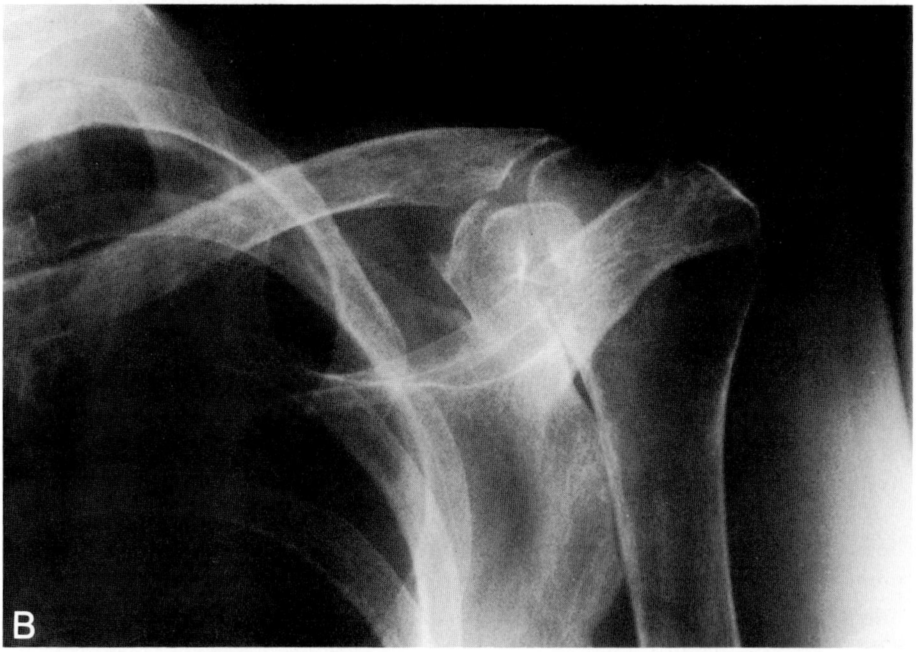

Fig 1-4. *A,* Preoperative x-rays of a patient with severe destruction of the shoulder and bone loss of the glenoid and impingement of humerus on the glenoid. *B,* Postoperative glenoidectomy. There was not enough bone stock and rotator cuff present to do a total shoulder.

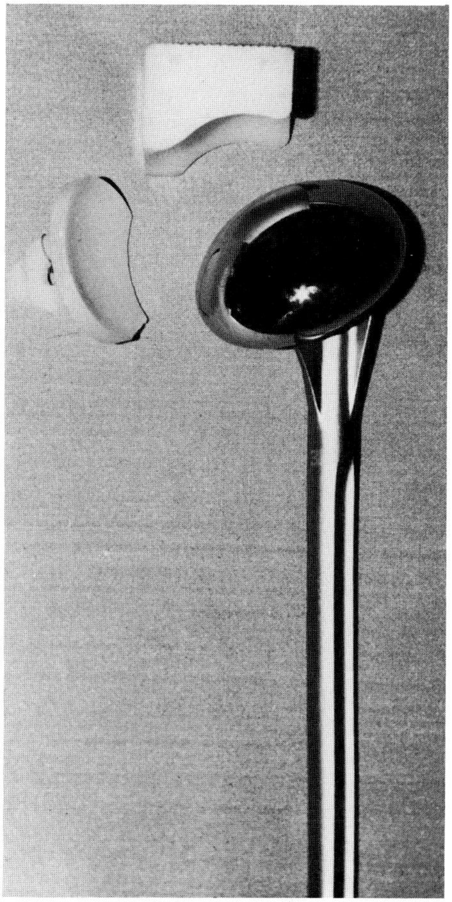

Fig 1-5. Neer total shoulder replacement with subacromial spacer.

any other devices. It was designed to depress the humeral head, thereby giving the deltoid a better mechanical advantage, enabling this muscle to initiate abduction and act as a rotator cuff. In addition, the spacer changes the relative position of the articular surfaces, similar to performing an osteotomy. This spacer is now used only in conjunction with the Neer humeral prosthesis in cases of an irreparable rotator cuff. The glenoid component completing the total shoulder was then developed.

The Denver Orthopedic Clinic has divided shoulder prosthetic arthroplasties into three groups: In group I are those in which the Neer humeral replacement was used alone; in group II are those in which the humeral replacement was used in conjunction with a subacromial spacer; and in group III are those with the humeral component and the glenoid replacement. The glenoid component has been used in all of the recent humeral implants in rheumatoid arthritis because of the erosion of the glenoid occasionally seen after several years when the vitallium humeral head has been left to articulate with the articular cartilage of the glenoid.

Operative Technique

A deltopectoral incision extending from the acromioclavicular joint to the axilla is made. The deltoid is not released from its bony origin. The tendinous portion of the subscapularis is divided, leaving enough tendon attached distally for later repair.

If the shoulder has an internal rotation contracture, the subscapularis is divided by beveling the tendon so that it can be lengthened when closing. The capsule of the shoulder joint is opened.

The decision should be made whether to use the subacromial spacer. If the rotator cuff is not torn or can be repaired, the coracoacromial ligament is excised and an anterior acromionectomy is carried out by removing a minimal wedge of bone. If there are arthritic changes in the acromioclavicular joint, the distal clavicle is excised. A synovectomy is carried out if boggy synovium is present. The bicipital tendon helps to stabilize the shoulder and is left in place if possible, but if it has already torn, the intra-articular portion is excised and the distal end stabilized onto the humerus. The proximal end of this tendon can sometimes be used to aid in the repair of a rotator cuff tear. If the spacer is to be used, the coracoacromial ligament and the acromion must be present. The humeral head is then dislocated and the articular surface excised. At this point we have to make our final decision as to what type of arthroplasty is needed. If the glenoid articular surface is uninvolved, we prepare the intramedullary canal of the humerus with rasps. Trial reductions begin with a small-stemmed humeral component. Once we have determined the proper size, a larger-stemmed component is used. This may result in a tight press-fit, but we do not hesitate to use cement fixation if there is any question of component stability. All of our recent cases of rheumatoid arthritis have undergone total shoulder replacement. In this situation, the humeral implantation is the last step in our procedure.

The spacer is attached to the coracoacromial ligament by two #2 Dacron sutures (Fig 1-6). This fixation is adequate and allows the spacer to seek the best mechanical position following surgery.

Osteophytes are trimmed as necessary, allowing visualization of the true glenoid. A high-speed bur prepares the glenoid surface. The surgeon defines the scapular neck with the fingers and carefully burs a seating hole in a position to accept the stem of the glenoid component. Only the cartilage is removed from the remainder of the glenoid, and the subchondral bone is not removed. The component is cemented in place under pressurization. The humerus is prepared and trial reductions of both components are completed. If cement is to be used, as in most cases, the humerus is plugged just distal to the stem. The cement is injected and the humeral component cemented. If the rotator cuff must be repaired, the long head of the biceps tendon may be taken down from its glenoid insertion and used for repair. It can be widened by longitudinal splitting if the defect requires a larger graft. The biceps stump is reattached distally. The subscapularis can also be used for rotator cuff reinforcement by dividing a portion and advancing it superiorly and distally, or it can be length-

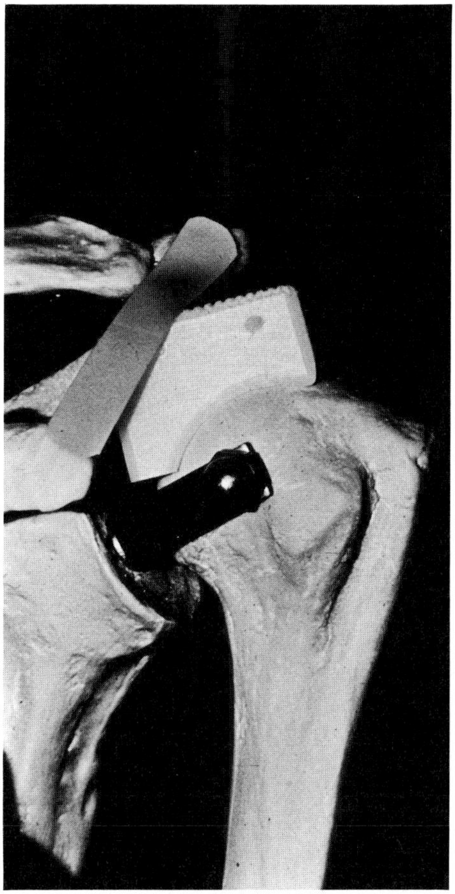

Fig 1-6. Subacromial spacer in position against the coracoacromial ligament. This polyethylene component is designed to be used with a Neer prosthesis.

ened if the internal rotation contracture limits external rotation to the neutral position. The wound is closed and the patient placed in a sling and swathe, unless it was necessary to perform an extensive rotator cuff repair. In these cases, a humeral foam-rubber splint or an airplane splint is used to keep the arm in 60° of forward flexion.

Postoperative Rehabilitation

Patients are encouraged to perform hand, wrist, forearm, and elbow motion in the first 3 days following surgery. Therapy is divided into three stages. Stage I lasts from 4 days to 3 weeks. In this stage, only passive and gentle assisted exercises are done. Pendulum exercises and passive range of motion are begun on the 4th day. Motion is limited only by the integrity of the repair when tested at the time of surgery. This is especially true for external rotation exercises. The subscapularis repair is protected by internally rotating and adducting the arm

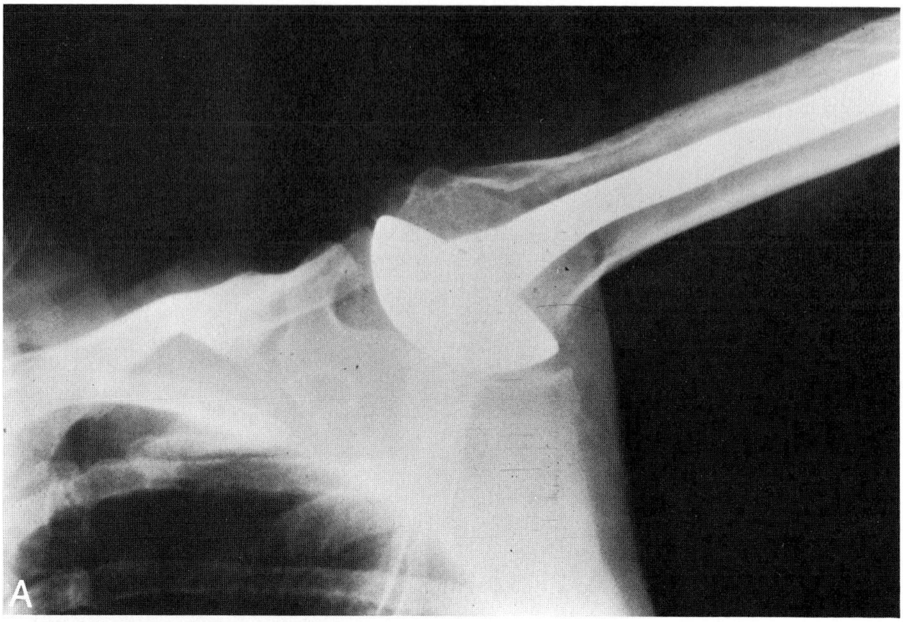

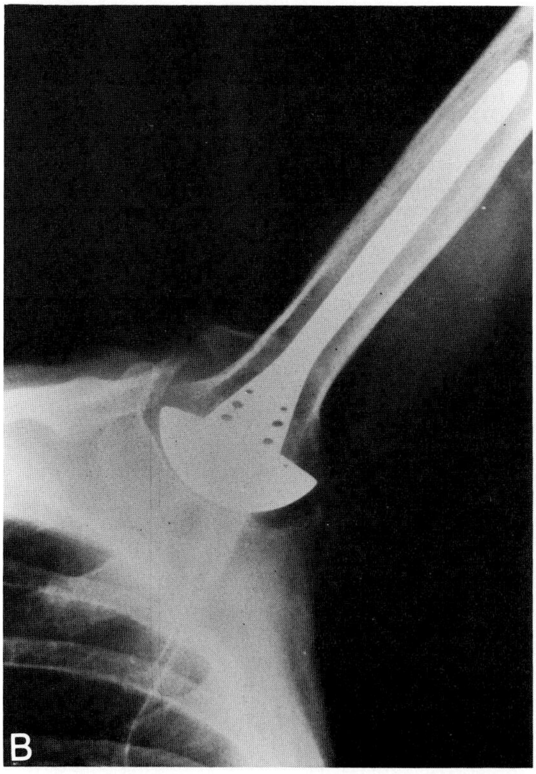

Fig 1-7. *A,* Immediate postoperative x-rays showing position of the prosthesis in relationship to the glenoid. *B,* Five-year postoperative x-rays showing erosion of the glenoid.

for all forward flexion exercises. At the end of 1 week the sling may be discarded during the daytime and active assisted exercises are begun.

Stage II lasts from 4 to 6 weeks. In addition to active assisted exercises, gentle active exercises may be added, depending on the patient's musculature, needs, and strength of repair. Active motion is started at the beginning of the 4th postoperative week. If the deltoid muscle has not been detached at the time of surgery, active motion quickly progresses.

Stage III starts 6 weeks after surgery. Active resistive exercises are added to the active exercise program. It is *important* to treat each patient as an individual and adjust the rehabilitation schedule according to the specific surgical repair.

Results

Good pain relief can be expected and was found in 85% of our patients followed for a minimum of 2 years. There may be a limited increase in motion, however. Therefore, if replacement arthroplasty is done for the painless, stiff shoulder, the end result may turn out to be a very disappointed patient.

Shoulders with a hemiarthroplasty fared about as well as those with a total replacement at 2 years, but we have seen cases in the rheumatoid patient where the glenoid eroded after this procedure and became painful several years later (Fig 1-7).

Motion was less in the shoulder with the spacer than in those in which the glenoid was used, but in the latter group the tissues were of poorer quality. Pain relief was the same (Fig 1-8).

In our series there were no infections, nerve problems, or cases of clinical loosening, in spite of the presence of radiolucent lines around the cement and the fact that some of the humeral components were not cemented in place. Two patients with only the humeral head replaced showed erosion of the glenoid 5 years later, and one of these developed arthritis- type pain. One patient had a recurrent dislocation of the humeral head. Further surgery was recommended.

One should expect the results from limited surgery to the shoulder for rheumatoid arthritis to be quite satisfactory if done for the proper indications, such as resection of the distal clavicle for limited acromioclavicular disease or anterior acromioplasty for impingement condition or synovectomy for early disease. Rheumatoid arthritis is a progressive disease, and one should expect that the eventual outcome in the shoulder will lead to replacement arthroplasty. Therefore, limited surgery that will preclude replacement arthroplasty at a later time should not be done.

Conclusion

Few operations are done on the shoulders of patients with rheumatoid arthritis. This is not because surgery is not successful, but because problems in other

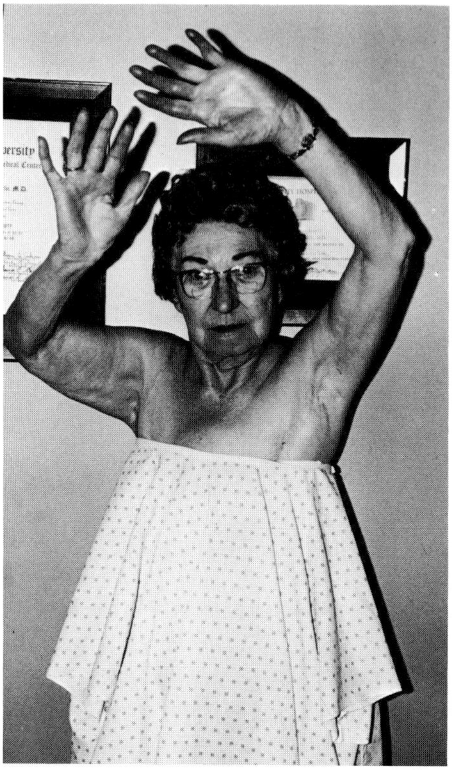

Fig 1-8. Range of motion 8 years after shoulder replacement with a subacromial spacer and Neer humeral replacement.

joints take precedence, and conservative treatment is often successful. The emphasis in treatment has been on replacement arthroplasty, which has been quite effective in the control of pain in the shoulder with severe destruction due to rheumatoid arthritis. Lesser operative procedures, such as synovectomy, partial acromionectomy, or bursa resection, may also give good results in earlier stages of the disease.

References

1. Clayton ML, Ferlic DC, Jeffers PD: Prosthetic shoulder arthroplasties. *Clin Orthop Rel Res* 1982;164:184.
2. Averill R, Sledge C, Thomas WH: Neer total shoulder arthroplasty. *Orthop Trans* 1980;4:287
3. Cofield RH: Status of total shoulder arthroplasty. *Arch Surg* 1977;112:1088.
4. Cofield RH, Morrey BF, Bryan RS: Total shoulder and total elbow arthroplasties: The current state of development. *JCE Orthop* 1978; (pt 1, December):14.
5. Marmor L: Hemiarthroplasty for the rheumatoid shoulder joint. *Clin Orthop* 1977;122:201.

6. Neer CS II: Articular replacement for the humeral head. *J Bone Joint Surg Am* 1964;46A:1607.
7. Neer CS II: The rheumatoid shoulder, in Gruess RE, Mitchell N (eds): *Surgery of Rheumatoid Arthritis.* Philadelphia, JB Lippincott Co, 1971.
8. Neer CS II: Replacement arthroplasty for glenohumeral osteoarthritis. *J Bone Joint Surg Am* 1974;56:1.
9. Neer CS II, Gruess RL, Sledge CB, et al: Total shoulder replacement: A preliminary report, abstracted. *Orthop Trans* 1977;1:244.
10. Neer CS II, Watson KC, Stanton FJ: Recent experiences in total shoulder replacement. *J Bone Joint Surg Am* 1982;64A:319.
11. Post M, Jablon H, Singh M: Constrained total shoulder joint replacement. A critical review. *Clin Orthop* 1979;144:135.
12. Post M, Haskell S, Jablon M: Total shoulder replacement with a constrained prosthesis. *J Bone Joint Surg Am* 1980;62A:327.
13. Clayton ML, Ferlic DC: Surgery of the shoulder in rheumatoid arthritis. *Clin Orthop* 1975;106:166.
14. Cooney WD, Bryan RS: Rheumatoid arthritis in the upper extremity. Treatment of the elbow and shoulder joints. *American Academy of Orthopaedic Surgeons Instructional Course Lectures* 1979;247.
15. Linscheid RL: Surgery for rheumatoid arthritis—timing and techniques: The upper extremity. *J. Bone Joint Surg Am* 1968;50A:605.
16. Smith-Petersen MN, Aufranc OE, Larson CB: Useful surgical procedures for rheumatoid arthritis involving joints of the upper extremity. *Arch Surg* 1943;46:764.
17. Hammond G: Complete acromionectomy in the treatment of chronic tendinitis of the shoulder. *J Bone Joint Surg* 1962;44A:494.
18. Neer CS II, Marberry TA: On the disadvantages of radial acromionectomy. *J Bone Joint Surg Am* 1981;63A:416.
19. Neer CS II Anterior acromioplasty for the chronic impingement syndrome in the shoulder. *J Bone Joint Surg Am* 1972;54A:41.
20. Benjamin A, Herschowitz D, Arden, GP: The treatment of arthritis of the shoulder joint by double osteotomy. *Int Orthop* 1979;3(3):211.

2

Rotator Cuff Tear: Diagnosis and Treatment

Melvin Post

Rotator cuff disease has been recognized for 150 years since Smith[1] in 1834 first described defects in the capsule joint at the insertion of the supraspinatus tendon. Many others have specifically described rupture of the supraspinatus, which is a major cause of painful shoulder.[2-6] The pathology and pathogenesis of the condition have been defined.[4,7-11] More recently Neer[12] showed that the vast majority of chronic tears of the rotator cuff resulted from an impingement of the rotator cuff tissue primarily against the anterior edge of the acromion and the coracoacromial ligament. Nevertheless, treatment for rotator cuff disease remains a problem.

Small tears are easily repairable, whereas much larger tears are often neglected or misdiagnosed. Many surgeons question the advisability of repairing larger and massive tears. The fact is that most large and massive tears are repairable by a variety of means, and most obtain good functional results in shoulders that often are painfree if certain principles are followed.[10]

Blood Supply and Function of the Rotator Cuff

Lindblom and Palmer[8] showed that there are areas of relative avascularity in the supraspinatus tendon close to its insertion and a similar zone of avascularity in the long head of the biceps near its origin. Others have shown the importance of the anterior humeral circumflex artery and proved that arterial branches perforated the head via the region of the rotator cuff attachment.[13] Codman[4] described a "critical portion" of the rotator cuff located 1 cm medial to the attachment of the supraspinatus tendon, which was later termed the "critical zone."[14] Rothman and Parke[15] showed that the critical zone is hypovascularized in relation to the rest of the cuff. They concluded that it was this region that was most prone to degenerative changes. Rathbun and Macnab[16] found a constant avascularity in this region and suggested that the position of the rotator cuff tendon predisposed it to constant pressure from the humeral head, which squeezed blood from the vessels when the arm was in the resting position of adduction and neutral rotation. Later, Post et al[17] found that when the external rotators were weakened and the deltoid was strong during abduction, there was a greater degree of tension exerted on the rotator cuff tendons with a corresponding increase in the upward displacement of the humeral head. In this case, the capillaries of the rotator cuff are further compressed, and blood flow to the tissues and attendant damage to the fibers may explain in part the pathological condition. A large rotator cuff tear does not preclude the loss of active abduction if deltoid function is good to excellent and impingement in the subacromial space is relieved by a decompression operation that includes a partial anterior acromionectomy described by Neer.[10,12]

Supraspinatus action permits abduction of the arm and is initiated by supraspinatus contraction which continues throughout abduction. Saha[18] described the "zero position" as the position of the arm when the humerus is 165° overhead and 45° anterior to the coronal plane. In this position the short rotator muscles are ineffective, and active rotation is lost. Normal abduction of the shoulder is still possible, because these structures create a fulcrum by depressing the humeral head and holding it against the glenoid while the deltoid exerts its action. Inman et al[19] described the complex interrelationships of the four articulations that constitute the harmonious motion of the shoulder girdle. Poppen and Walker[20] showed that the average excursion of the humeral head on its glenoid surface in the superoinferior plane is less than 1.5 mm between each 30° arc of motion in a normal subject with a normal compressive force. Thus, if rotator cuff function is impaired for any reason or the external rotators are weakened, the corresponding normal fulcrum of the humeral head will be abnormal and an upward translation of the humeral head allowed. The evidence shows that if there is a greater degree of tension, which most likely increases the symptoms, an impingement syndrome can result and will eventually lead to rotator cuff tear.

Classification

Bosworth[21] and McLaughlin[9] employed a classification to treat patients with rupture of the rotator cuff. The lesions can be divided into complete tears of various sizes and incomplete tears. Incomplete tears do not involve the entire thickness of the rotator cuff. Surface tears may cause irregularities and irritation of the bursal floor and are almost always associated with severe impingement. When a direct communication occurs between a subdeltoid or subacromial bursa and the joint cavity, a complete tear is present. These tears may be arbitrarily divided into various sizes as measured in the longest diameter. A small tear is defined as one measuring less than 1 cm, a medium-sized tear as less than 3 cm, and a large tear as less then 5 cm, whereas a massive tear measures more than 5 cm in diameter, usually with retraction of the torn cuff edge.

Surgical Technique

A variety of surgical approaches may be used to repair rotator cuff tears. The author prefers a saber incision starting 1.5 cm medial and slightly anterior to the posterior corner of the acromion and extending forward and slightly medially and laterally over the region of the acromioclavicular joint. Full-thickness skin flaps are raised both medially and laterally. The deltotrapezius aponeurosis is opened transversely with the use of a pointed coagulation needle, and entry into the acromioclavicular joint is avoided unless a resection of the lateral clavicle is planned in advance. The deltoid is elevated from the region of the acromioclavicular joint extending laterally along the anterior and anterolateral acromion. The deltoid muscle is split anteriorly but never more than 3 to 5 cm, depending upon the extent of the pathologic lesion, to avoid injury to the axillary nerve.

Preoperative x-rays and a thorough examination at operation should exclude an os acromiale. If this congenital condition is present it may be removed, if small, and the deltoid reattached to the remaining acromion following repair of the rotator cuff tear. Larger ossa acromiales should be fused if they are unstable and internally fixed with threaded pins bent at the ends because removal of a significant portion of the acromion produces results similar to a total acromionectomy and destroys the fulcrum of the deltoid muscle, giving very poor functional results.

In any event, a Neer partial anterior acromionectomy is performed during this procedure, and the coracoacromial ligament is resected. Bone spurs that may be present at the undersurface of the acromioclavicular joint and impinge upon the rotator cuff are removed. If there is associated severe degeneration of the acromioclavicular joint, especially if the preoperative arthrogram shows a "geyser" sign, the lateral clavicle is resected distal to the coracoclavicular ligament. A total acromionectomy or any other acromionectomy that shortens the acromial process is to be avoided. A subacromial and subdeltoid bursectomy is performed and the tear exposed. As much cuff tissue is mobilized as necessary in large and massive tears to permit effective coverage of the humeral head, although a watertight seal is sought. This is not as important as achieving the proper tension in the rotator cuff tendon that will permit optimum function in the corresponding muscles. The cuff edges are freshened by resecting severely degenerated tissue, but not to the extent of creating a more significant defect. The internal rotator cuff is carefully inspected for significant intimal tears. Intimal tears are repaired, and if the glenohumeral ligament is also torn the edge is freshened and tacked down in situ using 2-0 Vicryl absorbable sutures if the glenohumeral ligament cannot be pulled down to its anatomic position. This is recommended to avoid further tearing and retraction of this portion of the rotator cuff. When the rotator cuff is avulsed, pulled, or retracted from the bone at the anatomic neck, the bone is rongeured to create raw, bleeding bone but not to the extent of creating a large bony defect. This allows restoration of the freshened cuff edge to heal to bone. Heavy nonabsorbable sutures are inserted directly through drill holes in the peripheral bone if needed. The arm is abducted and the sutures are tied, to obviate tearing and undue tension at the repair line. Occasionally, when there is excessive tension at the repair site, one or two staples are required to protect the repair. In exceptionally large and massive tears the supraspinatus muscle may be advanced by opening the superior portion of the capsule and elevating the supraspinatus a few centimeters with a blunt elevator from its fossa. However, the supraspinatus is not advanced as recommended by others.[22] The surgeon must be careful not to overstretch the muscle fibers, or muscle function may be lost. In other cases, the superior portion of the subscapularis may have to be utilized to achieve an adequate closure over the humeral head. In this case, the tendon should be separated from the capsule. Similarly, the teres minor may be advanced to achieve adequate closure of the cuff tissues.

The deltoid and the deltoid tendon are then firmly reattached to their bony origin by means of drill holes placed through the lateral clavicle and the anterior and lateral acromion. The deltotrapezius aponeurosis is restored. Large tears require up to 80° abduction using a foam pillow to protect the repair site. The following day all tears greater than 3 cm are treated with plaster of Paris spica cast with the arm in the desired abduction position especially if there is tension upon the repair. After 21 to 25 days the arm is lowered slowly to the side. It may have to be lowered over a period of hours or days to avoid severe pain. Active assistive and passive motion exercises are then started and gradually increased for as long as 4 to 6 months. The muscles of the shoulder girdle are gently strengthened during this period. If the repair is secure, then motion exercises may be started after several days following surgery.

Indications for Operation

Surgery is recommended if a tear is known to be present and there is unremitting pain and loss of function. Very small tears may sometimes be treated conservatively. However, it a tear is thought to be extensive and function decreases, surgery is recommended. With acute tears operation is recommended in the first 7 to 10 days to avoid increasing shoulder muscle girdle atrophy. The earlier such surgical treatment is performed, the better is the functional result. In addition, a congruous, nonarthritic joint must be present. If severe cuff arthropathy is known to exist, the surgeon must be prepared to perform a prosthetic replacement of the shoulder rather than merely performing a repair of a rotator cuff tear that will most certainly fail.

Diagnosis

Every patient who is diagnosed as having a rotator cuff tear usually has severe pain and weakness of the external rotator and deltoid muscles to varying degrees. Preoperative muscle strength testing is not always objective because pain often precludes full testing of muscle strength. Many patients have crepitus and pain when elevation is tested against resistance. Forceful flexion against the anterior acromion (positive impingement sign) causing pain is ordinarily relieved by the injection of 10 ml of 1% lidocaine into the subacromial space. When there has been a long-standing, extensive tear a greater degree of muscle atrophy is present than with medium-sized tears.

Routine x-rays often show a decrease in the normal space between the superior humerus and the undersurface of the acromion to less than 5 mm in older large and massive tears.[11,23] Cyst formation at the insertion of the supraspinatus tendon into the humerus, irregularity and sclerosis of the greater tuberosity, exaggeration of the groove between the greater tuberosity and the peripheral articular surface, and sclerosis of the undersurface of the acromion may be observed.

Arthrograms, either single contrast or double contrast using air, are recommended as a means of confirming full-thickness rotator cuff tears. When there is degeneration of the acromioclavicular joint a geyser sign may be present. In any event, there is no specific correlation between the amount of dye leakage and the extent of the tear observed at surgery. The physical examination is considered more reliable in correlating the extent of the tear than the arthrogram.

Results

Patients with small and medium-size tears that are correctly repaired usually achieve excellent results. Even large and massive tears give excellent results if the rotator cuff tear is adequately closed and there is residual muscle function. Pain relief is significant if impingement is relieved.

In some cases with very large and massive rotator cuff tears the use of polylactic acid-carbon filament ribbon may be used to close large cuff defects. Healing will not result between the torn rotator cuff and its bony insertion if a gap is present because cells do not jump gaps. The flat carbon stent is woven in and out of the rotator cuff and placed through holes large enough (3.2 mm) in diameter to accept the carbon stent so as not to injure the multiple filaments, thereby weakening the material. Carbon filament should be handled with plastic jaw-protected hemostats or forceps and a flat knot obtained. In some cases carbon buttons may be used to protect the repair site and anchor the two ends of the carbon filament into bone. The polylactic acid-carbon filament stent is biodegradable and biocompatible. Preliminary results show that good results can be achieved if the principles of any other rotator cuff repair are followed.

Second operations ordinarily do not give the same good results as initial operations. Patients who have second operations, particularly when a total acromionectomy has been done or there is permanent muscle damage, are advised that the results may be poor with regard to both relief of pain and restoration of function.

Elderly patients and those patients in poor health who can tolerate their pain are advised not to have surgery. Thus, age alone is not the deciding factor as to whether or not a patient should be operated upon.

Conclusion

Early surgical repair of rotator cuff tears with a partial anterior acromionectomy is recommended as a means of achieving a painfree shoulder and restoring function. It is more important to obtain adequate tension in the cuff tissue than to obtain a watertight closure. Patients with chronic complete tears may have good results from a reconstruction of a torn rotator cuff. However, merely closing a rotator cuff tear will not permit a good functional result if the ability of the muscles to contract adequately is lost forever. In those patients who have very significant impingement and need to perform heavy laboring activities, external rotator strength must be restored to near normalcy. Otherwise, many of these patients may have to be retrained for lighter work activities not involving heavy lifting in the overhead position in a repetitive manner, as these are the kinds of patients who often develop impingement symptoms again postoperatively. Finally, a very carefully supervised postoperative rehabilitation program is essential for best results.

References

1. Smith JG: Pathological appearances of seven cases of injury of the shoulder joint, with remarks. *London Medical Gazette* 1834;14:280 (reported in *Am J Med Sci* 1834;16:219.
2. Codman EA: Complete rupture of the supraspinatus tendon. Operative treatment with report of two successful cases. *Boston Med Surg J* 1911;164:708.
3. Codman EA: Obscure lesions of the shoulder: Rupture of the supraspinatus tendon. *Boston Med Surg J* 1927;196:381.
4. Codman EA: *The Shoulder.* Boston, Thomas Todd, 1934.
5. Codman EA: Rupture of the supraspinatus, 1834 to 1934. *J Bone Joint Surg* 1937;19:643.
6. Codman EA, Akerson IB: The pathology associated with rupture of the supraspinatus tendon. *Ann Surg* 1931;93:348.
7. Lindblom K: On pathogenesis of ruptures of the tendon aponeurosis of the shoulder joint. *Acta Radiol* 1939;20:563.
8. Lindblom K, Palmer F: Rupture of the tendon aponeurosis of the shoulder joint—The so-called supraspinatus rupture. *Acta Chir Scand* 1939;82:133.

9. McLaughlin HL: Lesions of the musculotendinous cuff of the shoulder. I. The exposure and treatment of tears with retraction. *J Bone Joint Surg* 1944;26A:31.
10. Post M, Silver R, Singh M: Rotator cuff tear: Diagnosis and treatment. *Clin Orthop Rel Res* 1983;173:78–91.
11. Weiner DS, Macnab I: Superior migration of the humeral head. A radiological aid in the diagnosis of tears of the rotator cuff. *J Bone Joint Surg* 1970;52B:524.
12. Neer CS II: Anterior acromioplasty for the chronic impingement syndrome in the shoulder. A preliminary report. *J Bone Joint Surg Am* 1972;54A:41.
13. Laing PG: The arterial supply of the adult humerus. *J Bone Joint Surg Am* 1956;38A:1105
14. Moseley HF, Goldie I: The arterial patterns of the rotator cuff of the shoulder. *J Bone Joint Surg* 1963;45B:780.
15. Rothman RH, Parke WW: The vascular anatomy of the rotator cuff. *Clin Orthop* 1965;41:176.
16. Rathbun JB, Macnab I: The microvascular pattern of the rotator cuff. *J Bone Joint Surg Br* 1970;52B:540.
17. Post M, Jablon M, Miller H, et al: Constrained total shoulder joint replacement: A critical review. *Clin Orthop* 1979;144:135.
18. Saha AK: Mechanism of shoulder movements and a plea for the recognition of "zero position" of glenohumeral joint. *Indian J Surg* 1950;12:153.
19. Inman VT, Saunders JB, Abbott LC: Observations on the function of the shoulder joint. *J Bone Joint Surg Am* 1944;25A:1.
20. Poppen NK, Walker PS: Normal and abnormal motion of the shoulder. *J Bone Joint Surg Am* 1976;58A:195
21. Bosworth DM: Analysis of 28 consecutive cases of incapacitating shoulder lesions radically explored and repaired. *J Bone Joint Surg* 1940;22:369.
22. Debeyre J, Patte D, Elmelik E: Repair of rupture of the rotator cuff of the shoulder. With a note on advancement of the supraspinatus muscle. *J Bone Joint Surg Br* 1965;47B:36.
23. Cotton RE, Rideout DF: Tears of the humeral rotator cuff. A radiological and pathological necrosy survey. *J Bone Joint Surg Br* 1964;46B:314.
24. Hammond G: Complete acromionectomy in the treatment of chronic tendinitis of the shoulder. A follow-up study of 90 operations on 97 patients. *J Bone Joint Surg Am* 1971;53A:173.

3

Constrained Total Shoulder Arthroplasty

Melvin Post

The vast majority of patients with disease of the glenohumeral joint who can benefit from a prosthetic arthroplasty can be well managed by employing an unconstrained prosthesis with or without a plastic liner.[1,2] A small number of patients will not fare well with an unconstrained prosthesis because the stability needed by these prostheses and provided by the soft tissues for satisfactory results cannot be achieved.[3] These patients are candidates for a fixed-fulcrum or constrained prosthesis.

Although a constrained prosthesis causes highly abnormal stresses on the contiguous bony parts and is much more likely to fail than an unconstrained replacement, this method is still worthwhile under special circumstances. Certain criteria must be met, and the patient must be informed of the attendant risks. First, those patients must be prudently selected who have the most to gain and the least to lose. The operation is a salvage procedure used when glenohumeral motion is desired and other standard operations are not likely to be effective. If a constrained prosthetic replacement fails and is removed, the patient is left with a flail shoulder resembling a resection arthroplasty.

Indications and Contraindications for a Constrained Prosthesis

The chief reason for a prosthetic arthroplasty, with rare exceptions is pain relief. The four anatomic prerequisites for considering a patient as a candidate for a constrained prosthesis are:

1. an intact glenoid face and glenoid vault.
2. strong serratus anterior and trapezius muscles to stabilize the scapula against the chest wall

3. an adequate release of soft-tissue contractures.
4. a strong deltoid muscle if active overhead motion is desired.

A weak or absent deltoid does not preclude the use of a constrained prosthesis if passive motion is acceptable to the patient. However, if a goal of treatment is active elevation, then a relatively strong deltoid muscle is needed.

A constrained prosthesis provides a fixed fulcrum and does not depend on the rotator muscles. It permits a stable range of lateral rotation, abduction, and forward flexion. The indications for constrained joint arthroplasty are:

- the arthritides
- osteonecrosis of the humeral head
- old severe humeral head fracture
- resectable tumor of the proximal humerus, with or without pain
- symptomatic old dislocation or fracture-dislocation
- capsular insufficiency

If the rotator cuff tissues are functional or can be surgically restored, as is the case in many patients, an unconstrained rather than a constrained prosthesis should be performed, especially in patients with osteoarthritis. If a proliferative, florid synovitis is present in the capsular tissue and the tissues are of poor quality as in a cuff arthropathy, especially in an older patient a constrained prosthesis may be considered in exceptional cases. Even in cases of cuff arthropathy an unconstrained prosthesis can still be performed, or at least the prosthesis can be covered well enough to allow some active motion and considerable passive motion. In the last category of capsular insufficiency, it is understood that when the rotator cuff is not salvageable under any circumstances and will not permit active use of an unconstrained prosthesis, then a constrained prosthetic device can be considered as a last resort. The functional loss of the stabilizing short rotator muscles that dynamically fix the humeral head on its glenoid may be caused by an unrepairable massive tear of the rotator cuff wherein the capsular tissues are not present or cannot be identified; by nonunion of the proximal humerus; by excessive resection of the proximal humerus, leading to a flail shoulder; or by severe scarring of the soft tissues whether due to multiple operations, trauma, or radiation treatments. Accordingly, each patient must be carefully assessed before operation to determine the need for a constrained prosthesis.

Equally important is the need to study the contraindications of constrained prosthetic arthroplasty, to minimize a high failure rate and various complications of the surgery. The contraindications include:

- previous or active local infection
- complete paralysis of the shoulder caused by a neural lesion including stroke
- loss of an adequate amount of scapular bone tissue
- psychiatric disorders including senility and alcoholism
- a Charcot lesion of the glenohumeral joint.

The surgeon should also be wary of the "cured" alcoholic who has promised not to inbibe in the future. Any patient who fails to live up to this commitment may incur unnecessary complications.

Prosthetic Design

Various constrained designs have been successfully employed. However, the design of the Michael Reese total shoulder replacement is such that the glenoid must be preserved, meticulous surgical technique must be used to minimize failure, and following a dislocation of the humeral component the shoulder is capable of being revised.

A hemispheric metal humeral head component fits into a polyethylene socket that is assembled from halves. The internal diameter of the plastic cavity is the same as the diameter of the metal head, whereas the diameter of the peripheral lip of the assembled plastic halves is slightly smaller. This feature permits a fixed fulcrum while allowing a controlled dislocation of the metal head from its plastic socket when the humeral head component is forced beyond its maximum range of motion. This protects the scapula from fracturing through the suprascapular notch that may occur in a permanently fixed fulcrum design. Controlled dislocation decreases the risk of loosening. Although 275 inch-pounds is the average torque beyond which the scapula fractures in vitro, a value of 150 inch-pounds has been arbitrarily selected to control dislocation to protect a large variety of scapulae from fracturing.

The assembled polyethylene parts fit precisely into the metal glenoid component that is attached to the scapula. A self-locking metal ring is placed first about the metal of the humeral component, and then the plastic pieces are fitted within the metal head and the parts assembled. The metal locking ring is tightened about the glenoid component, thereby completing the assembly. The metal glenoid component is truncated 10° and permits the arm to hang away from the side slightly, thereby reducing the impingement of the humeral neck on the plastic rim.

New series II components are made of cobalt-chromium. The humeral head and humeral neck have diameters of 8 mm and 22 mm, respectively. The yield strength of the metal neck is 4,970 pounds. Series II components have been used since January 1976, and none have bent or broken to date as occurred in series I models that were made of stainless steel, type 316L, with a humeral neck diameter of 4 mm. Series I models had a high failure rate because the metal neck, having a yield strength of 824 pounds, often bent or broke.

It is essential to preserve the glenoid subchondral bone and the internal supporting spongy cancellous bone. The region of greatest trabecular density is located beneath the subchondral plate of the glenoid face. It provides the greatest support for the metal glenoid component. For this reason it should not be removed or damaged in any manner. It also permits a homogeneous dispersion of methylmethacrylate cement in the early stage of curing throughout the vault. Laboratory studies and clinical experience have shown that the placement of the needed 6.3- and eccentric 3.2-mm holes for the metal glenoid post and screws embedded in this system with the bone cement pressurized throughout the vault is the best method of attaching the glenoid component and minimizes loosening. Even unconstrained plastic or plastic-metal glenoid liners used in unconstrained replacements should be mounted in this manner. The cortical cover or cancellous vault is compromised by severe osteoporosis, destructive tumor tissue, surgical excavation, or severe erosion. In these cases the attachment of the metal glenoid to the vault will be tenuous at best. Thus, the chance of failure of a constrained prosthesis is enhanced under these circumstances. Accordingly, these conditions should serve as contraindications for a constrained prosthesis. A true axillary view of the glenoid is frequently needed to study the contours of the vault width.

Humeral Attachment

The metal stem is available in various widths. The largest possible stem width should be used. When there is an excessive loss of the proximal humerus, a custom-made prosthesis may be needed. Its size is determined from roentgenograms. However, shortening of the humerus by as much as 2.5 cm will not cause loss of function in the upper extremity. Methylmethacrylate cement is forced under pressure into the intramedullary canal after a plug has been inserted. The humeral component is inserted in 25° of retroversion by means of a special guide holder. It is important to achieve the proper retroversion angle of 25° so that external rotation of the arm is obtained during activities of daily living. The surgical technique has been described.[3,4]

Results

A result is considered a failure if the metal humeral neck breaks or if the prosthesis is permanently removed for any reason. When traumatic dislocation occurs the prosthetic parts behave according to the design. In any event, a revision procedure is needed in these situations.

In series I patients operated from 1973 through 1975 (24 shoulders), 11 patients were not revised. The metal necks of this early series were made of stainless steel and had a diameter of 4 mm. Many bent or broke. In these cases pain relief was excellent in eight patients, good in two, and poor in one. Of these 11 cases, 3 patients eventually died, one from a myocardial infarction after riding a motorcycle, and two from metastatic malignancy. However, their long-term follow-ups were known. Table 3-1 shows the distribution of their failures. Of the series II (74 patients with 78 replacements) protheses, which are made of chromium-cobalt and whose metal necks have an 8-mm diameter, none have failed because of metal failure. In both series I and II, intractable pain was the chief reason for prosthetic replacement. One patient whose long-term data are

Table 3-1 Complications of Constrained Total Shoulder Replacement

Complication	*Series I*	*Series II*
Traumatic dislocations	3	8
Traumatic bent neck	2	0
Broken humeral neck	8	0
Allergy	1	0
Infection	0	2
Traumatic loose stem	0	3
Traumatic loose glenoid	2	7
Broken glenoid screws	2	3

known eventually was lost to follow-up examination. Five patients died of myocardial infarction and cancer. Their long-term data are also known. Among the series II unrevised cases 20 patients had excellent results, 30 had good results, and 17 were fair, whereas 3 were considered poor results. Table 3-1 shows the various complications encountered in these patients since January 1976.

Functions

Among series I cases, 22 patients had a severe loss of rotator cuff function. Many of these patients had had multiple procedures before constrained joint arthroplasty was performed. In the unrevised series I patients, there was an 83.5% overall improvement in active function and an 89.6% improvement in passive function compared with preoperative levels. In one patient who had a recurring giant-cell tumor with normal function and no pain prior to operation, the patient lost function because of the nature of surgery which required an extensive excision of the tumor and surrounding soft tissues. The proximal humerus was replaced with a custom-made prosthesis.

In series II cases rotator cuff degeneration was advanced and resembled cuff arthropathy. None of the remaining rotator cuff tissues were reattached to the humerus in these patients. In these cases there was a 60% overall improvement in active function and a 65% gain in passive function. As a group, these patients had exceptionally poor deltoid muscle strength. In 70 series II patients 41 procedures were performed, before the patients underwent a constrained joint arthroplasty.

Complications

Table 3-1 shows various complications that have occurred in series I and II patients. A more recent complication has related to metal fatigue in screws made of chromium cobalt that were cast initially and hold the glenoid. These screws have a yield strength of 65,000 psi. They are now made from a cold rolled process and have a yield strength of 140,000 psi. Only one such patient, operated elsewhere, is known to have had a failure of the later-model screws that broke. It is important to have the screws fit at right angles to the metal cup and glenoid to minimize excessive stress on the midsection of the screw after countless rotations relating to arm movement. In two other patients the metal cup pulled away from the glenoid following metastases to the glenoid 2 years after their operations, resulting in a weakening of the bone.

Radiolucency

Two years after operation 50% of the patients show radiolucency of 1 to 2 mm about the stem, and 30% of the shoulders show radiolucency of 1 mm about the screws and central posts. The significance of these findings is not known. Some of the components may eventually loosen and require revision.

Discussion

If the rotator cuff is functional or can be made reasonably functional, an unconstrained prosthesis should always be considered first as a method of alleviating pain and restoring function in a damaged shoulder. Constrained total shoulder replacement is truly a last-resort operation. Good shoulder function permits the hand to be placed in a variety of positions that depend upon the shoulder, which is the pivotal point of the upper extremity. If the rotator cuff mechanism is markedly ineffective, the use of a constrained prosthesis can be considered primarily in an older person. When a total shoulder replacement fails, particularly a constrained joint, the prosthesis can be removed and the patient is left with a resection-type arthroplasty that is, in effect, a flail shoulder.

The chief causes of failure in constrained replacements are: 1) poor patient selection (incorrect indication), 2) inadequate surgical technique, and 3) material failure. Patients who have constrained total shoulder replacements should be forewarned that the shoulder will not accept heavy laboring activity and excessive stress and may eventually fail if the patient abuses the prosthetic device. In selecting patients for constrained arthroplasty it is essential that the integrity of the glenoid be well maintained for secure fixation of the metal glenoid component. Previous local infection, advanced osteoporosis, and tumor of the bone with attendant loss of bone in the glenoid vault preclude the use of a constrained prosthesis. Patients must be capable of cooperating at all times after operation. Those who are senile or have psychiatric problems including alcoholism should be excluded from having a constrained replacement.

An advantage of constrained joint arthroplasty is that it avoids postoperative subluxation and overstretching of the soft tissues, especially the deltoid muscle. An excellent, supervised postoperative rehabilitation program is essential for best results, especially if the surgeon hopes to restore active muscle function. The replacement should not be forced beyond its motion limits because it may dislocate. In fact, several of the dislocations in series II patients noted in Table 3-1 occurred because either the therapist or someone close to the patient had forced the shoulder beyond its motion limits. These patients required revision surgery.

Conclusion

Constrained total shoulder arthroplasty is a salvage procedure to be used when other standard operations including an unconstrained replacement cannot be performed. These patients either have a destruction of the proximal humerus because of tumor or an ineffective rotator cuff mechanism that cannot be used to stabilize an unconstrained replacement. Many complications can be expected from constrained replacements. However, the results can be gratifying if such a replacement is correctly used.

References

1. Neer CS II: Replacement arthroplasty for glenohumeral osteoarthritis. *J Bone Joint Surg Am* 1974;56A:1.
2. Neer CS II, Watson KC, Stanton FJ: Recent experience in total shoulder replacement. *J Bone Joint Surg Am* 1982;64A:319.
3. Post M, Haskell SS, Jablon M: Total shoulder replacement with a constrained prosthesis. *J Bone Joint Surg Am* 1980;62A:327.
4. Post M, Jablon M, Miller H, et al: Constrained total shoulder joint replacement: A critical review. *Clin Orthop* 1979;114:135.

4

Surgery in Rheumatoid Arthritis: The Elbow

Mack L. Clayton and
Donald C. Ferlic

Anatomy and Function

The elbow joint is made up of the distal humerus articulating with the proximal ulna and radius, which also articulate together. These articulations are enclosed in a common fibrous sheath. The synovial lining is continuous with all components of the joint, so that a synovitis presenting in the radiohumeral portion of the joint will not be limited only to that area. The bones about the elbow are held together by a ligamentous network with a particularly strong anterior band of the medial collateral ligament.

The elbow is commonly thought of as strictly a hinge joint, with the radius rotating about the capitellum and the radial notch of the ulna. Detailed studies have attempted to define the kinematics of the elbow, some in an attempt to explain directly the high incidence of loosening of uniaxial total elbow replacements.

Ewald[1] and Morrey and Chao[2] described a pathway of instant centers near the center of the trochlea for flexion and extension. Forearm rotation has likewise been said to involve only the radial-capitellar articulation, but Ray et al[3] have shown that there is some motion of the ulna with rotation of the forearm, with 8° to 9° of lateral abduction of the distal end of the ulna in full supination and pronation.

Extra-articular Considerations

Rheumatoid elbows often have superficial problems, such as olecranon bursae which become painful and inflamed. The olecranon bursa does not normally communicate with the elbow joint, but in rheumatoid arthritis it occasionally does, and infection of the joint occasionally presents as a draining olecranon bursa; one should be suspicious of joint involvement with copious drainage. Bursae tend to recur or drain after excision. To prevent this, we insert a drain and splint the elbow 10 to 14 days after surgery. Prominent rheumatoid nodules about the bony surface of the olecranon may also be painful and ulcerate. Although these may require removal, it is important to warn the patient that these nodules frequently do recur and that small ones should be left alone. Rheumatoid arthritic patients are hypersensitive to pressure, and most nodules are related to pressure. Protective padding helps prevent recurrence. Antecubital cysts in the rheumatoid elbow are similar to Baker's cysts in the knee and occasionally do have to be removed because of pain or nerve impingement.

There is a linkage between elbow and hand/wrist problems, and therefore when a patient is examined for a hand problem, it is always necessary to consider the elbow as well. One should keep three things particularly in mind: forearm rotation, ulnar nerve problems, and posterior interosseous nerve palsy resulting from elbow synovitis. Seventy-five percent of our patients who have undergone elbow synovectomy and radial head resection have also had distal ulnar resection and synovectomy of the wrist. Elbow problems are also closely linked to shoulder problems. Good elbow function often provides compensation for limited shoulder motion. The general function of the shoulder and elbow is to position and move the hand in space.

When a rheumatoid patient presents with inability to extend the fingers, the pathology may be in the hand, the wrist, or the elbow, and there may very well be a problem in differentiating between posterior interosseous nerve palsy at the elbow, subluxation of the extensor tendons off the metacarpophalangeal joints in the hand, or even ruptured extensor tendons at the wrist. This problem can be correctly diagnosed only if one is aware of all these possibilities. A hand with posterior interosseous nerve palsy can often be differentiated by demonstrating a positive tenodesis effect. When the wrist is flexed, the intact extensor tendons should extend the fingers, but if the wrist or metacarpophalangeal joints are stiff, the tenodesis effect will not be apparent, and this may present an additional problem in diagnosis.

An arthrogram of the elbow may reveal a large antecubital cyst pressing on the posterior interosseous nerve. A steroid injection into the elbow may resolve the inflammation, but synovectomy and nerve decompression may also be necessary.

The rheumatoid patient may also develop ulnar neuritis at the elbow. Bony deformities, erosions, or synovitis may contribute to its cause. The patient may present with numbness and paresthesias in the ulnar nerve distribution in the hand or with weakness. This is often interpreted merely as symptoms of arthritic involvement of the hand, but one needs to consider neuropathy of the ulnar nerve at the elbow. Usual treatment is by rerouting of the nerve anteriorly.

Laine and Vainio[4] found two thirds of their patients with rheumatoid arthritis to have elbow involvement. Elbow problems necessitating surgery arise later in the disease because 1) the onset of elbow symptoms is insidious; 2) disability is often not noted until destruction is advanced, because the range of motion is aided by gravity, which helps to maintain extension, and the activities of daily living help to maintain flexion; 3) loss of pronation may be compensated by shoulder motion; and 4) the elbow frequently responds well to conservative measures such as rest, splinting, and analgesics.

Elbow Synovectomy and Débridement

Indications for surgery are pain, swelling (synovitis), reasonable range of motion (40° to 110° minimum), and preservation of ulnohumeral cartilage (stage II or early stage III). Painful crepitus over the radial head with rotation but smooth ulnohumeral motion with minimal crepitus is a favorable sign.

Operative Technique

A posterior lateral incision is made extending from the posterior border of the ulna 4 cm distal to the top of the olecranon to a point 2 cm proximal to the lateral epicondyle of the humerus (extending to the triceps tendon), keeping the forearm pronated to protect the radial nerve[5] (Fig 4-1). A fascial incision is made along the line between the anconeus and the common extensor tendon origins and to the triceps tendon posteriorly. The common extensor tendons are detached by sharp subperiosteal dissection from the lateral condyle and retracted upward, maintaining a continuous ligamentous-tendinous-fascial layer. The radial head is excised, synovectomy carried out, and the ulna subluxed to remove the synovium from the posterior and medial sides. By flexing the elbow, the anterior recess can be cleared, and with the elbow in extension the olecranon fossa can be cleared. A rongeur is used to remove the synovium. The coranoid process is partially excised if it limits flexion, and bone from the tip of the olecranon can also be excised to gain extension.

A silicone radial head prosthesis is then inserted in selected cases in an attempt to prevent proximal migration of the radius and modulate the forces across the elbow. Use of a radial head implant has not been proven to give better results. Many rheumatoid patients have quite lax joints, and the radial head is important in preventing extremes of valgus angulation about the elbow, particularly if the medial collateral ligament is unstable. The radial head implant acts as a spacer and "shock absorber" to help unload the ulnohumeral joint.

If there is ulnar neuropathy, a medial incision is made. The ulnar nerve is isolated and transferred anteriorly; medial capsular incision allows further synovectomy if necessary. A bulky dressing with a posterior splint is applied postoperatively, and active and passive motion is begun in 3 or 4 days.

In our series of 47 patients we have performed 56 procedures. This group includes 41 females, age range 21 to 74 years, with an average age of 48 years.

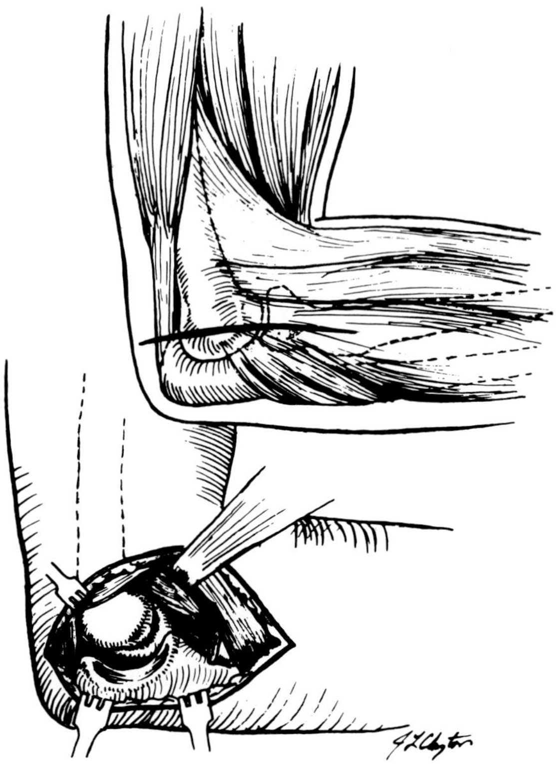

Fig 4-1. Lateral skin incision for synovectomy and débridement of the elbow. Good exposure is obtained after subperiosteal release of the femoral condyle and excision of the radial head and subluxation of the elbow.

Six patients were juvenile rheumatoids, and 36 of the 40 patients had suffered from the disease for more than 10 years (average 7½ years).

Pain relief was over 80% for 5 years. There was a slight gain in flexion-extension (9°) and a moderate gain in rotation (22°). Seventy-eight percent still had satisfactory to excellent results at 7+ years. Also, synovectomy does not burn any bridges. The results of synovectomies in the elbow are the best for any joint. This is probably due to the non-weight-bearing status and the decompression effect obtained with radial head excision.

Case Report

A 56-year-old woman with long-standing chronic rheumatoid arthritis of 8 years' duration complained of pain on motion of her elbow. Examination revealed that hers was the "loose" type of rheumatoid disease with full rotation of the right elbow and motion from 0° to 150°. There was painful crepitation around the radial head, and there were nodules over the olecranon. X-rays showed slight narrowing of the articular space with some mild irregularity.

The patient underwent synovectomy of the elbow, débridement, radial head resection, and excision of the rheumatoid nodules in 1967. Postoperatively she was relieved of pain and could flex from 0° to 135° and had full rotation. X-rays shortly after the surgery showed the amount of bone resected. Seven years later she had motion from 10° to 135° with full rotation and minimal medial pain in the elbow. X-rays done 11 years after the surgery showed some destruction of the joint, but her surgical result remained excellent. She had had multiple lower extremity operative procedures done for rheumatoid deformities and was able to use a walker or crutches during much of the time.

Arthroplasty

For the elbow with more advanced disease, fascial interpositional arthroplasty has been used in the past with varying results. We have not used this procedure in the past 7 years as a failure makes total elbow arthroplasty more difficult.

Total Elbow Arthroplasty (With Prostheses)

There have been numerous reports of total elbow arthroplasty resulting in a high complication rate and frequent withdrawal of the components for redesign. Silicone hinge arthroplasty at the elbow has been tried elsewhere but has been abandoned because of breakage.

The Mayo Clinic[6] obtained satisfactory results in 75% of cases of total elbow replacement for rheumatoid arthritis but with only a 2-year follow-up. The rheumatoid patients again showed better results than the patients with post-traumatic arthritis. As in the knee, nonconstrained elbows have been introduced in hopes of alleviating the loosening problem.

We have performed 19 total elbow replacements, all on rheumatoid patients. Four were done with rigid hinges, three with GSB, and one with a Coonrad. The first of these was performed in 1971, and two are still excellent results. Flexion and extension arc is between 104° and 140°, and all have had full rotation. We chose the GSB initially because we felt that its small size would preserve bone stock, so that if the device had to be removed, a fascial arthroplasty with stability was still possible. These four patients were followed between 22 and 84 months. One of the elbows loosened after 6 years and is painful now. One GSB elbow did well for 7 years before developing a deep wound infection which necessitated operative treatment; this elbow is still functioning well 6 months later.

We are now using the Ewald elbow because of the high rate of hinge loosening that has been associated with the original, rigid GSB. (The GSB has been modified and is a "lax" hinge.) If there are adequate ligaments and bone stock, the nonconstrained elbow is indicated. We have performed 15 Ewald[1] total elbow replacements since 1977 in 11 patients with rheumatoid arthritis, and all were done for severe pain. Two patients had had a synovectomy, débridement, and radial head resection previously. Postoperative motion ranged from 95° to 125° of flexion-extension and 90° to 100° of rotation. The complications in the earlier cases were numerous but usually did not jeopardize the final result.

Complications

Only one half of our 19 cases experienced no complications. The complications that we have encountered are listed in Table 4-1. In spite of these complications, only one patient claims to be a failure. Eighty percent of the patients are pleased with their relief of pain and good range of motion (Fig 4-2), and one patient is too early to rate. The future is bright for the nonconstrained surface replacement of the elbow inserted with proper stability of the medial collateral ligament.

Arthrodesis

Arthrodesis of the elbow in the rheumatoid patient is not indicated. This procedure relieves pain but markedly interferes with function of the upper extremity. The single exception may be an infected or otherwise failed total elbow arthroplasty where there is not enough bone stock for another procedure or where resection arthroplasty is not acceptable.

Conclusion

Synovectomy of the elbow with radial head resection gives good to excellent results in stage II and early stage III involvement, so relatively few total elbow replacements are necessary.

The results of total elbow replacement are improving, but this procedure has had a high complication rate. As in the knee, a nonconstrained prosthesis is

Table 4-1. Complications of Total Elbow Replacement

Complication	*No. of Cases*
Subluxation (mild)	4
Ulnar neuropathy	1
Noise in the prothesis	1
Skin necrosis	2
Failure due to infection (late)	1
Rupture of triceps repair	1

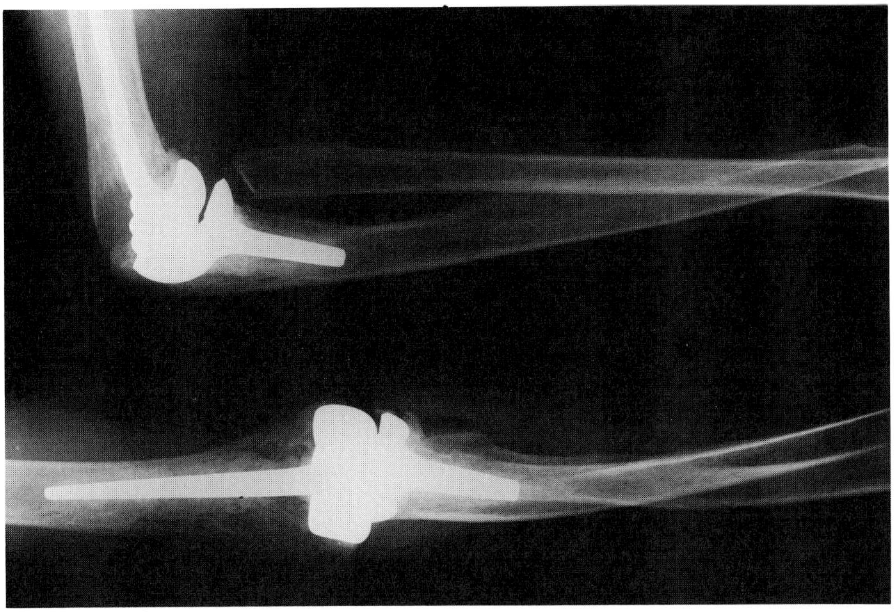

Fig 4-2. Nonconstrained total elbow replacement (Ewald). The polyethylene component is within the metal tray of the ulna. Patient had motion from 25° to 135° with full pronation and supination.

preferred, but if there is an excessive amount of bone or ligament destruction, a constrained, nonrigid (lax or sloppy) prosthesis may be necessary.

The overall results of elbow replacement will improve with perfection of surgical technique and component design.

References

1. Ewald FC, Scheinberg RD, Poss R, et al: Capitello-condylar total elbow arthroplasty. *J Bone Joint Surg Am* 1980;62A:1259.
2. Morrey BF, Chao EYS: Passive motion of the elbow joint. A biomechanical analysis. *J Bone Joint Surg Am* 1976;58A:501.
3. Ray RD, Johnson RJ, Jameson RM: Rotation of the forearm: An experimental study of pronation and supination. *J Bone Joint Surg Am* 1951;*33A*:993.
4. Laine V, Vainio K: The elbow in rheumatoid arthritis, in Hijmans WDP, Herschel H (eds): *Early Synovectomy in Rheumatoid Arthritis. Proceedings of the Symposium on Early Synovectomy in Rheumatoid Arthritis, Amsterdam, April 12–15, 1967* Amsterdam. Excerpta Medica Foundation, 1969, p 112.
5. Ferlic DC, Clayton ML, Parr PL: Synovectomy and arthroplasty of the elbow in rheumatoid arthritis. *Ortho Dig* 1977;5:11.
6. Cooney WP III, Byron RS: Rheumatoid arthritis in the upper extremity. Treatment of the elbow and shoulder joints. *American Academy of Orthopaedic Surgeons Instructional Course Lectures* 1979;28:247.

5

Injuries of the Capitular Epiphysis

Thomas G. Wadsworth

Injury to the capitular epiphysis is fairly common in children between the ages of 3 and 14 years. The injury is potentially serious in view of the disturbance it causes in the important developing area at the lower end of the humerus; in many of the injuries there is disruption of the osseous link between the capitular epiphysis and that of the trochlea (Fig 5-1). Ulnar nerve damage may ensue later in life.

Types of Injury

The author has described four types of injury to the capitular epiphysis[1,2] (Fig 5-2). The line of fracture and the area of separation in the first three types are in the metaphysis (Fig 5-3). In the unstable or displaced injury the fracture line is through the epiphyseal cartilage and thus into the joint at the junction of the trochlear and capitular centers, which are consequently separated, the lateral lip of the trochlea coming away with the capitulum. Less frequently, there is a fracture through the inner part of the ossification center itself. Typically, the metaphyseal fragment is triangular, but many type I cases have a thin rim of metaphysis lying above the epiphyseal center, and it is uncertain whether the unstable cases of this type more often have a triangular or a rim metaphyseal fragment. Late displacement of the type I injury occurs when there is disruption of the preosseous cartilage medial to the capitular epiphysis, most likely if the lateral fracture gap is 3 mm or more on radiography[3]; in the stable injury the preosseous cartilage is intact, and the lateral fracture gap is likely to be 2 mm or less (Fig 5-4). Type IV injury is most often the result of repeated impingement of the radial head against the capitulum, the articular surface being damaged; this injury is sometimes seen in young baseball players in the United States.

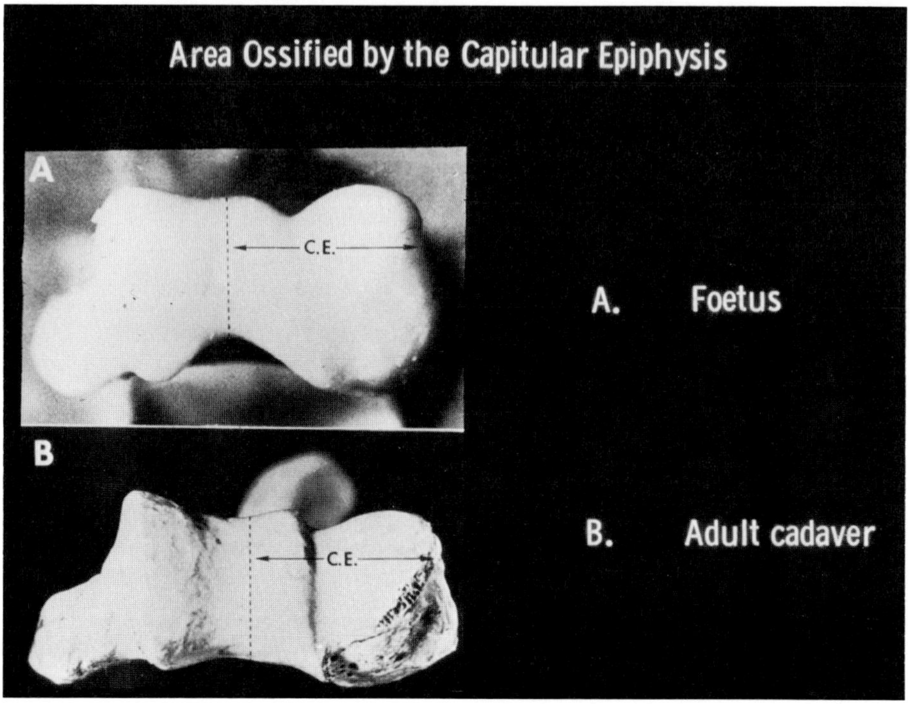

Fig 5-1. The capitular epiphysis (CE) accounts for ossification of the lateral lip of the trochlea as well as the capitulum. *A*, Fetal specimen; *B*, specimen from adult cadaver. Source: Reprinted with permission from *Clinical Orthopaedics and Related Research* (1972;85). Copyright © 1972, JB Lippincott Company.

The majority of type I injuries heal rapidly, and immobilization of the elbow with a collar-and-cuff sling, perhaps combined with a posterior plaster of Paris (POP) splint with the elbow at 90°, results in union of the metaphyseal fracture within 4 weeks. If there is doubt about stability, and particularly if there is much soft-tissue swelling over the outer aspect of the elbow, it is wise to take lateral radiographs with the elbow in as much flexion and extension as can be obtained to make sure that there is no instability; also, it is necessary to x-ray the elbow at 1, 2, and 4 weeks postinjury in all cases where stability remains in doubt. Operative fixation is required for the unstable case.

In type II injury there is subluxation of the epiphysis with its metaphyseal fragment. In these cases it is always necessary to reduce the epiphysis accurately and to provide adequate internal fixation of the fracture.

In type III injury, besides displacement in the coronal plane, the capitular epiphysis hinges on the intact lateral ligament of the elbow, and the medial margin of the fragment is often rotated forward. As with types I and II, the mechanism of the injury is debatable, but most often it would appear that force is taken on the hand and forearm; the radial head impinges on the capitular

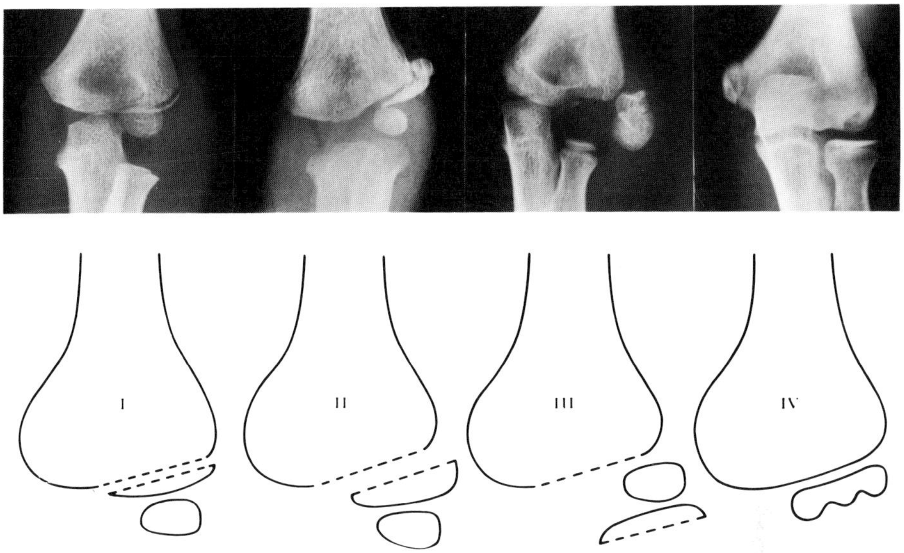

Fig 5-2. Four types of capitular epiphyseal injuries. (See text for description.) Source: Reprinted with permission from *Clinical Orthopaedics and Related Research* (1972;85). Copyright © 1972, JB Lippincott Company.

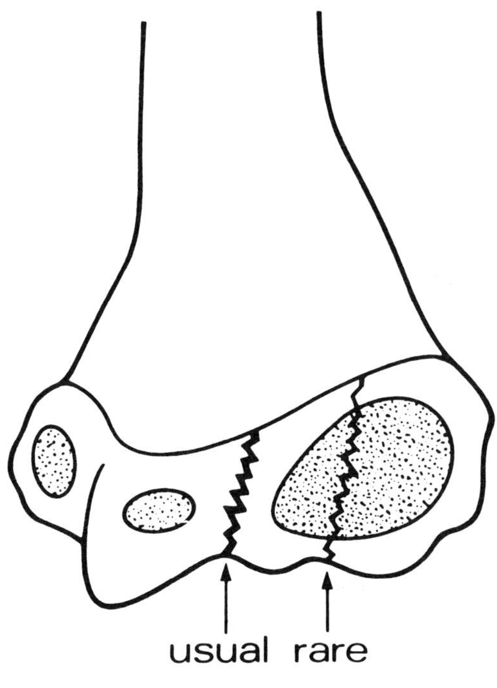

Fig 5-3. Location of capitular epiphyseal injuries. In types I to III, the fracture is medial to the capitular ossification center; rarely, the fracture passes through the area of ossification. Source: Reprinted from *The Elbow* by TG Wadsworth with permission of Churchill Livingstone Inc, © 1982.

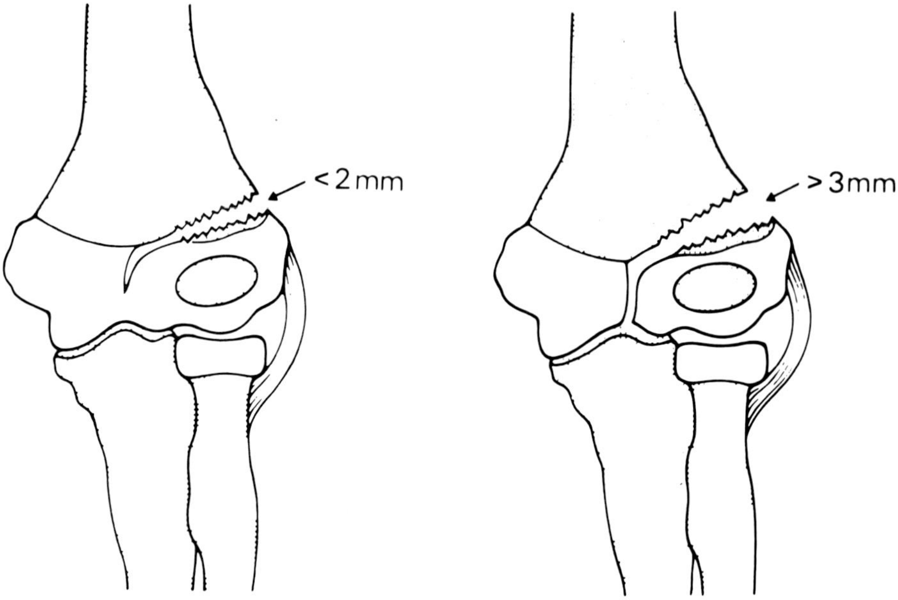

Fig 5-4. Displacement in type I injury is more likely if the lateral gap at the fracture is 3 mm or more; in such patients, there is a complete fracture through the preosseous cartilage at the inner aspect of the capitular epiphyseal center. Stability is more likely if the gap is 2 mm or less. Source: Reprinted from *The Elbow* by TG Wadsworth with permission of Churchill Livingstone Inc, © 1982.

epiphysis, thus producing the metaphyseal fracture and the fracture through the epiphyseal cartilage, or ossification center, into the joint. Tearing of fascia and muscle on the lateral side of the elbow, together with contraction of the forearm extensor muscles, produces the gross deformity. Open reduction and secure fixation are always required.

Pitting of the articular cartilage and chondromalacia may be difficult to diagnose in the early stages of the type IV case, and radiographic evidence will usually only be present when an osteochondral fragment becomes detached. Characteristically, there are patchy zones of rarefaction in the subarticular zone of the capitulum, giving a cystlike appearance, and sometimes a crater that can be detected radiologically. Not all loose bodies are seen in the radiograph as some of them are fragments of articular cartilage and are radiolucent.

Arthroscopic examination may in the future be useful in these patients. Operative treatment is indicated when loose bodies are present or suspected and particularly when symptoms persist despite an adequate period of rest to the joint.

Rarely one sees a displaced capitular epiphysis with a very large metaphyseal fragment (type II). This injury occurs typically in the older child not long before epiphyseal closure. A displaced capitular epiphysis may also be part of a T shaped supracondylar fracture. In these patients a posterior approach is most useful for open reduction and internal fixation.

Operative treatment is necessary for the unstable type I case and all type II and type III cases[1,2,4] (Fig 5-5). The objective is to restore the developing osseous link between the trochlear and capitular centers and so maintain a congruous joint surface and an adequate lateral lip of the trochlea. Accurate reduction of the metaphyseal fracture eliminates the risk of nonunion. Malunion and nonunion result in a deficient lateral trochlear lip, with the result that lateral shift of the ulna and cubitus valgus occur, the sequel being poor articulation, limited movement, and considerable risk of ulnar palsy in later life.

A lateral approach under general anesthesia and pneumatic tourniquet control is usual. Two Kirschner wires or a screw are preferable; however, the size of the metaphyseal fragment varies considerably, and only if it is sufficiently large can a screw be used.

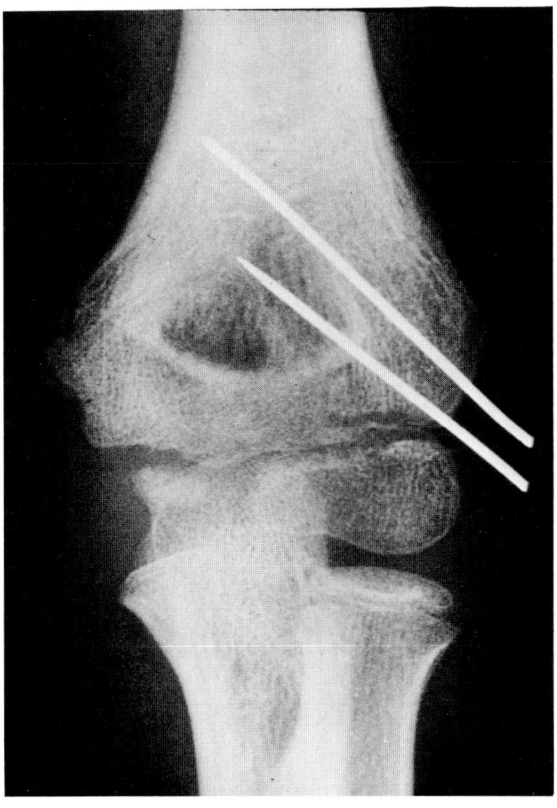

Fig 5-5. The unstable injury must be reduced and fixed. This method of Kirschner wire fixation is recommended, the wires being removed after 6 weeks. All type II and III injuries and the unstable type I injury require internal fixation. Source: Reprinted from *The Elbow* by TG Wadsworth with permission of Churchill Livingstone Inc, © 1982.

Complications

There are several complications of injuries to the capitular epiphysis.

Malunion

Malunion is the inevitable complication of an unreduced or redisplaced type II injury or unstable type I injury with subsequent displacement of the capitular epiphysis. Unreduced type III cases will almost inevitably result in nonunion, but if reduction is not perfect or displacement recurs with the fracture surfaces still in contact, malunion will be more unusual. The important osseous link between the trochlear and capitular centers is lost, with production of a "fish-tail" deformity; as a result of loss of the lateral lip of the trochlea, lateral shift of the ulna occurs and so valgus deformity is produced. Poor articulation of the ulna with the trochlea usually results in impaired elbow motion. Overgrowth of the lateral aspect of the lower humeral metaphysis, in the form of a spur, is a constant feature of type I, II, and III injuries, whatever the severity; it is unimportant. Deformity from incomplete union occurs at the articular surface when there has been an unreduced fracture through the inner part of the capitular ossification center. In the type IV case, enlargement of the radial head and medial epicondyle as well as deformity of the articular surface of the capitular epiphysis are commonly seen.

Premature Epiphyseal Fusion

Premature epiphyseal fusion has been observed after type I, II, and III injuries. It can also occur after the type IV lesion in the young baseball pitcher where there is accelerated growth and premature closure of the epiphyses in the throwing arm. The author has described two types of premature fusion[5] (Fig 5-6). In the first type the capitular epiphysis alone fuses prematurely to the metaphysis and, as this epiphysis accounts for ossification of the outer part of the trochlea, disturbance of growth, commonly referred to as fishtail deformity, results. In the second type of premature fusion the normal pattern of fusion is followed, the capitular and trochlear epiphyses first fusing together and then to the metaphysis; however, the capitular epiphysis is sometimes in advance of that of the trochlea. Outward shift of the ulna can follow premature fusion of either type and can result in cubitus valgus. The observation that premature fusion and even valgus deformity can result from a stable type I injury indicates that it is an inevitable complication in some cases. It is likely that its effect, particularly in the first type of premature fusion, may be diminished by always obtaining an anatomical reduction with stable fixation in the unstable injury. Even with perfect treatment, one cannot always give an optimistic prognosis with regard to valgus deformity and tardy ulnar palsy; this has some legal and practical importance. There is considerable variation in the appearance and normal fusion of the lower humeral epiphyses, and adequate long-term follow-up is necessary to demonstrate this complication.

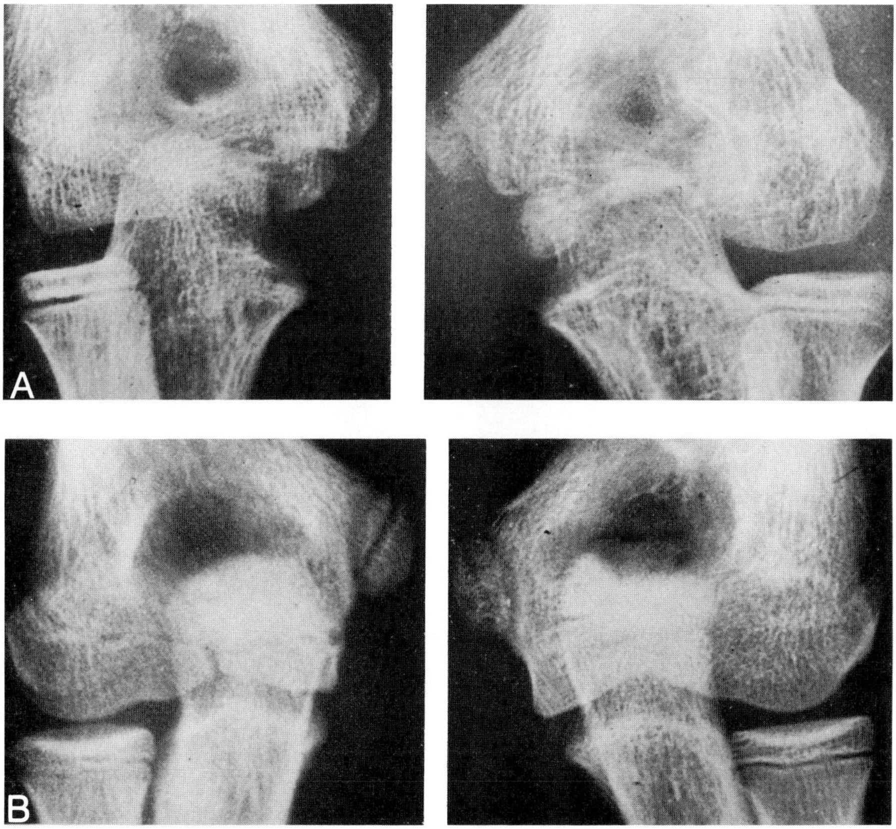

Fig 5-6. Premature epiphyseal fusion can occur in two ways.[5] In *A,* the capitular epiphysis alone fuses prematurely and there is "fishtail" deformity. In *B,* the normal pattern of fusion occurs, but it is sometimes accelerated on the lateral side. Cubitus valgus can occur with either type of premature fusion. Source: Reprinted with permission from *Journal of Bone and Joint Surgery* (1964;46B). Copyright © 1964, Journal of Bone and Joint Surgery, Inc.

Avascular Necrosis

Avascular necrosis is usually an avoidable condition. During operative reduction, great care should be taken to preserve the attachment of the soft tissues to the capitular epiphysis and its metaphyseal fragment in order to preserve the blood supply.

Nonunion

Nonunion is the inevitable consequence of the untreated type III case where all contact is lost between the fracture surfaces, but it has also been observed even in the type I case with late displacement and in the type II injury (Fig 5-7).

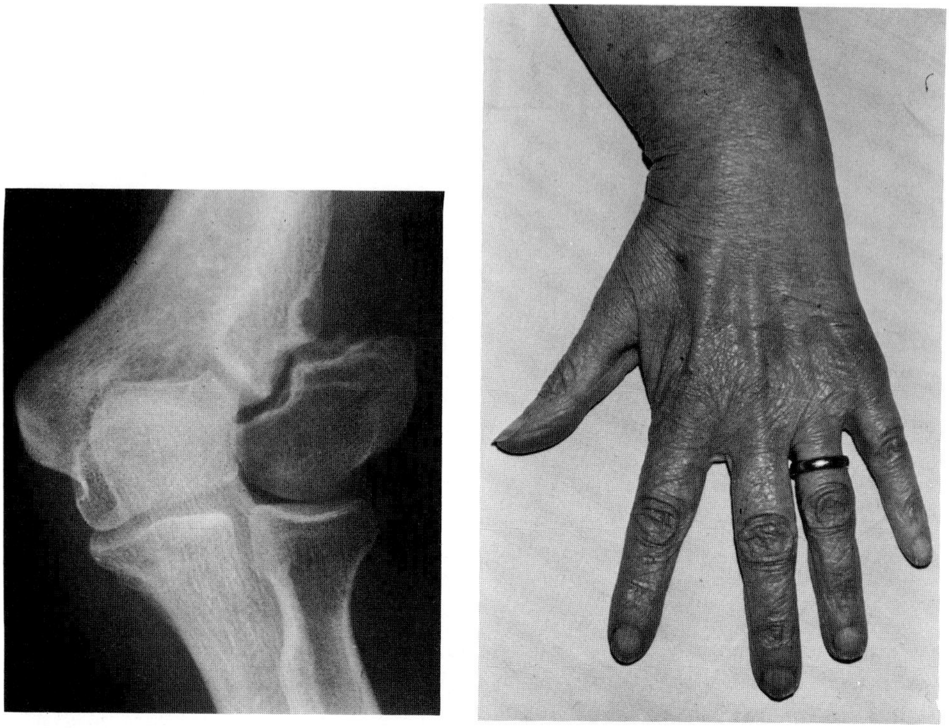

Fig 5-7. Nonunion of the lateral condyle with wasting and weakness of ulnar-innervated muscles in the hand. In such patients neurological deficit varies from sensory loss alone to a combination of sensory and motor deficit. Source: Reprinted from *The Elbow* by TG Wadsworth with permission of Churchill Livingstone Inc, © 1982.

Imperfect fixation is felt to be an important factor in determining this complication, and one should avoid closed reduction and POP fixation or soft-tissue suture alone in the unstable case. To obtain union, the two fracture surfaces must be placed in accurate contact, any interposed soft tissue must be removed and stripping of the displaced epiphysis and its metaphyseal fragment has to be avoided in order to preserve its blood supply. Nonunion is accompanied by a varying amount of lateral displacement of the capitular epiphysis and disruption of its osseous link with the trochlear epiphysis; the consequences of all this are lateral shift of the ulna, limited movement, and frequent onset of ulnar compression neuritis in adult life. Drilling of the metaphyseal fragment, packing of the fracture area with cancellous bone, and screw fixation can be considered in the child exhibiting this complication.

Valgus Deformity

Valgus deformity can result from union in malposition, nonunion, avascular necrosis, or premature fusion of the capitular epiphysis. The normal "carrying angle" is commonly greater in the female, but this sex difference does not appear until puberty; in the adult, the angle averages between 10° and 15°. Abduction of the ulna is due to the varying but greater depth of the inner lip of the trochlea compared with the outer lip. The fact that the inner lip is much deeper distally than anteriorly accounts for the diminishing angle in flexion. A few people exhibit cubitus rectus, that is, no carrying angle and some cubitus varus. Valgus deformity results from disturbance of the important osseous link between the trochlear and capitular centers; this may be gross in the first type of premature fusion, in malunion, or in nonunion, all of which result in loss of the outer lip of the trochlea and fishtail deformity. Less serious disturbance of growth leads to a shallow outer lip of the trochlea. Whether the deficient outer lip of the trochlea is absolute or of a minor nature, lateral shift of the ulna and an increased carrying angle are the inevitable consequences.

Ulnar Compression Neuropathy

Ulnar compression neuropathy in the final analysis is the most important complication of injuries to the capitular epiphysis.[6,7,8] Tardy ulnar palsy has been recognized as a consequence of elbow injury in childhood, the effects of which are seen in the adult, since it was first described by Panas in 1878.[6] In these cases, the roof of the cubital tunnel, the arcuate ligament, approaches more closely than normal the floor of the tunnel; obvious cubitus valgus is usually present. Once ulnar palsy is present with weakness of the hand, surgical relief is necessary. One should bear in mind the various other possible causes of ulnar neuropathy when faced with the problem of the ulnar intrinsic minus hand; in most cases it will be obvious that the pathology lies at the level of the elbow. In addition to sensory and motor deficit, there is local tenderness over the cubital tunnel, often with referred paresthesias into the forearm and inner aspect of the hand. A confirmatory clinical finding is the positive elbow flexion test.[2,8] The elbow is held fully flexed for 1 to 5 minutes. The test is positive when paresthesias are initiated or aggravated; the test is explained by the fact that the arcuate ligament, forming the roof of the cubital tunnel, is slack in extension and taut in full elbow flexion, while bulging of the medial ligament of the elbow in the flexed position also leads to diminished volume of the cubital tunnel (Fig 5-8). The osseous part of the cubital tunnel is well seen in the cubital tunnel radiograph.[2,8] Swelling of the ulnar nerve can frequently be palpated just above the proximal edge of the arcuate ligament at the cubital tunnel in these patients.

Several surgical procedures are available for relief of the cubital tunnel syndrome.[2,8] The Osborne procedure consists of dividing the arcuate ligament along the length of the ulnar nerve and then sewing the ligament deep to the nerve. Another popular procedure is to transpose the ulnar nerve anteriorly

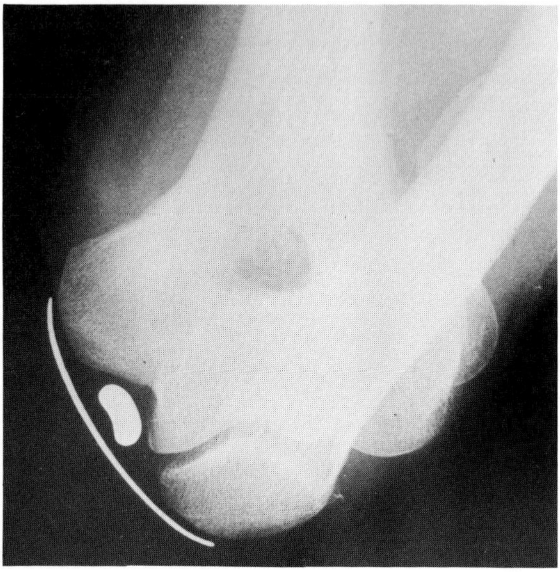

A

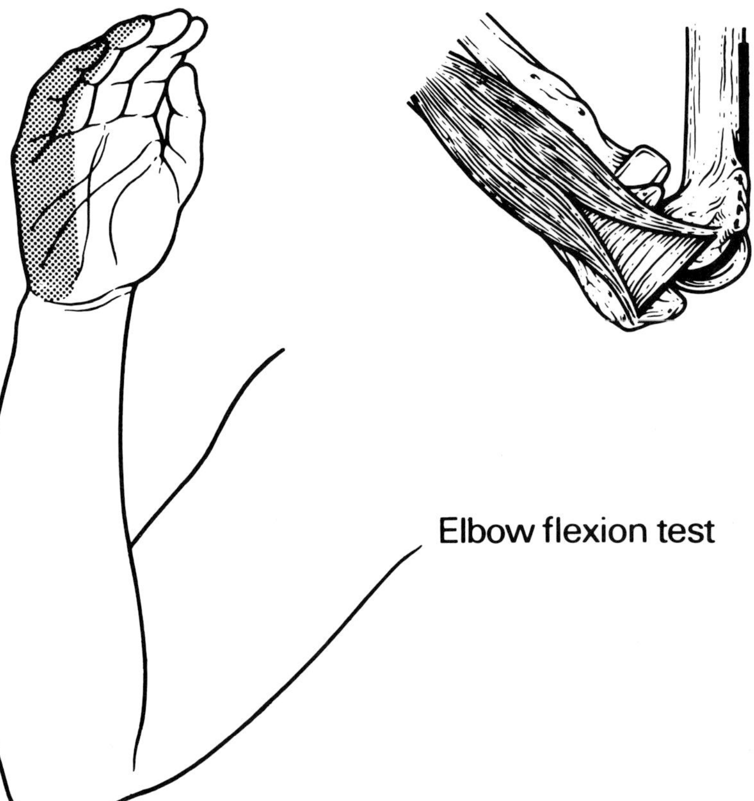

B

Fig 5-8. *A,* The cubital tunnel radiograph is useful for demonstrating the osseous floor of the tunnel. *B,* The elbow flexion test[2,8] is positive when paresthesias are initiated or aggravated after full elbow flexion, which should be maintained from 1 to 5 minutes. Source: Reprinted from *The Elbow* by TG Wadsworth with permission of Churchill Livingstone Inc, © 1982.

deep to the common flexor musculature. A third, less common procedure is to perform medial epicondylectomy. Whatever one's approach, the earlier surgical treatment is performed once ulnar nerve palsy has commenced, the better the result will be. In the later stages a cure is unlikely, and only prevention of further crippling of the hand can be expected.

References

1. Wadsworth TG: Injuries of the capitular (lateral humeral condylar) epiphysis. *Clin Orthop Rel Res* 1972;85:127–142.
2. Wadsworth TG: *The Elbow*. Edinburgh, Churchill Livingstone, 1982.
3. Jakob R, Fowles JV, Rang M: Observations concerning fractures of the lateral humeral condyle in children. *J Bone Joint Surg Br* 1975;57B:430–436.
4. Flynn, JC, Richards JF, Saltzman RI: Prevention and treatment of non-union of slightly displaced fractures of the lateral humeral condyle in children. *J Bone Joint Surg Am* 1975;57A:1087–1092.
5. Wadsworth TG: Premature epiphysial fusion after injury of the capitulum. *J Bone Joint Surg Br* 1964;46B:46–49.
6. Panas J: Sur une cause peu connue de paralysie du nerf cubital. *Arch Gen Med Paris* 1878;2:5–22.
7. Mouchet A: thesis. Paris, 1898.
8. Wadsworth TG: The external compression syndrome of the ulnar nerve at the cubital tunnel. *Clin Orthop Rel Res* 1977;124:189–204.

6

Management of Ulnar-Sided Wrist Pain

D. C. R. Ireland

The diagnosis of ulnar-sided wrist pain can be particularly elusive as many different conditions affect this relatively small area. This difficulty is compounded when there is no clear history of acute injury, when the examination findings are equivocal, and when radiographic studies are apparently normal. The diagnosis may be further confused when there is gross discrepancy between all of the above factors and a severity of subjective symptoms, as seen in many secondary gain situations, for example, where workers' compensation is involved.

A knowledge and understanding of the surface anatomy and kinematics of the wrist and the radioulnar joint will usually enable localization of the pathology. Local anesthetic infiltration is an aid in separating intra-articular from extra-articular lesions. Modern radiological techniques, including wrist arthrography, computed tomography (CT) scanning, radioisotope scanning, and fluoroscopic video recording, in addition to motion-study radiographs and special views, are indispensable tools.

Some of the conditions that cause pain on the ulnar side of the wrist are listed in Table 6-1. The more obvious painful conditions that follow acute injury and in which radiographic findings on plain views are usually obvious have been excluded.

Lunotriquetral Instability

Lunotriquetral ligamentous injury varies from sprain to disruption with frank instability. The mechanism of injury is obscure. Wristache is constant and exacerbated by radial-to-ulnar deviation. Tenderness is well localized to the dorsum of the lunotriquetral joint. The ballottement test (D.S. Reagan, MD: written communication, 1984)[1a] causes pain and a click when the triquetrum

Table 6-1. Conditions Causing Ulnar-Sided Wrist Pain

Lunotriquetral instability
Triquetrohamate instability
Ulnocarpal abutment
Distal radioulnar joint subluxation
Triangular fibrocartilage complex–ulnar styloid avulsion
Extensor carpi ulnaris tenosynovitis/tendonitis/subluxation
Triquetrohamate impaction
Radiolunate impaction syndrome
Ulnar compression neuropathy–Guyon's canal
Fractured hook of the hamate
Pisotriquetral joint sprains/malacia/arthrosis

pisiform bones, pinched between the thumb and index of one hand, are moved in a dorsalvolar plane on the lunate, which is fixed between the thumb and index of the other hand. Frank ligamentous disruptions are best confirmed by arthrography, where dye injected into the midcarpal joint is seen leaking between the lunate and the triquetrum into the radiocarpal joint. In many cases, dye will also leak across the triangular fibrocartilage complex into the distal radioulnar joint, in which case the lunotriquetral leak may be the effect rather than the cause, which is ulnocarpal abutment syndrome.[1] In such cases, treatment should be directed to ulnar recession rather than lunotriquetral limited wrist arthrodesis, which I find the most effective treatment for chronic lunotriquetral instability. Arthrodesis is performed as a corticocancellous, iliac crest inlay bone graft.

Triquetrohamate Instability

Triquetrohamate instability presents as a dynamic loss of power and collapse of the wrist on dorsiflexion and ulnar deviation, rather than with pain. A "clunk" can be seen and heard as the triquetrum pops like a pea out of its pod, from the volar low position in radial deviation to the dorsal high position on ulnar deviation of the wrist.[2] The head of the capitate appears as a dorsal prominence on ulnar deviation because of excessive volar flexion of the capitate with an increase in reciprocal midcarpal (lunate-capitate) rotation. It is difficult to capture this dynamic instability on plain films, but fluoroscopic video recording may reveal a snapping triquetrum and midcarpal lunate-capitate instability on ulnar deviation, as the lunate dorsiflexes and the capitate flexes volarward, subluxating the capitate head from the concavity of the lunate. Of the limited wrist arthrodeses available for wrist instability, I have found triquetrohamate fusion for triquetrohamate instability the most reliable, because it blocks ulnar deviation past the neutral position, preventing excessive triquetral rotation and the normal reciprocal midcarpal break. As with lunotriquetral instability, this operation is performed as a corticocancellous, iliac crest inlay bone graft.

Ulnocarpal Abutment

Ulnocarpal abutment has been eruditely termed and explained by Palmer.[1] Patients with this condition present after the third decade and complain of episodic ulnar-sided wrist pain during power gripping. The pain is due to malacia of the lunate and triquetrum induced by chronic abutment against the ulna; this pain is exacerbated by ulnar deviation of the wrist. This condition is more commonly seen in patients with ulna plus and neutral variance, but it has also been demonstrated in association with the ulna minus variant.

The perforated and fragmented triangular fibrocartilage complex (TFCC) can be demonstrated by arthrography; however, treatment should be directed at the cause, which is the relatively long ulna, rather than the effect, (the perforated disk). The relatively long ulna is shortened by transverse osteotomy and fixed with a six-hole dynamic compression plate. Owing to the high torque that is developed on forearm rotation, failure of the fixation device can occur when the plate is of inadequate length and size.

Distal Radioulnar Joint Subluxation

Dislocations of the distal radioulnar joint are quite obvious clinically and radiographically, but subluxations often present as poorly localized wrist pain and clicking with apparently normal radiographs. Dorsal subluxation of the ulna is more common than volar subluxation and follows a pronation injury. It is often associated with Galeazzi's fractures and malunited fractures of the distal radius. Dorsal subluxation of the distal ulna relative to the radius causes pain on supination, which may be blocked in the midrange until the ulna is passively manipulated volarward, enabling further full supination. Objective confirmation of the diagnosis may require CT scanning through the distal radioulnar joint. Acute injuries are treated by immobilization of the reduced distal radioulnar joint in full supination for 6 weeks, and provided the initial reduction is complete, the prognosis is good. Chronic dorsal subluxation can be treated by a volar tenodesis using a distally attached slip of the flexor carpi ulnaris.[3] The less common volar subluxation is treated by dorsal tenodesis using a slip of the extensor carpi ulnaris. When dorsal ulna subluxation is associated with a malunited, dorsally angulated fracture of the distal radius, corrective osteotomy of the radius is required to effect reduction of the subluxated distal radioulnar joint. In this situation I have not found the flexor carpi ulnaris tenodesis procedure necessary; however, excessive radial shortening due to the initial fracture impaction may necessitate concomitant ulnar shortening to restore radioulnar joint congruity and prevent ulnocarpal abutment.

Triangular Fibrocartilage Complex–Ulnar Styloid Avulsion

Chronic pain, clicking, and instability may be due to a tear of the TFCC at its apical attachment at the base of the ulnar styloid process. Alternatively, the styloid may be avulsed by the TFCC as a transverse basal fracture. This condition is differentiated from a TFCC degenerative perforation by fluoroscopic arthrography. Avulsions show dye leaking peripherally under the TFCC, rather than centrally as with perforations.

Very occasionally, more distal styloid fractures cause pain on ulnar deviation, due to styloid-triquetrum impaction, whereas the vast majority of ulnar styloid fractures are quite asymptomatic. With the styloid-triquetrum impaction syndrome, tenderness is well localized over the styloid fragment, pain is reproduced by ulnar deviation, crepitus may be elicited against the ulnar side of the triquetrum, and degenerative cavitation may be evident on the ulnar side of the triquetrum radiographically. If this condition warrants surgical exploration, simple excision of the styloid fragment will alleviate the symptoms.

Extensor Carpi Ulnaris Tenosynovitis, Tendonitis, and Subluxation

Of the wrist's prime movers, only the extensor carpi ulnaris (ECU) has a variable moment arm, as it moves around the head of the ulna on forearm rotation.[4] This dynamic nature of the ECU renders it susceptible to injury, ranging from inflammation to gross fibrillation and rupture of its compartmental septum.[5] This condition is seen in a younger age group of workers who engage in prolonged, repetitious forearm rotation and in athletes who engage in racquet sports such as badminton, squash, and tennis. When conservative measures such as rest, splinting, and anti-inflammatory medication and local corticosteroid infiltration fail to alleviate the symptoms satisfactorily, the tendon is surgically explored. I have seen a 25-year-old female process worker with a 90% rupture of the ECU accompanied by gross fibrillation and inflammatory tenosynovitis. Her job was inspecting confectionery wrappings for imperfections on a rapidly moving conveyor. This work involved forearm rotation at a rate of approximately 80 times per minute for 4 hours at a time. I have also consulted on a case involving a 45-year-old lawyer and social tennis player who presented with neuritis of the overlying dorsal cutaneous branch of the ulnar nerve due to underlying gross inflammatory swelling of the ECU sheath. At surgical exploration in such cases, inflamed tenosynovium is excised, together with fibrillated tendon material. The septum is reconstructed and the tendon tethered dorsally using a slip of the extensor retinaculum.[5]

Triquetrohamate Impaction

The triquetrum normally glides along the helical proximal surface of the hamate to assume the so-called volar position, where it is dorsiflexed on ulnar deviation and ascends to the high dorsal position, where it is relatively volarly flexed on radial deviation. Sudden, forced ulnar deviation and dorsiflexion can impact the triquetrum against the proximal surface of the hamate, causing triquetrohamate chondromalacia. Severe, acute impaction may split the triquetrum or the hamate. The common dorsal chip fracture of the triquetrum may be an impaction rim fracture rather than an avulsion fracture, initiated by this mechanism. Patients with this condition complain of pain on ulnar deviation and have tenderness well localized to the distal and ulnar aspects of the triquetrum. They complain of weakness and instability on power gripping. When conservative measures fail, surgical exploration is indicated. Severe, degenerative changes between the triquetrum and the hamate are best treated by triquetrohamate limited wrist arthrodesis.

Radiolunate Impaction Syndrome

The radiolunate impaction syndrome (R.L. Linscheid, MD: written communication) like the radioscaphoid impaction syndrome, is seen as a repetition stress injury in patients such as Olympic-style gymnasts, who repeatedly force the wrist into dorsiflexion under a load. Eventually, shearing of articular cartilage causes chondromalacia, and dorsal contiguous osteophytes develop, causing pain and limiting dorsiflexion. Clinically these patients have well-localized tenderness to the dorsal pole of the lunate. The differential diagnosis is Kienböck's disease, which is readily diagnosed radiographically, and occult intracapsular ganglion cyst, which arises from a degenerate adjacent scapholunate ligament within the wrist capsule. When the usual conservative measures fail to give sustained relief, surgical débridement becomes necessary, removing the dorsal rim of overhanging radius as well as the dorsal lunate and scaphoid osteophytes. The dorsal capsule is carefully repaired. This procedure alleviates pain but seldom increases the range of dorsiflexion.

Ulnar Compression Neuropathy in Guyon's Canal

Pain in the volar-ulnar aspect of the wrist may be caused by compression neuropathy of the ulnar nerve in Guyon's canal. This may be due to a ganglion cyst arising from a degenerate pisotriquetral joint.[6] Ulnar nerve compression may also be due to inflammatory swelling following fracture of the pisiform or the hook of the hamate. Because of its subcutaneous location in Guyon's canal, ulnar neuritis may be caused directly by occupational trauma, as described in gold polishers, oyster shuckers, and motorcyclists.[6] ulnar artery diseases such as arteritis and thromboangiitis can also directly affect the adjacent nerve.[7] The radial wall of Guyon's canal is closely related to the flexor tendons of the little finger. I have seen localized tenosynovitis of these tendons compressing the ulnar nerve through this radial wall.

Patients with ulnar nerve compression neuropathy in Guyon's canal complain of volar-ulnar wrist pain with paresthesias radiating into the two ulnar digits. The ulnar nerve is tender and percussion causes a positive Tinel's sign. If the deep motor branch is affected, there is weakness and wasting of the ulnar intrinsics of the hand. Surgical decompression of Guyon's canal and neurolysis of the ulnar nerve are the treatment of choice.

Fractured Hook of the Hamate

The hook of the hamate provides an ulnar attachment to the volar carpal ligament. Falls on the outstretched hand or direct blows may strain this ligament, causing well-localized pain and tenderness when the wrist is dorsiflexed. The same symptoms and findings follow fracture of the hook of the hamate, which is difficult to diagnose on plain films. Oblique views and/or carpal tunnel views may be necessary. Sprains of the hamate ligament attachments are treated conservatively. Chronic nonunions of the hook of the hamate are best excised.

Pisotriquetral Joint Sprains, Malacia and Arthrosis

The pisiform is a mobile sesamoid bone within the tendon of the flexor carpi ulnaris. Gliding movement at the pisotriquetral joint is easily elicited by springing the pisiform radially, enabling tenderness and crepitus at this joint to be easily localized. The joint is prone to chondromalacia following direct compression injuries, and arthrosis here is not uncommon. The joint is best viewed on an oblique radiograph of the wrist. Sprains, malacia, and early arthrosis respond well to local corticosteroid infiltration. When this fails, excision of the pisiform is curative with minimal morbidity.

Traumatic calcific tendonitis may involve the flexor carpi ulnaris superficial to the pisiform following repetitious trauma against the volar-ulnar aspect of the wrist, as seen in "hubcap thumpers" (new car detailers). Acute calcific tendonitis of the flexor carpis ulnaris occasionally develops as exquisite, acute volar-ulnar wrist pain without antecedent trauma. This condition is analogous to acute calcific tendonitis of the rotator cuff at the shoulder and is treated similarly by aspiration of the liquid calcific material and infiltration of local anesthetic, in addition to splinting and narcotic medication during the acute phase.

References

1a. Regan DS, Linscheid RL, Dobyns JH. Lunotriquetral sprains. *J Hand Surg* 1984; 4:502–514.

1. Palmer AK, Werner FW: The triangular fibrocartilage complex of the wrist—anatomy and function. *J Hand Surg* 1981;6:153–162.
2. Weber ER: Biomechanical implications of scaphoid waist fractures. *Clin Orthop* 1980;149:83–89.
3. Hui FC, Linscheid RL: Ulnotriquetral augmentation tenodesis: A reconstructive procedure for dorsal subluxation of the distal radioulnar joint. *J Hand Surg* 1982;7:230–236.
4. Youm Y, Ireland DC, Sprague BL, et al: Moment arm analysis of the prime wrist movers, in Komi PV (ed): *Biomechanics V-A*. Baltimore, University Park Press, 1976, pp 355–365.
5. Burkhart SS, Wood MB, Linscheid RL: Post-traumatic recurrent subluxation of the extensor carpi ulnaris tendon. *J Hand Surg* 1982;7:1–3.
6. Shea JP, McClain EJ: Ulnar nerve compression syndromes at and below the wrist. *J Bone Joint Surg Am* 1969;51A:1095–1103.
7. Buck-Gramcko D, Hoffmann R, Neumann, R. *Der handchirurgische Notfall.* Stuttgart, Hippokrates Verlag, 1983.

7

The Rheumatoid Wrist: Natural Course in Absence of Treatment

L. Mannerfelt

The wrist joint is very often involved in rheumatoid arthritis. The distal radioulnar joint, the radiocarpal joint, and the intercarpal joints work together in a kinesiological chain. According to Fick[1] the controlling ligaments have an important role in the movements of this chain. Synovitis first stretches and lengthens the ligaments of the wrist joint and later destroys them. This mechanism helps explain articular collapse situations as seen in the rheumatoid wrist. When untreated, the rheumatoid wrist ends in a weak, painful, and often totally insufficient hand.

Two ligamentous complexes in particular are known to play a role in the sequence of deformities of the rheumatoid wrist. In the first, the capsular band apparatus in the distal radioulnar joint is first distended and then destroyed by the synovitis. The synovitis affects the ulnar head as well, eating away bony structures at the border between cartilage and bone and leaving spurs, which are dangerous for the gliding mechanism of the extensor tendons. In some cases the extensor tendons on the ulnar aspect of the rheumatoid wrist can rupture. These have been called attrition ruptures,[2] and the condition has also been called caput ulnae syndrome.[3]

In the second condition, an invasive and destructive synovitis in the radiocarpal joint causes the radioscapholunate ligament[4] to distend and eventually rupture. The rheumatoid granulations between the scaphoid and lunate bones use this ligament for their proximal propagation, following the vessels through a foramen nutritium in the distal palmar central part of the radius (Fig 7-1). As a result, a so-called radius crypt[5] is often visible (Fig 7-2). In cases of untreated rheumatoid wrist one sees a progressive destruction of the wrist joint (Fig 7-3).

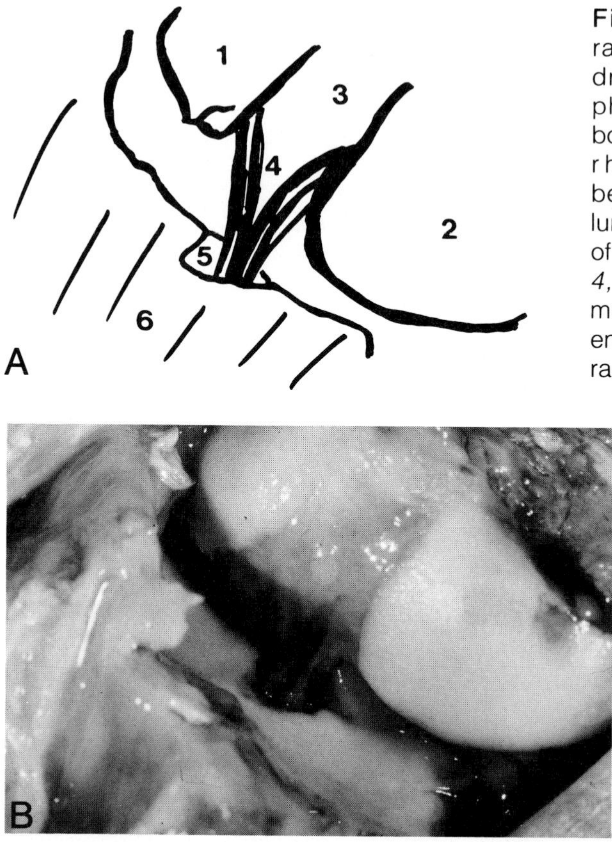

Fig 7-1. Evolution of the radius crypt. *A*, schematic drawing; *B*, intraoperative photograph. *1*, scaphoid bone; *2*, lunate bone; *3*, active rheumatoid synovitis between the scaphoid and lunate bones with elongation of the scapholunate ligament; *4*, radioscapholunate ligament (Testut's ligament); *5*, entrance to the crypt; *6*, distal radius.

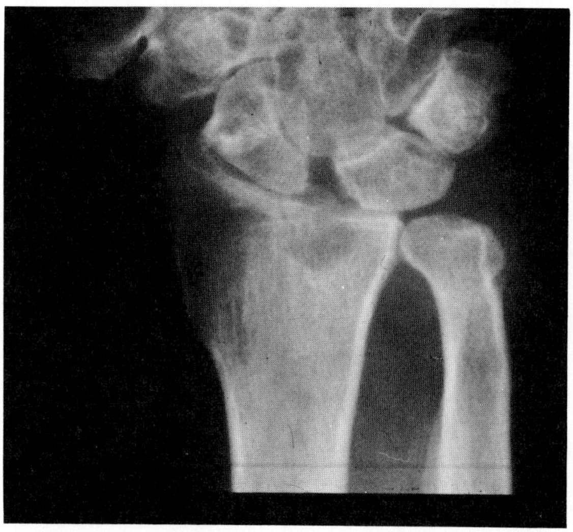

Fig 7-2. The radius crypt is facing the distended scapholunate joint. Note the dissociation between the scaphoid and the lunate.

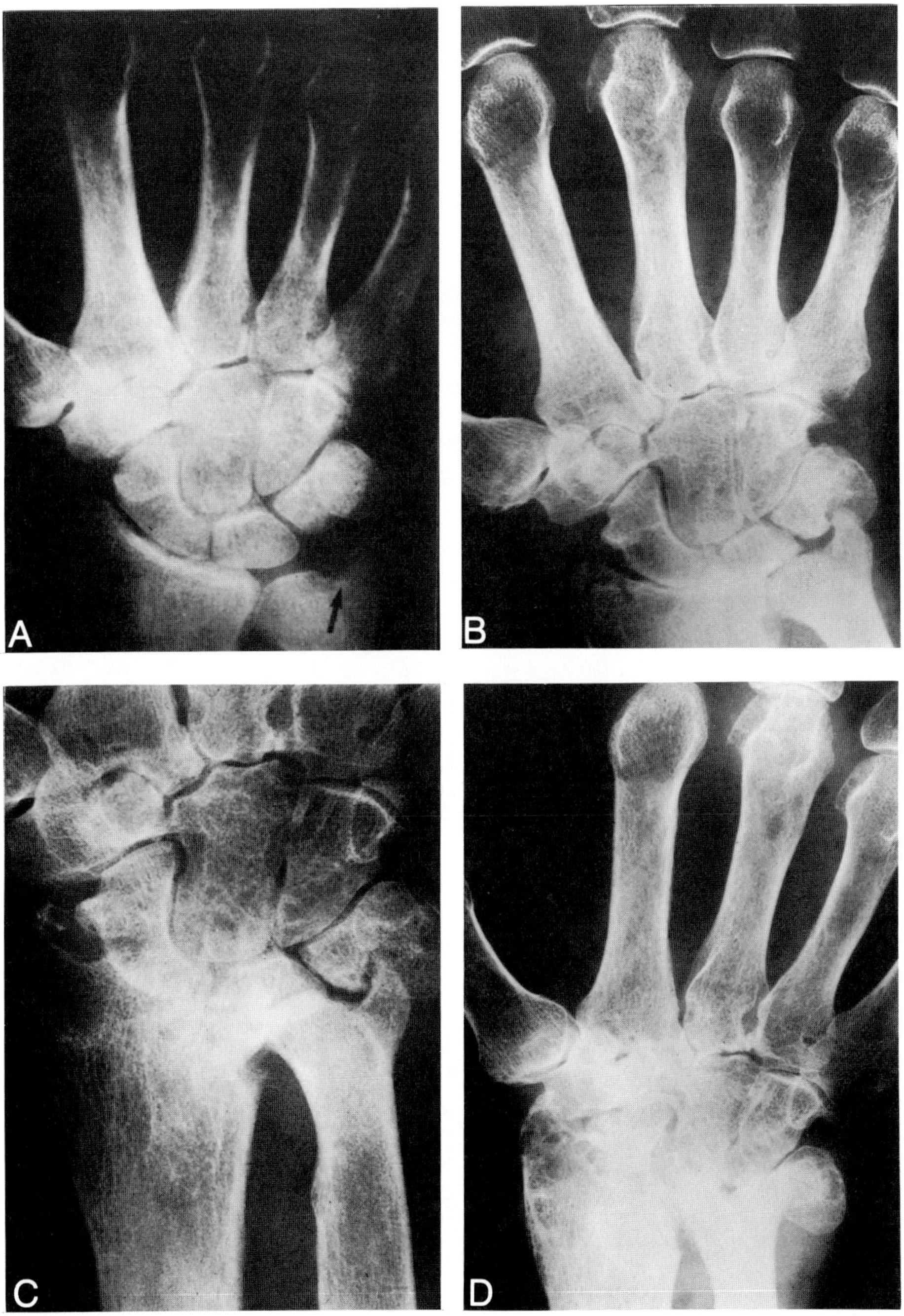

Fig 7-3. Progressive destruction of an untreated rheumatoid wrist joint. *A,* Early stage of the disease with erosion distal to the ulnar head; *B,* ulnar rotation of the first carpal row around an axis situated on the proximal third of the capitate bone, with significant cartilage reduction in the corners of the radius, scaphoid, and lunate; *C,* beginning of collapse; *D,* terminal collapse situation.

The Progressive Destruction of the Rheumatoid Wrist

The progressive deterioration of the radioscapholunate ligament is of great importance for understanding the factors producing collapse situations in the rheumatoid wrist joint. It is known that this ligament possesses vessels and that inflammatory tissue follows vessels into the bones.[6] Moberg and co-workers[7] and Mannerfelt and Norman[8] showed how the rheumatoid tissue could give rise to destruction of bone just at the border between cartilage and bone. The rheumatoid granulations also follow vessels through foramina nutritia into the bone.

The proliferative rheumatoid granulations between the scaphoid and lunate bones enlarge and proliferate in a proximal direction following the vessels through a foramen nutritium at the distal palmar central part of the radius at the border between cartilage and bone. The granulations use the vessels on the radioscapholunate ligament as a transport path into the distal radius. In active cases the granulations destroy the spongy tissue internally at the distal end of radius. On x-ray one can most often see a round cyst, which we call the radius crypt[5] (Fig 7-2).

Early in the disease, the radioscapholunate ligament will be elongated, and later on it ruptures. The proximal carpal row (scaphoid, lunate, and triquetrum) slides in an ulnar direction. This is the so-called *glissement carpien*[9] and results from rotation around a dorsopalmar axis situated in the proximal third of the capitate bone. This axis of rotation was first described by the Swedish roentgenologist Forssell in 1901.[10] These findings were confirmed by Flatt and co-workers in 1978.[11]

When the first carpal row rotates in an ulnar direction, logically, a secondary radial rotation of the distal carpals and metacarpals is noted. In this radial deviation of the middle part of the hand, one often sees a progressive ulnar deviation of the fingers. This is a typical collapse situation (collapse of the intercalated bone segment according to Landsmeer[12]). Such a collapse mechanism in the rheumatoid hand has been called "hand scoliosis"[5] (Fig 7-4).

Fearnley[13] divided the ulnar deviation into three degrees:

- Degree I, in which the patient can reduce the deformity actively
- Degree II, in which the ulnar deviation can be reduced passively
- Degree III, in which the ulnar deviation is fixed and reduction is impossible.

Treatment

It has been shown[14] that treatment with dorsoradial traction orthoses reduces the hand scoliosis. Therefore, in conservative postoperative treatment of ulnar

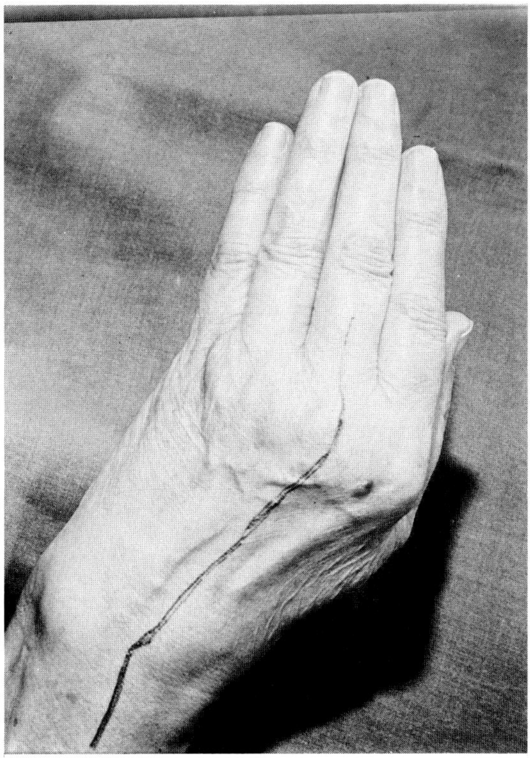

Fig 7-4. Hand scoliosis with radial deviation of the middle of the hand in relation to the radius and ulnar deviation of the fingers in the metacarpophalangeal joints.

deviation of the fingers the wrist joint should be placed in a slight ulnar deviation (Fig 7-5). Likewise, when performing a wrist arthrodesis in rheumatoid arthritis, the arthrodesis should be placed in a slight ulnar deviation, which is possible with the technique of Mannerfelt and Malmsten[15] using as internal fixation a rush-pin equipped with compression staples to prevent rotation and maintain compression. Techniques using Steinman pins are inferior because no elective position of the wrist joint can be achieved.

The question of what is primary and what secondary in the pathogenesis and the pathomechanics of ulnar deviation of the fingers in rheumatoid arthritis is not quite solved. The work of Shapiro[16] and Pahle and Raunio[17] nevertheless indicates that hand scoliosis plays an important role in the development of ulnar deviation of the fingers. Logically, therefore, wrist deformations with ulnar deviation of the four ulnar fingers should be treated as early as possible by dynamic orthosis in which the wrist joint is placed in a slight ulnar deviation.

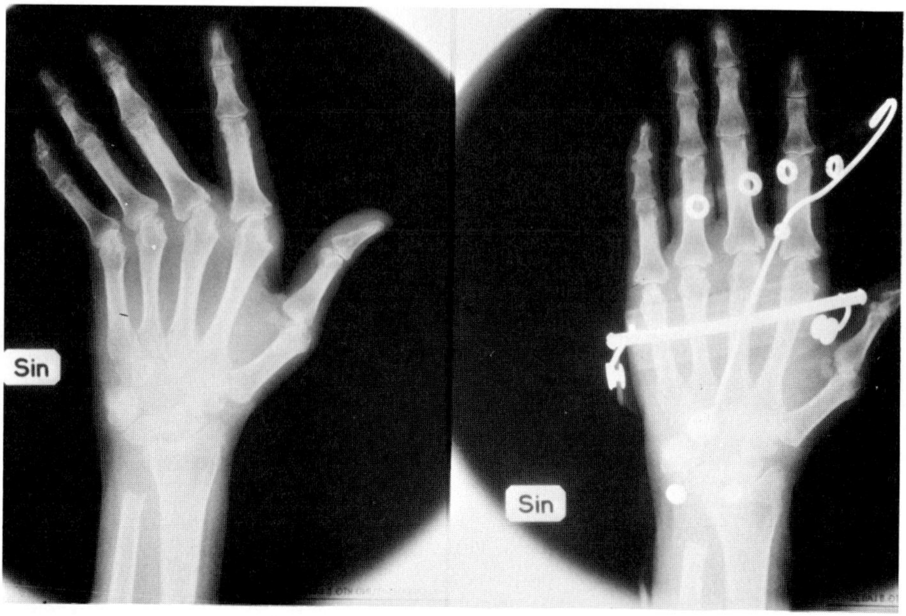

Fig 7-5. A rheumatoid hand after wrist synovectomy and excision of the ulnar head without *(left)* and with *(right)* a dorsoradial traction dynamic orthosis. In the dynamic splint the hand scoliosis is eliminated.

References

1. Fick L: *Physiologische Anatomie des Menschen.* Leipzig, Verlag von Christian Ernst Kollmann, 1845.
2. Vaughan-Jackson OJ: Rupture of extensor tendons by attrition at the inferior radio-ulnar joint. *J Bone Joint Surg Br 1948;30B:528.*
3. *Bäckdahl M: The caput ulnae syndrome in rheumatoid arthritis. Acta Rheumatol Scand* 1963(suppl 5).
4. Testut L, Latarjet A: *Traité d'anatomie humaine.* Paris, Gaston Doin & Cie, 1928.
5. Mannerfelt L, von Raven M: Die Ätiologie und Bedeutung der Radiuskrypte im rheumatischen Handgelenk. *Verh Dtsch Ges Rheumatol* 1978;5:94–96.
6. Lexer E: Die Entstehung entzündlicher Knochenherde und ihre Beziehung zu den Arterienverzweigungen der Knochen. *Arch Klin Chir* 1903;71:1.
7. Moberg E, Wassén E, Kjellberg SR, et al: The early pathologic changes in rheumatoid arthritis. *Acta Chir Scand* 1966(suppl 357):142.
8. Mannerfelt, Norman O: Attrition ruptures of flexor tendons in rheumatoid arthritis caused by bony spurs in the carpal tunnel. *J Bone Joint Surg Br* 1969;51B:270–277.
9. Isemin L, Fournier AM: *La polyarthrite chronique évolutive.* Paris, Masson et Cie, 1956, pp 91–114, 138–140.
10. Forssell G: Über die Bewegungen im Handgelenk des Menschen. Eine röntgographische Studie. *Scand Arch Physiol* (special issue), 1901;12.

11. Flatt AE, cited in Youm Y, McMurtry RY, Flatt AE, et al: Kinematics of the wrist. *J Bone Joint Surg* 1978;60A:423.
12. Landsmeer JMF: Studies in the anatomy of articulation, I. The equilibrium of the "intercalated bone." *Acta Morphol Neerl Scand* 1960;3:288.
13. Fearnley GR: Ulnar deviation of the fingers. *Ann Rheum Dis* 1951;10:126–136.
14. Mannerfelt L, Fredriksson K: *The effect of commercial orthoses on rheumatically deformed hands. Clinical-technical testing and evaluation of commercially available orthotic appliances for ulnar drift in rheumatoid arthritis* (STU-s Informationssektion, STU-Report no 47-1976). Stockholm, Liber Tryck, 1976.
15. Mannerfelt L, Malmsten M: Arthrodesis of the wrist in rheumatoid arthritis. A technique without external fixation. *Scand J Plast Reconstr Surg* 1971;5:124–130.
16. Shapiro JS: The etiology of ulnar drift: A new factor. *J Bone Joint Surg* 1968;50A:634.
17. Pahle J, Raunio P: The influence of wrist position on finger deviation in the rheumatoid hand. *J Bone Joint Surg* 1969;51B:664.

8

Injuries of the Wrist

Neville R. M. Kay

Injuries to the wrist are a common occurrence. Most emergency physicians are aware of the clinical and legal penalties associated with missing a fracture of the scaphoid; however, it is a sad reflection on the general level of knowledge of the anatomy, function, and dysfunction of the wrist after injury that all too frequently perilunar dislocations of the wrist are still regularly missed on initial presentation to the emergency department. Although the function of the hand and the significance of particular injuries have attracted the attention of surgeons for many years, it was not until comparatively recent times that injuries to the wrist attracted attention. Lambrinudi[1] was one of the first to recognize the key function of the scaphoid in the mechanics of the wrist, and his initial concepts of carpal stability have been expanded and amplified by many others, notably Linscheid et al,[2] Fisk,[3] Taliesnik et al,[4] and others. Although this Cinderella-like lack of interest has now been superseded, understanding of the complex mechanics of the normal wrist, let alone the disabled wrist, is far from perfect.[5] This chapter briefly reviews the surgical anatomy of the wrist, with particular reference to the ligaments of the wrist and relates this to the common injuries of the carpus.

Surgical Anatomy of the Wrist

A standard anatomical text[6] describes the carpus as "consisting of eight small irregular bones arranged in two rows, proximal and distal." It is noted that there are four bones in each row, and that each bone, with the exception of the pisiform, articulates with its neighbors in its own row and with the bones above and below it. The large dorsal articular surface of the scaphoid is understood to allow for extension of the wrist, which takes place mainly at the radiocarpal articulation, whereas flexion of the wrist is principally a function of the midcarpal joint. However, the key function of the scaphoid in linking the two rows of carpal bones receives little attention in anatomical texts.

That movements of the wrist are complex and difficult to analyze is well recognized. In an effort to simplify these movements the capitate can be regarded as the central pivot of wrist movements, but it is essential to recall that the physiological axis of wrist movement in normal daily activities is not simple dorsiflexion and palmar flexion of the wrist, but extends along a line from dorsiflexion in radial deviation to palmar flexion in ulnar deviation. It is this axis of movement that allows an artisan—or a surgeon—to throw a hammer onto a chisel.

To simplify the anatomical relationships of the carpal bones for practical and clinical purposes, the "rule of three" has definite advantage. Clinically, the importance of the three C's of the lower end of the radius, the lunate and the capitate being absolutely in line in the lateral radiograph, will prevent perilunar dislocations being missed. Anatomically, the functional concept of three vertical rows of carpal bones stabilized by ligaments arranged in three layers is a useful mnemonic and relates to the complex problem of carpal instability.

The Carpal Rows

Fig 8-1 is a diagrammatic representation of the carpus. It will be seen that three columns of carpal bones can be identified. First, the radial or lateral column carries the thumb and is the most freely mobile column of bones. This row consists of the scaphoid, the trapezoid, and the trapezium, and being the most mobile it is perhaps the most vulnerable to injury and degenerative changes. Interestingly, collapse of this row necessarily induces changes in the other carpal rows (discussed later in this chapter). The central row consists of the lunate and the capitate. Although the capitate can be regarded as the axis of wrist movements in general, the central row is principally concerned with dorsiflexion and palmar flexion of the wrist. Excessive mobility of the lunate on the capitate secondary to trauma to the scapholunate articulation is a potent cause of carpal instability. The third column, the ulnar or medial column, consists of the triquetrum and the hamate, with the pisiform perched on top of the triquetrum. Direct trauma to this column sustained by direct blows to the pisiform and small avulsion flake fractures from the dorsum of the triquetrum are well-recognized wrist injuries. The principal function of the ulnar or medial column is to serve as an axis that translates rotatory movements of the forearm to the wrist.

The Ligaments of the Wrist

Again, the rule of three has a practical application, as the ligaments of the wrist are essentially arranged in three layers, namely, the volar and dorsal carpal ligaments, the extrinsic ligaments, and the intrinsic ligaments of the wrist. The volar carpal ligament can be regarded as a continuation of the antebrachial

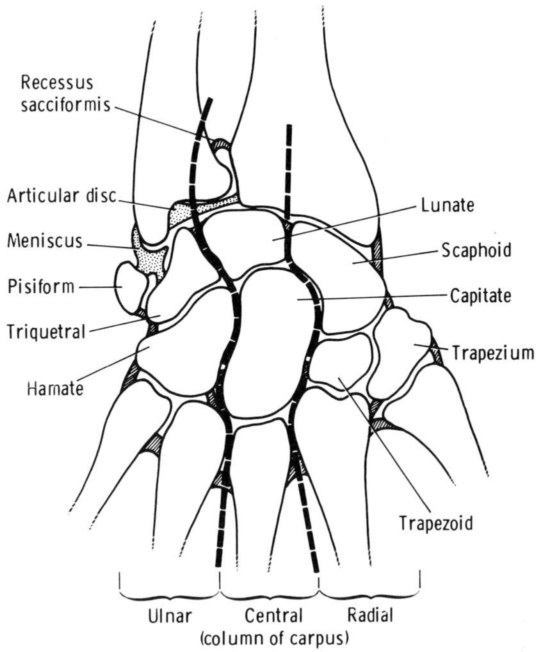

Fig 8-1. The three columns of carpal bones—radial, central, and ulnar—and the arrangements of the intrinsic ligaments of the carpus.

fascia, whose principal function is to prevent the flexor tendons from bowstringing. Curiously, surgical division of this ligament seems to produce only beneficial effects although Fisk[7] has shown ulnar subluxation of the pisiform on the triquetrum following carpal ligament division. The dorsal carpal ligaments have a similar function in retaining the extensor tendons in situ and have some clinical importance in the etiology of tenosynovitis of the extensor tendons.

The second or middle layer of extrinsic ligaments forms the capsular ligaments. The radial collateral ligament attaches to the distal pole of the radius and continues onto the trapezium. Anteriorly, the radial collateral ligament merges with the volar radiocarpal ligament, which is much stronger than the dorsal radiocarpal ligament, and is in two layers.

The ulnar collateral ligament is attached to the styloid process and divides into two fasciculi, one of which attaches to the medial side of the triquetrum, the other to the pisiform bone.

The intrinsic ligaments of the wrist consist of the ligaments between the individual carpal bones. From the point of view of function the articular disc between the lower end of the ulna and the lower end of the radius and the ulnocarpal "meniscus" can be considered as intrinsic ligaments of the carpus, for one of the characteristic features of the intrinsic carpal ligaments is that traumatic rupture of the ligaments results in some degree of carpal malfunction.

Injuries to the Bones of the Carpus

The articular surface of the lower end of the radius is an integral part of the carpus, and logically a Colles' fracture should be considered as the most common of all carpal injuries. Surprisingly, satisfactory wrist function seems to be preserved remarkably well following Colles' fractures. Fractures of the lower end of the radius of the Colles' or Smith's variety need no special mention. However, the practical importance of the relatively weak dorsal radiocarpal ligament is worth recalling in those highly comminuted fractures of the dorsal lip of the radius. In such fractures internal fixation is not a realistic possibility, but frequently the capsule is structurally intact, and manipulation and volar flexion will realign the comminuted fragments of the radius.

Fractures of the Scaphoid

Fractures of the carpal scaphoid have rightly attracted considerable attention from physicians and lawyers. The scaphoid is the most commonly fractured of all the carpal bones, and the mechanism of injury—a fall on the outstretched hand—is a common accident in working life, sporting activities, and military maneuvers. The penalty of missing a fractured scaphoid is so inculcated into the minds of emergency physicians that any patient with pain on the radial side of the wrist tends to be treated as a suspected fractured scaphoid and placed in an appropriate cast. All too frequently, elderly patients with a little carpometacarpal arthritis, or younger patients with de Quervain's stenosing tenovaginitis, have to be rescued from plaster immobilization inflicted on the suspicion of a fractured scaphoid. The clinical differentiation of these conditions from a painful fractured scaphoid is worth noting in the hope of preventing unnecessary repetition of this error (Fig 8-2). Most fractures of the scaphoid can be seen on the first radiographs taken, provided they are of good quality.

Although the mechanism of scaphoid injuries (forced dorsiflexion) is well documented, and it is agreed most patients are best treated conservatively by adequate immobilization, there is no universal agreement as to the ideal method of immobilization or how long it should be maintained. Surprisingly, in a recent review of carpal scaphoid injuries[8] no mention is made of the blood supply of the scaphoid and its effect on healing. Obletz and Halbstein[9] drew attention to the variations in blood supply of the scaphoid and their effect on healing potential. Two principal types of blood supply to the scaphoid were identified, namely, those in which the blood supply was evenly distributed throughout the length of the bone (comprising approximately 70% of subjects) and those (Fig 8-3) in which the blood vessels entered the distal half only (approximately 30%). Clearly, fracture in the former type will not automatically devitalize part of the scaphoid, whereas in the latter type fracture through the waist or the proximal pole may effectively infarct the proximal segment of the scaphoid. In these circumstances, nonunion is highly likely. Although the

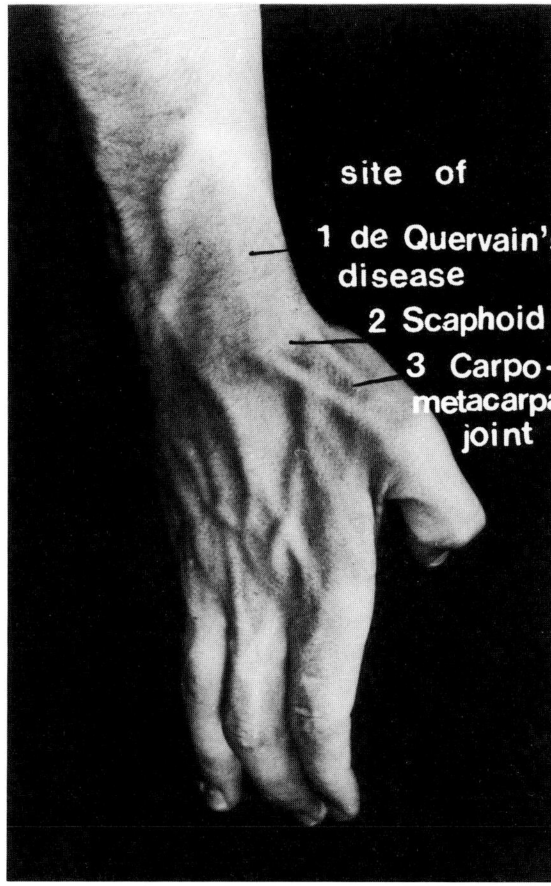

Fig 8-2. The different diagnostic sites of pain on the radial side of the wrist, which are clinically and radiographically differentiated from injuries to the scaphoid.

vascular anatomy of an individual scaphoid will not be known at the time of fracture, the anatomy of the fracture line and any associated rotary deformity of the fragments can be determined from the radiographs.

In simple, uncomplicated fractures of the scaphoid a fixed or standard period of immobilization is illogical. Nonetheless, the dangers inherent in individualizing treatment in busy fracture clinics have to be recognized and some practical compromise reached. Most authorities recommend a period of immobilization of approximately 9 weeks; however, increasing experience with electromagnetic therapy, combined with immobilization of fractures at all sites that prove slow to unite, has reinforced the value of immobilization in achieving union of fractures. For this reason, it is recommended that any fracture of the scaphoid should have a minimum period of immobilization of 9 weeks. Fractures of the waist and proximal pole should be immobilized for 12 weeks in

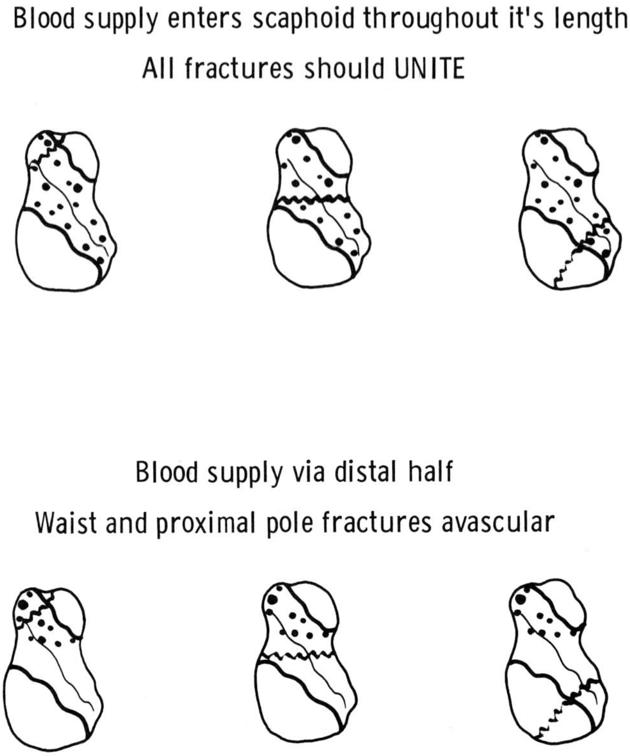

Fig 8-3. The different types of blood supply to the scaphoid. Note that the vessels enter the scaphoid principally on its dorsal surface. Source: Adapted from *Journal of Bone and Joint Surgery* 1938;20:424 by BE Obletz, BM Halbstein with permission of the publisher, © 1938.

---

the hope that those 30% of patients in whom the fracture has amputated the blood supply to part of the bone will unite and so allow natural revascularization of the bone.

The position of immobilization is by no means clearly established. London[10] drew attention to the many methods of immobilizing a fractured scaphoid, and although the position of supination and ulnar flexion (the so-called "wine waiter's" position) has been recommended by Squire,[11] the most common technique of a close-fitting, below-the-elbow cast, with the wrist slightly dorsiflexed and the proximal phalanx of the thumb included in the plaster, proves satisfactory in over 90% of patients. More recently, particularly with the advent of the Herbert scaphoid screw, primary internal fixation of the fractured scaphoid has been advocated.[12]

However, the insertion of the Herbert screw is not without operative trauma to the capsule and ligaments. It is difficult therefore to justify primary internal fixation of simple fractures of the scaphoid unless there are strong overriding indications: for example, in athletes in whom a period of some 9 to 12 weeks of immobilization of the wrist may effectively curtail their professional careers. Fractures of the scaphoid associated with ligamentous injuries such that rotation of the fragments persists despite conservative immobilization, as well as fractures of the scaphoid associated with perilunar dislocation or other carpal injuries, are probably best treated by internal fixation of the scaphoid with the Herbert screw.

Nonunion of the Scaphoid

Nonunion of the scaphoid is a frequent and recognized complication of fractures of the scaphoid. The importance of the fracture anatomy and the blood supply has been discussed, and displacement of the fracture is a recognized cause of nonunion. The real incidence of nonunion of the scaphoid is difficult to assess, because many of the fractures that subsequently go on to nonunion never present for primary treatment. Nonetheless, in patients presenting for treatment an incidence of approximately 5% is documented. The standard method of treating established nonunion of the scaphoid is by anterior bone grafting as described by Russe.[13] Fisk prefers an anterolateral wedge graft and claims the advantage that such a graft not only corrects the deformity in the scaphoid but effectively brings the bone out to length and so tightens up the carpal ligaments. It also has the added advantage of removing the radial styloid.[14]

The treatment of late, established fractures of the scaphoid (10 to 15 years after the injury) is essentially the treatment of arthritis of the wrist. It is surprising how many patients can tolerate an ununited fracture of the scaphoid for 20 years or more only to have disabling wrist pain after some trivial trauma to the wrist (Fig 8-4). Usually at this late stage there are well-established arthritic changes in the scaphoradial articulation, and if there has been effective collapse of the scaphoid, degenerative changes in the radial column of bones and in the radiolunate articulation are by no means rare. If the symptoms are sufficiently severe, localized intercarpal arthrodesis or, not infrequently, formal arthrodesis of the wrist will be necessary.

Lunate Dislocations

The lunate is the linchpin of the wrist. The normal anatomical relationship of the lunate to the lower end of the radius with the wrist in the neutral position has already been noted, but it is worth recalling that the lunate is also cone shaped, broader volarly than it is dorsally. The common mechanism of injury to the wrist is forced dorsiflexion, and if this is combined with supination the lunate may be squeezed out of the carpus like a pea from a pod (Fig 8-5). A proper examination of the radiographs will always reveal the nature of the dislocation, but in any wrist in which there is huge swelling, marked pain, and symptoms of

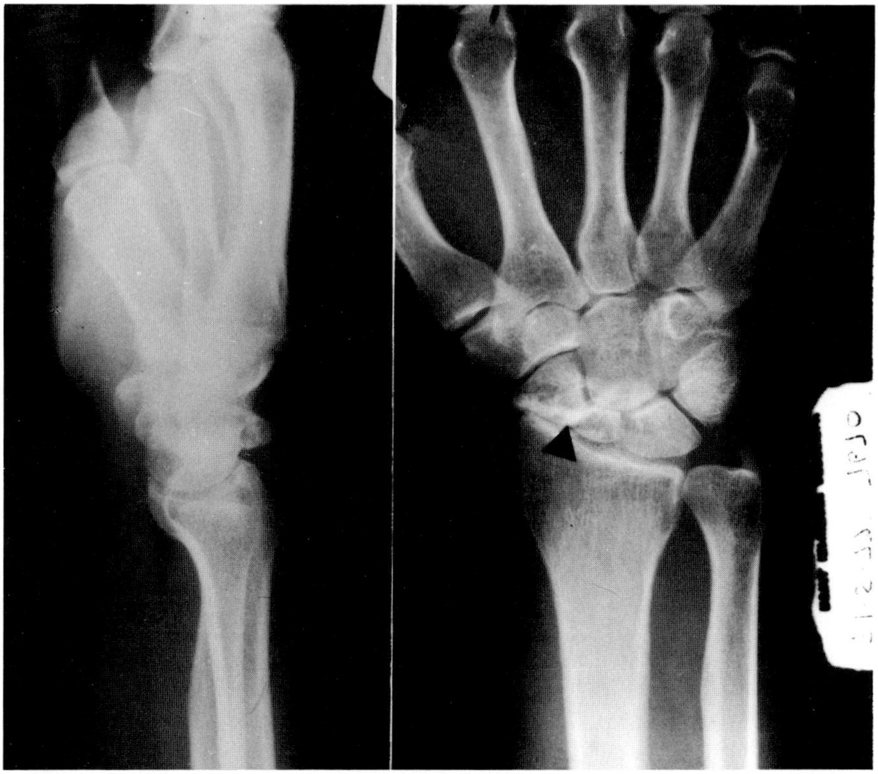

Fig 8-4. Lateral *(left)* and anteroposterior *(right)* views of an old, ununited fracture of the scaphoid now symptomatic after minor trauma.

median nerve compression without an obvious radiographic fracture, dislocation of the lunate must always be suspected. Seniority and experience are no guarantee against missing lunate dislocations, and if there is serious clinical doubt but inconclusive radiographic evidence, further x-rays and, if necessary, screening under the image intensifier will help elucidate the diagnosis.

Simple perilunar dislocations are usually reducible by closed manipulative techniques. The reduction should be stabilized by a single Kirschner wire, and complicated lunate dislocations (ie transscaphoid perilunar dislocation or scaphoperilunar dislocations) always require stabilization. In many of these cases primary internal fixation of the scaphoid and stabilization of the lunate offer the best hope of a functioning wrist.

Kienböck's Disease

In any discussion on injury to the carpus Kienböck's disease of the lunate has to be considered, for all too frequently its radiographic presentation is precipitated by some minor wrist injury.

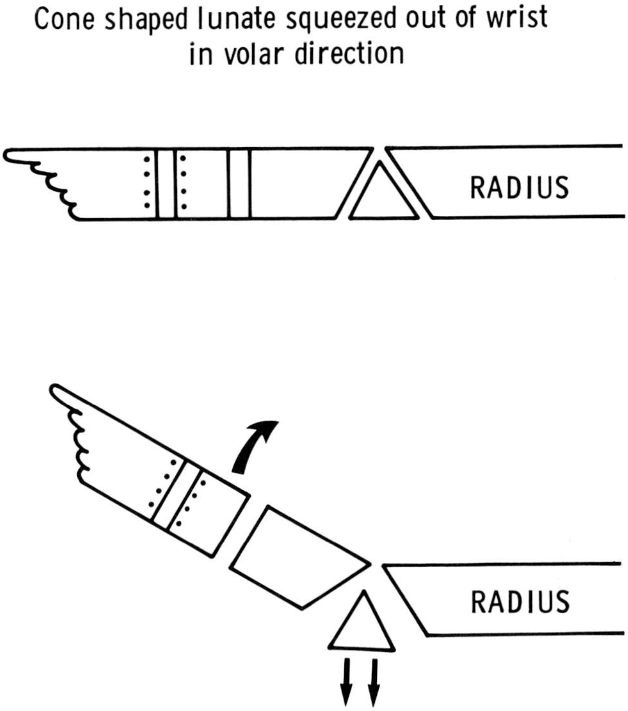

Fig 8-5. Schematic illustration of the lunate being squeezed volarly from the carpus in lunate dislocation.

The precise cause of Kienböck's disease is still unknown. Much has been written on the association of "ulnar minus" with Kienböck's disease, and this has resulted in enthusiastic lengthening of the ulna or shortening of the radius. A recent review[15] claims good results for this method of treatment, but doubt has been cast as to whether there is a true ulnar minus or merely a radiographic aberration. Certainly several patients with unilateral Kienböck's disease and apparent ulnar minus deformity show a similar ulnar minus deformity in the other wrist without the development of Kienböck's disease.

Repeated minor trauma at work is often cited as a cause of Kienböck's disease, but the probable cause is repeated episodes of transitory ischemia, as in Perthes' disease of the hip. This may be related to the fact that the intracapsular pressure is probably maximal in the lunate during gripping. Experimentally raising the intracapsular pressure has been shown as a possible cause of Perthes' disease in the hips of dogs.

The treatment of Kienböck's disease of the wrist is almost as enigmatic as its cause. There is no certain correlation between the radiographic signs and the patient's symptoms (Fig 8-6). Surgery at the time the patient first presents, in the form of excision arthroplasty and replacement of the lunate with either a

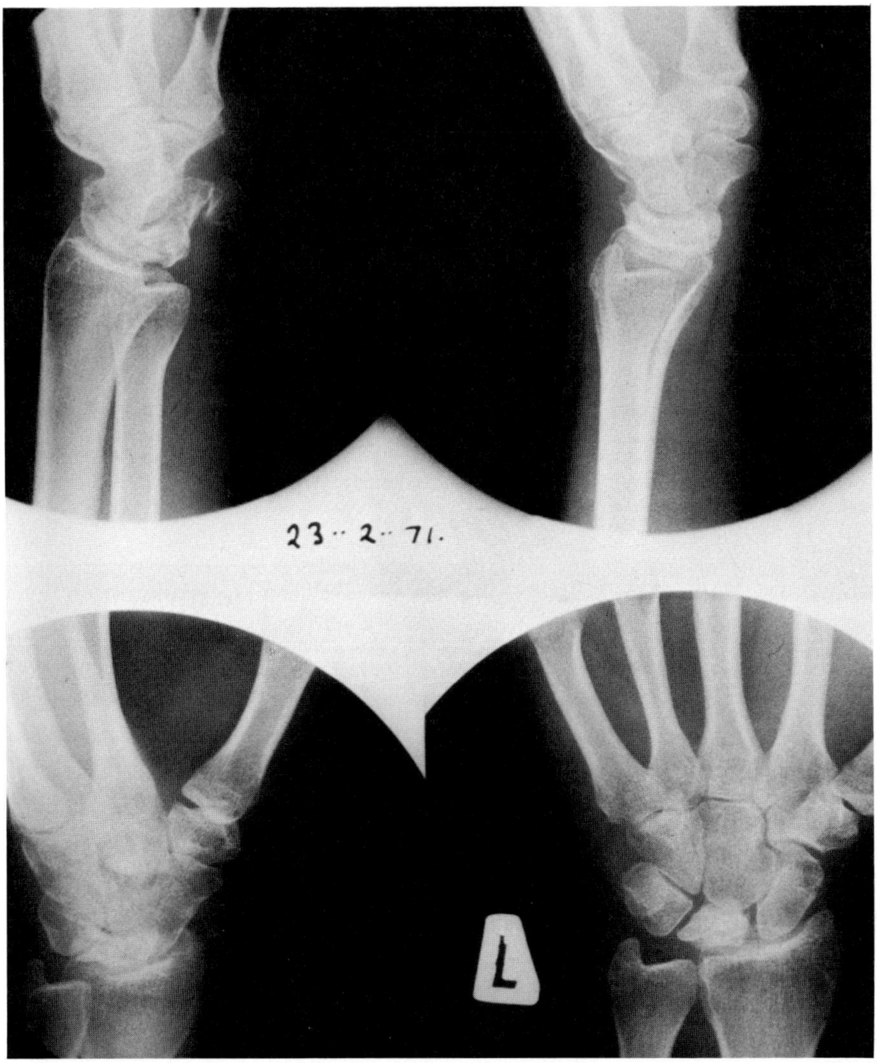

Fig 8-6. Established Kienböck's disease of the lunate. *Top,* lateral views; *bottom,* anteroposterior views.

rolled-up tendon or a Silastic prosthesis (Swanson's model), appears to give satisfactory results. On the other hand, some 60% of patients treated conservatively have good results. What appears to be critical is the collapse of the proximal row of the carpus. If the lunate loses height and the capitate intrudes between the scaphoid and the triquetrum, then whatever method of treatment is adopted the results are usually poor. This is the clinical dilemma. To operate early before collapse has occurred should in theory permit a good result—yet at the same time may be unnecessary. To wait too long and allow collapse to occur is an almost certain guarantee of a poor result. As yet, there appears to be no certain way of solving this clinical dilemma.

Ligamentous Injuries and Carpal Instability

Knowledge of the patterns of instability of the wrist has increased considerably since Lambrinudi's original work in 1943, and in an individual case the underlying cause may be identified with some precision; having identified the cause of the carpal instability, however, the results of logical surgical treatment of the underlying defect still leave much to be desired. Carpal instability can be defined as abnormal laxity of the ligaments of the wrist allowing subluxation of the bones of the carpus, which in turn allows buckling and malalignment. This occurs principally in the radial and central columns of the wrist, and the principle cause is trauma. The most common type of carpal instability results from hyperextension injury of the proximal row of the carpus on the lower end of the radius. There is buckling at the capitolunate joint surface such that the capitate assumes a hyperflexed position. This effectively shortens the central column of the carpus, and to accommodate for this shortening changes have to occur in the lateral (radial) column of the carpus, and the scaphoid is forced into flexion. If the interosseous ligament between the scaphoid and the lunate ruptures, a gap may be visible on the posteroanterior radiograph of the wrist, and the scaphoid may be so flexed that its longitudinal axis lies in a sagittal plane (Fig 8-7). This deformity has been described by Linscheid as dorsal intercalary carpal instability (DICI). The reverse deformity produced by flexion of the lunate and hyperextension of the capitolunate joint, although occurring less frequently, again forces the scaphoid into a hyperflexed position. This condition has been labeled volar intercalary carpal instability (VICI). A third, though much less frequent type of carpal instability affects the medial or ulnar column. Traumatic disruption of the interosseous ligament between the triquetrum and the hamate will allow excessive movement at the triquetrohamate joint, which occasionally results in a painful snapping of the wrist.

The treatment of carpal instability leaves much to be desired. Rarely is the instability noted at the time of the injury; the patient simply presents with a "sprained wrist." Because it is well recognized that ligamentous tissue takes some 3 weeks to heal and acquire some mechanical strength, there is much to be said for immobilizing badly sprained wrists in a close-fitting plaster for 3 weeks in the hope of maintaining the carpus in its correct position and allowing ligamentous healing to occur. Few patients are willing to tolerate such immobilization for a sprained wrist, and perhaps an unintentional spinoff from the overenthusiastic immobilization of the doubtful fractured scaphoid is the adequate conservative treatment of these unrecognized, unstable carpal injuries.

Once the instability is established and recognized, surgical treatment is disappointing. Fisk[7] recommends stabilization of the scaphoid by reinforcing

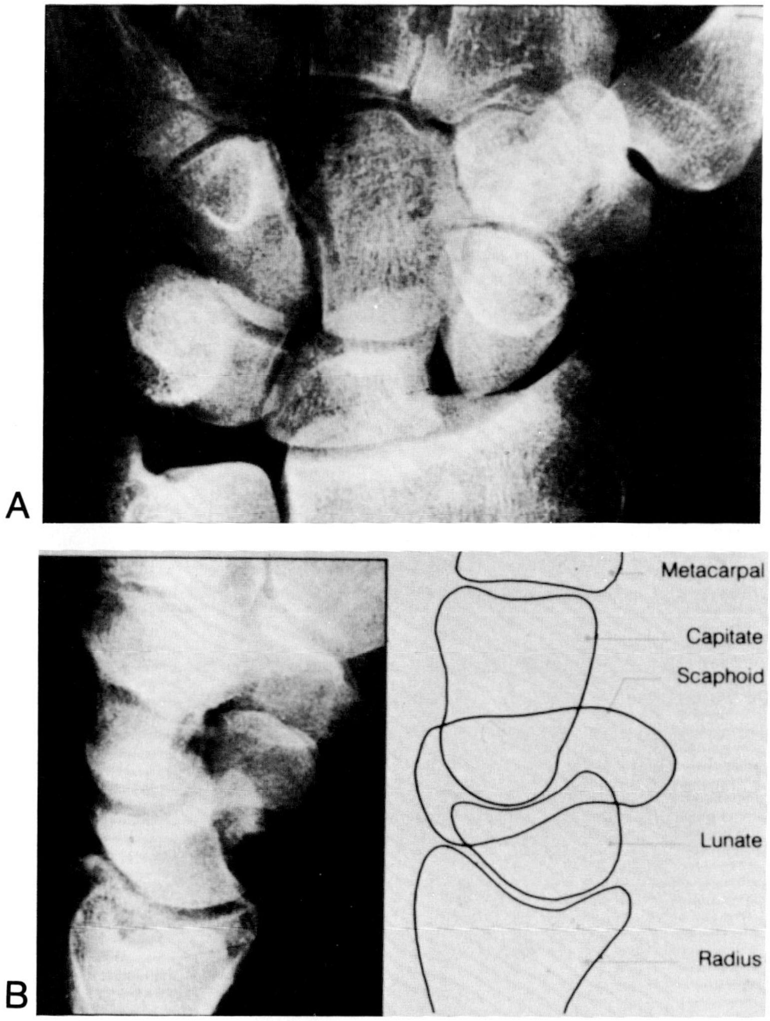

Fig 8-7. *A,* Posteroanterior view of the wrist shows the increased gap between the scaphoid and the lunate following a tear of the ligaments that normally hold these bones together. Freed of this restraint, the scaphoid has rotated into a more sagittal position and looks foreshortened. *B,* Lateral view of the wrist shows that the lunate has rotated into dorsiflexion, creating a Z-shaped deformity in the radius-lunate-capitate axis. The scaphoid has rotated the other way, and its long axis is almost at 90° to the axis of the arm (horizontal scaphoid). Source: Reprinted from *Surgery* 1983;1:62 by N Barton with permission of Medical Education (International) Ltd, © 1983.

the dorsal ligament, and various reconstructive ligamentous procedures have from time to time been advocated and subsequently abandoned.

Lesions of the Triangular Fibrocartilage

Interest has recently been revived in the triangular fibrocartilage between the lower end of the radius and the ulna. This is a structure of variable size but is one of the principal stabilizing structures between the lower end of the radius and the ulna, and as such should be regarded as an "intrinsic ligament" of the carpus. When the carpus is in flexion and ulnar deviation, this ligament forms a major part of the articular surface between the proximal carpal row and the inferior radioulnar articulation. Interestingly, degenerative changes with aging are reported in this meniscus. Not surprisingly, tears in this meniscus can be produced, and forced hyperextension injuries may rupture the ligament. Clinically, this will produce pain in the wrist, sometimes associated with a clicking noise, which when heard through the stethoscope can sound quite dramatic. Arthrography of the wrist is occasionally helpful in confirming the diagnosis, and excision of the torn articular disk may give symptomatic relief.

References

1. Gifford WW, Bolton RH, Lambrinudi C: Mechanism of wrist joint with specific reference to fractures of the scaphoid. *Guys Hosp Rep* 1943;92:52–59.
2. Linscheid RL, Dobyns JH, Beaubout JW, et al. Traumatic instability of the wrist: Diagnosis, classification and pathomechanics. *J Bone Joint Surg Am* 1972;54A:1612–1632.
3. Fisk GR: Carpal instability and the fractured scaphoid. *Ann R Coll Surg Engl* 1970; 46:63–67.
4. Taliesnik J, Malerich M, Prietto M: Palmar carpal instability secondary to dislocation of the scaphoid and lunate: Report on the case and review of the literature. *J Hand Surg* 1982;7:602–612.
5. Mayfield JK, Johnson RP, Kilcoyne RK: Carpal dislocations: Pathomechanics and progressive perilunar instability. *J Hand Surg* 1980;5:226–241.
6. Frazer JE: *The Anatomy of the Human Skeleton.* London, J. A. Churchill, 1920, 101–120.
7. Fisk GR: The wrist. *J Bone Joint Surg Br* 1984;66B:396–407.
8. Leslie IJ, Dickson RA: The fractured carpal scaphoid: Natural history and factors influencing outcome. *J Bone Joint Surg Br* 1981;63B:225–230.
9. Obletz BE, Halbstein BM: Non union of fractures of the carpal navicular. *J Bone Joint Surg* 1938;20:424.
10. London PS: The broken scaphoid bone—The case against pessimism. *J Bone Joint Surg Br* 1961;43B:237–243.
11. Squire M: Carpal mechanics and trauma. *J Bone Joint Surg Br* 1959;41B:210.

12. Herbert TJ: Management of the fractured scaphoid bone using a new surgical technique. *J Bone Joint Surg Br* 1982;64B:633.
13. Russe O: Fractures of the carpal navicular. Diagnosis, nonoperative treatment and operative treatment. *J Bone Joint Surg Am* 1960;42A:759–768.
14. Fisk GR: Wedge grafting of the ununited fractured scaphoid, in Robb CG, Smith ER (eds): *Operative Surgery Orthopaedics Part II.* London, Butterworths, 1979.
15. Ovesen J: Shortening of the radius and the treatment of lunatomalacia. *J Bone Joint Surg Br* 1981;63B:231–232.

9

Carpal Kinematics

D. C. R. Ireland

Carpal kinematics is the study of the relative motion between individual carpal bones. This study enables analysis of the contribution of individual joints to a given range and arc of wrist motion and prediction of the same following limited wrist arthrodesis or localized carpal pathology. A knowledge of normal kinematics permits understanding and recognition of the pathokinematics of static and dynamic carpal instability patterns.

The carpus is a complex joint. It has eight separate links which enable true universal joint function. Not only can the carpus move in any direction and lock in any position, but through the carpus, the hand is able to move from one position to any other without first returning through the fixed axis of rotation. This requires the carpal bones to function variably as individual units and collectively as two horizontal rows and three vertical columns.[1]

The scaphoid is a convenient starting point. It stabilizes the midcarpal joint by connecting the proximal carpal row at the scapholunate joint to the distal carpal row at the scaphotrapezial joint. The scaphoid thus functions as a linkage in this three-link system,[2] the forearm being the proximal link, the proximal carpal row the middle link (intercalated segment), and the distal carpal row and the rigidly attached second, third, and fourth metacarpals the distal link. The stabilizing effect of the scaphoid prevents zigzag accordian collapse on compression loading.[3] Linscheid[4] has adapted the mechanical analogy of a slider-crank to the scaphoid, which allows synchronous, simultaneous movement at the proximal and distal carpal rows.

The scaphoid rotates from its neutral position of 45° into a more horizontal position on ulnar deviation, appearing in full profile in the posteroanterior (PA) plane. On radial deviation it rotates vertically, appearing foreshortened. Given that the radial side of the carpus is changing in height in radial-to-ulnar deviation and the overall shape of the carpus is constant, there being a fixed axis and center of rotation in the head of the capitate,[5] there must be: (a) a corresponding reciprocal change in height on the ulnar side of the carpus, and (b) midcarpal movement to allow for the changing vertical height of the scaphoid, without stressing its proximal and distal ligamentous attachments. The reciprocal ulnar-sided carpal motion is provided by the triquetrum. On full ulnar deviation, with the scaphoid at maximal height in the PA view (and horizontal in the lateral view), the triquetrum appears fully covered by the hamate in its volar low position, where it is dorsiflexed. This is seen in the lateral ulnar deviation view. As the wrist passes toward radial deviation (and the scaphoid rotates vertically, foreshortening the lateral mobile column), the triquetrum ascends along the helical proximal articular surface of the hamate to the proximal dorsal high position,[6] where it is relatively volarly flexed and appears radiologically uncovered by the hamate on the PA view.

The clinical application of this reciprocal rotating medial ulnar column and mobile lateral radial column motion in the normal wrist is the identification of ligamentous disruptions of the proximal row. If the PA view demonstrates a vertical scaphoid while the triquetrum assumes the volar low dorsiflexed position, covered by the hamate, then there must be a ligamentous disruption between either the scaphoid and the lunate or the lunate and the triquetrum. The same pathology exists when a horizontal (fully profiled PA view) scaphoid is associated with an uncovered triquetrum in the high dorsal proximal position, where it is volarly flexed. Whether the ligamentous disruption is between the scaphoid and the lunate, or between the lunate and the triquetrum, is determined by the position of the lunate on the lateral view. If the lunate remains with the triquetrum in the low dorsiflexed position while the scaphoid is vertical, then a scapholunate dissociation is present. If the lunate is volarly flexed with the scaphoid, while the triquetrum is in the low dorsiflexed position, then a lunotriquetral disruption exists. This has been described as a break in Shenton's line of the wrist,[1] where there is a disruption of the normal arc of the proximal carpal row.

The reciprocal midcarpal movement occurs at the lunocapitate midcarpal joint, which is spanned by the scaphoid, accommodating its changing height on radial-to-ulnar deviation by reciprocal midcarpal motion. On ulnar deviation the lunate dorsiflexes and the capitate flexes volarward, whereas on radial deviation the lunate flexes volarward while the capitate dorsiflexes. Taleisnik[1] has termed this normal reciprocal midcarpal motion between the lunate and the capitate the precollapse pattern, as it can permit excessive midcarpal motion to the point of dorsal subluxation of the head of the capitate from the concavity of the distal articular surface of the lunate on ulnar deviation, if the midcarpal ligaments are disrupted or attenuated, as is seen in triquetrohamate dynamic instability.

This study of radial-to-ulnar deviation indicates that although movement occurs at both the radiocarpal and midcarpal joints, the midcarpal joint movement is the intrinsic carpal movement which allows for predominantly radiocarpal motion of the wrist in this plane.

Carpal kinematics in the dorsiflexion-volar flexion plane is less complex than radial-to-ulnar deviation motion, and again the scaphoid plays the pivotal role. From the neutral position to dorsiflexion, midcarpal lunate-capitate motion occurs with synchronous radiocarpal motion, until the scaphoid rotates to its maximal horizontal inclination, tethered by the volar radioscaphoid ligaments.[7] This locks the midcarpal joints so that all further motion into dorsiflexion is radiocarpal. Sarrafian et al[8] have calculated that from the neutral position to dorsiflexion wrist motion is 34% midcarpal and 66% radiocarpal. From the neutral position to volar flexion, the scaphoid unlocks the midcarpal joint, allowing synchronous midcarpal and radiocarpal motion by the slider-crank mechanism effect.[4] Sarrafian et al[8] have estimated that volar flexion is composed of 60% midcarpal and 40% radiocarpal motion.

The clinical application of normal carpal kinematics and pathokinematics may help determine effective treatment for carpal instability. Personal experience indicates that frank carpal instabilities are most effectively treated by limited wrist arthrodesis of the unstable joint. A knowledge of normal carpal kinematics enables an accurate prediction of the anticipated loss of wrist movement following this treatment. When this is matched with the patient's vocational requirements, for example, power, stability, and freedom from pain in the dominant wrist of a young male boilermaker or welder, or maximal mobility for a cellist's wrist, I am inclined to choose scapholunocapitate limited wrist arthrodesis for scapholunate instability in the boilermaker or welder and scaphotrapeziotrapezoid limited wrist arthrodesis[9] for the cellist. The arc of movement rather than the range of movement may be a consideration in providing volar flexion for personal hygiene if the contralateral wrist is stiff, whereas dorsiflexion is preferable when power gripping is required.

The routine radiographic motion view series of the wrist includes the opposite plane, the clenched fist, radial deviation, and ulnar deviation. This study may indicate minimal motion in an arthritic intercarpal joint, in which case the patient can be assured preoperatively that the anticipated loss of pain will not be accompanied by loss of motion.

References

1. Taleisnik J: Post-traumatic carpal instability. *Clin Orthop* 1980;149:73–82.
2. Gilford WW, Bolton RH, Lambrinudi C: The mechanism of the wrist joint. *Guys Hosp Rep* 1943;92:52.
3. Fisk GR: Carpal instability and the fractured scaphoid. *Ann R Coll Surg Engl* 1970;46:2:63.
4. Linscheid RL, Dobyns JH, Beabout JS, et al.: Traumatic instability of the wrist. *J Bone Joint Surg Am* 1972;54A:1628.
5. McMurtry RY, Youm Y, Flatt AE, et al.: Kinematics of the wrist. *J Bone Joint Surg Am* 1978;60A:955–961.

6. Weber ER: Biomechanical implications of scaphoid waist fractures. *Clin Orthop* 1980;149:83–89.
7. Mayfield JK, Johnson RP, Kilcoyne RK: Carpal dislocations: pathomechanics and progressive perilunar instability. *J Hand Surg* 1980;5:226–241.
8. Sarrafian SK, Melamed JL, Goshgarian GM: Study of wrist motion in flexion and extension. *Clin Orthop* 1977; 126:153–159.
9. Watson HK, Hempton RF: Limited wrist arthrodeses. I. the triscaphoid joint. *J Hand Surg* 1980;5:320–327.

10

Bone Grafting for Scaphoid Nonunion Using a Volar Corticocancellous Inlay Bone Graft From the Iliac Crest

D. C. R. Ireland

The scaphoid may fail to unite following acute fracture for a number of different reasons. Inadequate immobilization is usually due to missed early diagnosis. Inadequate reduction, another cause of nonunion, does not necessarily preclude union; however, a malunited, foreshortened scaphoid may become more symptomatic, with arthritic pain and stiffness, than a chronic nonunion. Proximal-pole fractures are prone to develop avascular necrosis, which significantly diminishes the chances of osteosynthesis by conservative means. The unstable acute scaphoid fracture often fails to unite, even with cast immobilization, because compression loading across the carpus, as in power gripping, forces the unstable scaphoid into flexion, as the normal inclination of the scaphoid at approximately 45° to the vertical makes the volar surface the compressive load-bearing side and the dorsal surface the tensile load-bearing surface. This flexion deformity can rotate the fragments at right angles to each other. The effects of malrotation of the scaphoid fragments are multiple. Initially there is diminished bony contact between the two fragments, which minimizes the chances of osteosynthesis. Diminished bony surface contact causes a high, volar pressure point, which induces bone resorption with further compressive loading. This foreshortens the scaphoid, initiating carpal collapse and eventual wrist instability. Malrotation and foreshortening lead to radioscaphoid articular incongruity and eventual radioscaphoid osteoarthritis.

Scaphoid osteosynthesis with the two fragments in the derotated, reduced position is thus desirable. For established nonunion, this procedure requires a volar approach to derotate the fragments, a large bone graft to bridge and fill the volar resorption gap, and adequate fixation to stabilize the fracture. Metallic internal fixation may provide stability,[1] but it is bone graft that bridges the volar gap and provides the scaffold for osteosynthesis. A bone-grafting technique that provides both the nidus and scaffold and additionally the rigid fixation and stability required for osteosynthesis is ideal, as this obviates the necessity for an additional mechanical device, which reduces the volume and surface contact for bone graft, may damage joint surfaces, and may require a secondary procedure for removal.

Surgical Technique

A volar Russe[2] approach is made between the flexor carpi radialis and the radial vessels. There is a profusion of small vessels passing ulnarward which require electrocautery. This approach exposes the volar radial wrist capsule, which is divided in continuity with the periosteum of the distal radius and elevated carefully with the radiocarpal meniscoid. The fracture is often malrotated to a right angle, so that the distal pole is seen end-on. The fracture is reduced by dorsiflexion and ulnar deviation, which is maintained using the adjustable hand stand. The fracture may open volarly by up to 8 mm, exposing the resorbed margins. Obtaining and maintaining this reduction are the key to success, because the scaphoid height is restored, correcting carpal collapse; the scaphoid will mirror its shape on the radial facet and prevent pressure points, which cause osteoarthritis, and volar opening at the compression surfaces allows the graft to be firmly locked into position, obviating the need for additional internal fixation.

A trough is marked with ink on the volar surface of the scaphoid. This trough is cut with an oscillating minisaw. The trough is made 6 mm wide and 18 to 20 mm long. The two fragments are removed with a 5-mm osteotome, and the trough is deepened to the dorsal cortex, using a 6-mm, round-headed bur on a high-speed drill. The proximal and distal ends of the trough are undercut to take a slightly trapezoid-shaped graft, which becomes locked on compressive loading across the scaphoid, preventing extrusion. A side-cutting bur may next be used to square off the corners of the trough, permitting maximal contact between cancellous bone graft and recipient.

The graft is now cut from the iliac crest as a tricortical cancellous graft through the crest to include a full-thickness segment of ilium to the exact width of graft required (ie, 6 mm). The graft may be cut with two sharp, parallel osteotomes or a heavy-duty oscillating saw to yield a wedge of corticocancellous graft 20 to 30 mm long and 6 mm wide. The inner iliac table is slightly concave, resembling the shape of the scaphoid. The crest and outer table are now excised using the micro-oscillating saw to tailor the graft to the exact dimensions of the trapezoidal trough previously cut in the scaphoid. I do not believe such a graft can be "custom-cut" from anywhere but the ilium. The trabecular pattern and density of iliac cancellous bone are superior to those of the distal radius. The cortex acts as the internal fixation device, whereas the cancellous bone acts as the graft to stimulate osteosynthesis.

The graft is countersunk 1 mm below the surface of the scaphoid to prevent radioscaphoid impingement with volar flexion. The capsule is carefully closed, together with the periosteum over the distal radius. An absorbable subcuticular suture is used to close the wound. A below-the-elbow cast is applied, which prevents elbow flexion beyond 90° and extends distally to include the thumbnail. The cast is removed after 8 weeks and replaced by a removable splint worn 12 hours a day for a further 6 weeks. Proximal-pole fractures with avascular necrosis are immobilized in an above-the-elbow cast for a period of 12 weeks.

Material

I have used this technique on 52 wrists in 51 patients between 1977 and 1983. There were 50 males and 2 females. The average patient age was 25 years, and the average duration of symptoms was 39 months (if two patients, a 60-year-old farmer with a 40-year history of wrist instability due to scaphoid fracture and a 45-year-old housewife with a 20-year history, are excluded).

Follow-up

All of these patients have been personally treated, and none have been lost to follow-up. Eight of the 52 patients were excluded from the series, as follow-up from the time of surgery was less than 6 months. The 44 bone-grafted scaphoids have been followed for periods ranging from 6 months to 6 years, the average being 23 months.

As all of these patients had established nonunions of the scaphoid, rather than acute, unstable fractures, they have been simply classified as proximal-pole fractures, waist fractures, and distal-pole fractures. There were 8 proximal-pole fractures, 25 waist fractures, and 11 distal-pole fractures. Of the 44 nonunions, in 10 the proximal poles were avascular, as proven at the time of surgery. Five of these 10 had proximal-pole fractures, four had waist fractures, and one a distal fracture. In assessing the vascularity of the proximal pole radiographically, there were as many false negatives as false positives. The criteria for determining scaphoid union following bone grafting were diminished pain, increased grip strength, increased range of movement, and radiographic evidence of bone trabeculae crossing the previous fracture site.

Results

Forty-two of the 44 bone-grafted scaphoids have united. This includes three previously operated scaphoids, one of which had had three different prior procedures before this method proved successful. The two scaphoids that failed to unite had avascular necrosis in addition to fragmentation of the proximal pole, which had not been appreciated preoperatively.

This technique thus produced a rate of union of the scaphoid following volar corticocancellous inlay bone grafting in chronic nonunions of the scaphoid of

95%. Other series employing the volar bone-grafting approach have presented similar rates of union: Russe,[2] 90%; Dooley,[3] 87%; and Mulder,[4] 97%.

Conclusion

Ten percent of all scaphoid fractures go on to chronic nonunion.[5] These nonunions warrant treatment if they become either unstable and symptomatic or malrotated with the potential for carpal collapse and osteoarthritis. The technique of volar corticocancellous inlay bone grafting of the scaphoid enables correction of the malrotation, bridging of the fracture gap with cancellous bone, and rigid, stable fixation with cortical bone.

Whereas acute, unstable fractures require reduction and rigid internal fixation, chronic nonunions require reduction and bone grafting to stimulate osteosynthesis. The technique described is neither difficult nor lengthy, but it is exacting and requires power equipment. It is applicable to proximal-pole and avascular fractures of the scaphoid and has yielded a scaphoid union rate of 95%.

References

1. Herbert TJ, Fisher WE: Management of the fractured scaphoid using a new bone screw. *J Bone Joint Surg Br* 1984;66B:114–123.
2. Russe O: Fracture of the carpal navicular: Diagnosis, non-operative treatment and operative treatment. *J Bone Joint Surg Am* 1960;42A:759–768.
3. Dooley, BJ: Inlay bone grafting for non-union of the scaphoid bone by the anterior approach. *J Bone Joint Surg Br* 1968;50B:102–109.
4. Mulder JD: The results of 100 cases of pseudarthrosis in the scaphoid bone treated by the Matti-Russe operation. *J Bone Joint Surg Br* 1968;50B:110–115.
5. Fisk GR: Carpal instability and the fractured scaphoid. *Ann R Coll Surg Engl* 1970;46:63–76.

11

Total Wrist Arthroplasty

Robert G. Volz

In 1973 an articulated, semiconstrained, cementable total wrist prosthesis was developed at the Arizona Health Sciences Center.[1,2] Since 1974 this prosthesis has been in continuous clinical usage with only minor revisions in design and technique of insertion. In 1977 a design modification was made in the metacarpal component which allowed for a more accurate positioning of the prosthesis in a fashion that duplicated the normal instant center of motion for the wrist. Since 1977, 25 total wrist arthroplasties have been performed utilizing this newer design, the last 6 having been implanted without the use of methylmethacrylate cement about the metacarpal component.

Because the single most difficult aspect of total wrist arthroplasty is the postoperative balancing of soft tissues and musculotendinous forces crossing the wrist, it is essential that the surgeon be aware of several critical biomechanical features of the wrist. Essentially, only two planes of motion are observed at the wrist, these being flexion-extension and radial-ulnar deviation. All rotational movement of the hand, ie, supination and pronation, takes place through the proximal and distal radioulnar joints. The axis or instant center of motion for wrist motion is located within the proximal pole of the capitate at a position vertically in line with the long axis of the third metacarpal[3] (Fig 11-1). Of critical importance to the normal functioning of the wrist is the preservation of the metacarpal-carpal height ratio. This ratio is determined by comparing the length of the third metacarpal to the height of the carpal space as measured from the base of the third metacarpal to the supporting articular plate of the distal radius (Fig 11-2). Values of 1:0.54 ± .02 are considered within the normal range.[4] A decrease in this ratio brought about by loss of carpal height is reflec-

Source: Adapted with permission from *Clinical Orthopaedics and Related Research* (1984;187:112–120).

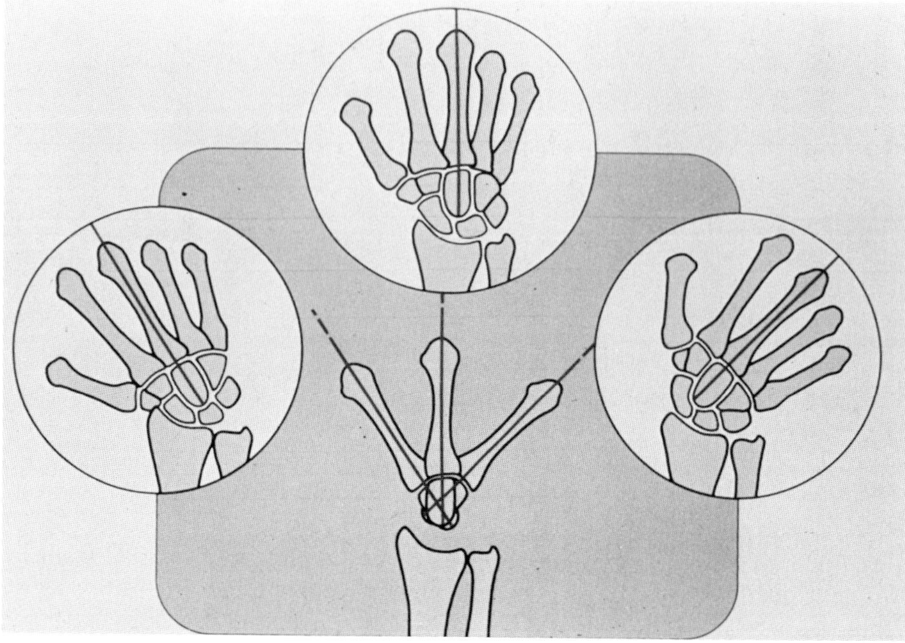

Fig 11-1. The instant center of motion of the carpus is located within the proximal pole of the capitate toward its volar surface. The instant center is not located in a single locus, but rather in a closely clustered group of focii. A vertical line drawn through the metacarpal of the long finger will transect the instant center of motion when the wrist is held in a neutral position. This vertical line then falls toward the ulnar border of the medullary canal of the radius.

tive of destructive changes to osseous and/or cartilaginous articular structures. When such changes occur, producing a collapse of the carpus, there is an associated relative lengthening of the musculotendinous structures crossing the wrist, thus giving rise to a compromise in grip strength and a decrease in active extension at the metacarpophalangeal joint.

Also of importance to the normal functioning of the wrist is the balance that exists between wrist flexor and extensor motors, for if any intrinsic imbalance exists preoperatively, the potential for the development of a postoperative deformity is greatly enhanced. The three palmar flexors and three dorsiflexors of the wrist are not intrinsically equal in their potential motor power.[5,6] The flexor carpi ulnaris is by far the strongest and most dominant wrist motor, whereas the extensor carpi ulnaris in most individuals is the weakest. When long-standing disease has existed at the wrist, such as with rheumatoid arthritis, patients frequently lose volitional control over the wrist extensors. Thus, many patients will grasp objects with a synergistic interplay of wrist flexors and finger flexors rather than with the customary combination of wrist extensors

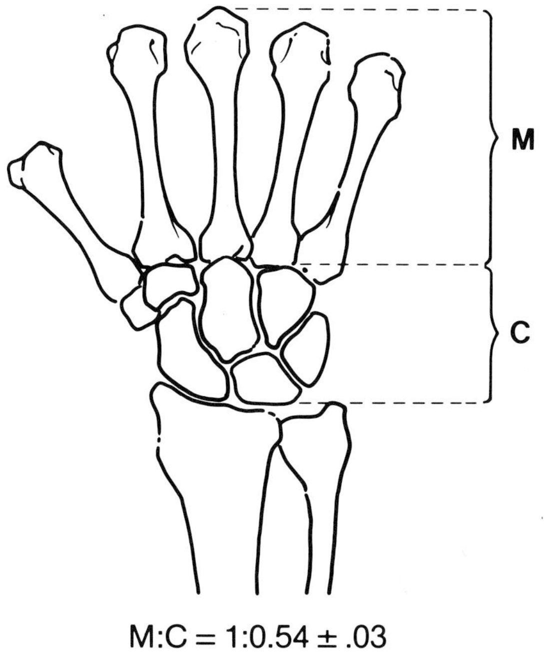

Fig 11-2. There is a fairly fixed relationship between the height of the carpus and the height of the long finger metacarpal. This measurement is helpful in identifying the degree of carpal collapse in the patient with far-advanced rheumatoid arthritis. One goal of reconstruction of the carpus with arthroplasty is to restore this carpal-metacarpal ratio so as to reconstitute the appropriate tension in the muscle forces crossing the wrist.

and finger flexors. This loss of volitional control over wrist extensors is felt to be due to pain inhibition, as observed also in patients undergoing arthrotomy of the knee who are unable voluntarily to contract the quadriceps muscle immediately postoperatively.[6] A dynamic imbalance between wrist flexors and extensors may also be provoked by spontaneous rupture of wrist extensors secondary to an active dorsal compartment tenosynovitis. As a result, the patient is left with a critical loss of extensor motion at the wrist, a loss that impairs fine motor control of the fingers and power grip. Eventually, if such an imbalance is allowed to continue, a contracture of the wrist flexors develops which may provoke deformity.

Lastly, any altered anatomy of the distal radioulnar joint can give rise to a disability of the radiocarpal articulation and to the arc of pronation and supination. The distal end of the ulna is stabilized at the distal end of the radius by the triangular fibrocartilage, a very strong tether which prevents upward displacement of the distal ulna with extremes of pronation.[6,7] This triangular fibrocartilage, which for all practical purposes serves as an interface between the proximal carpal row and the distal end of the ulna, also functions to absorb as much as 35% of the stress transmitted across the carpus to the forearm.[8] Thus, when a subluxation of the distal radioulnar joint exists, the stabilizing and load-sharing roles of the triangular fibrocartilage have been unquestionably compromised. As a result, forearm rotation, especially supination, may become limited, and the stress placed upon the joint formed by the scapholunate and the distal radius during grasping will be considerably increased. In the patient with rheumatoid arthritis, these biomechanical factors may accelerate the deterioration and instability of the radiocarpal articulation (Fig 11-3).

Prosthetic Design

The Arizona Medical Center wrist prosthesis is composed of a metacarpal and a radial component (Fig 11-4). The semiconstrained interface design allows for approximately 90° of palmar flexion and extension and 50° of radial-ulnar deviation; essentially no rotational movement is provided by the configuration of the interface. The concave/convex interface is sufficiently deep to eliminate the likelihood of dislocation provided the implant is properly inserted and soft tissues are placed under adequate tension. The intramedullary prongs of each component are offset 1½ mm dorsally, thereby placing the instant center of motion for flexion and extension more palmarward. This enhances the lever arm action of the extensors, thereby increasing their potential strength of action upon the carpus.

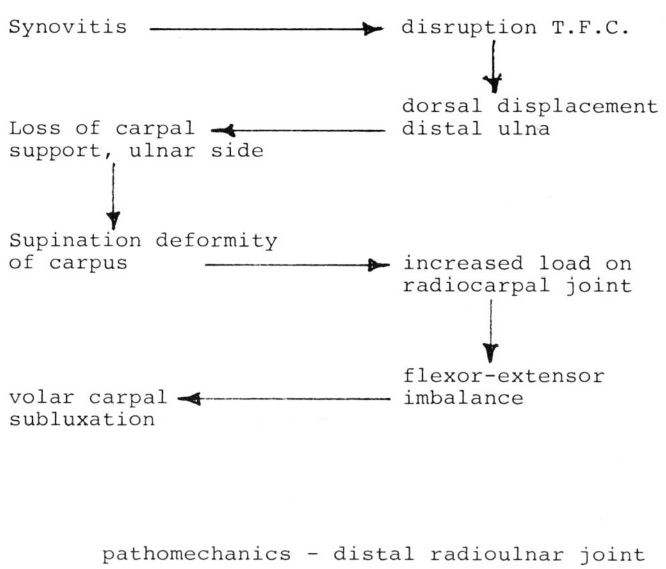

Fig 11-3. Sequence of events in rheumatoid arthritis involving the distal radioulnar joint. The process begins with an active synovitis which disrupts the triangular fibrocartilage, leading to instability between the distal ends of the radius and the ulna. This allows for an increase of stress mediated across the radiocarpal joint which eventually leads to subluxation of the carpus volarward, because of the greater intrinsic strength of the wrist flexors in relationship to the finger extensors.

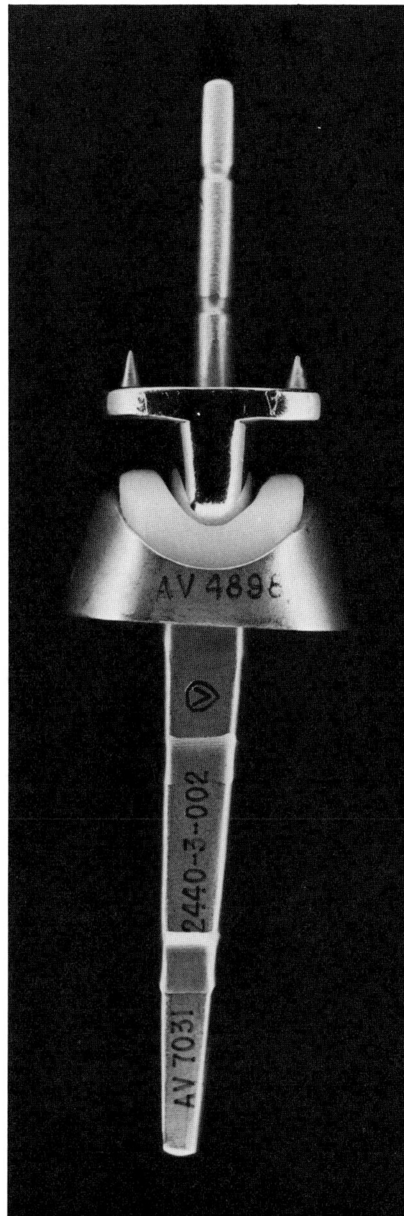

Fig 11-4. The Arizona Medical Center wrist prosthesis is composed of a metacarpal and a radial component. The single-pronged metacarpal component is designed for insertion within the medullary canal of the third metacarpal, whereas the radial component is secured within the medullary canal of the distal radius. The design of the interface, a toroidal sector, provides for 90° of flexion and extension and 50° of radioulnar deviation.

Methods and Materials

From 1977 until 1983, 22 patients have undergone 25 total wrist arthroplasties in which the modified Arizona prosthetic design was utilized; 3 patients returned for bilateral replacement. There were 19 patients who presented with the diagnosis of rheumatoid arthritis and 3 with degenerative osteoarthritis, 1 of whom had a failed arthroplasty for degenerative arthritis that had initially been treated elsewhere. In cases of sequential bilateral replacement, the decision as to which wrist was to be operated upon first was arrived at by a combination of factors including the degree of pain and disability in each wrist, dominance, and the presence or absence of associated hand, elbow, or shoulder disabilities. The age range of the 22 patients was from 26 to 72 years with a mean of 54 years. The longest follow-up was 6 years 7 months and the shortest 6 months, with a mean of 3 years 2 months (Table 11-1). All patients undergoing total wrist arthroplasty met the following criteria preoperatively:

- a functional or potentially restorable hand
- diffuse stage III or stage IV disease of the carpus
- a functional elbow
- intact dorsiflexors of the wrist
- healthy-appearing skin over the dorsal aspect of the wrist, ideally with some retained subcutaneous fat
- a highly motivated outlook, felt essential because of the intensive, 6-week postoperative therapy period required of most total wrist arthroplasties.

Operative Technique

Tourniquet hemostasis is considered mandatory in all cases. Placement of the incision should be in a straight line commencing from the base of the third

Table 11-1. Follow-up Period After Total Wrist Arthroplasty[a]

Postoperative Period (Months)	*No. of Patients*
72–84	1
60–72	7
48–60	2
36–48	1
24–36	7
12–24	3
6–12	4

[a]Mean follow-up was 3 years 2 months.

metacarpal and extending just proximal to the ulnar border of the distal radius. Care should be exercised in preserving all subcutaneous venous structures, as wound healing can be compromised by their sacrifice. If disease involves the distal radioulnar joint, this anatomical structure can be exposed without the need of a separate incision as follows: the dorsal compartment containing the extensor carpi ulnaris is entered by incising the extensor retinaculum. After careful dissection of all soft tissue about the distal ulna, 1 cm of this structure is excised by use of a microreciprocating saw. Stabilization of the distal ulna is carried out later, at the time of wound closure by tightly imbricating the dorsal capsule and overlying retinaculum, thus creating a snug sling about the distal end of the ulna.

Next, the dorsal retinaculum is incised in the third compartment, with care being taken not to injure the obliquely coursing extensor pollicis longus tendon. If necessary, a dorsal tenosynovectomy can be performed at this stage if a proliferative synovitis is encountered. The common extensor tendons are now retracted ulnarward and the extensor carpi radialis longus and brevis radialward. A U-shaped incision is made in the dorsal capsule with the base of the U directed radialward; the capsule is next carefully reflected radialward to expose the underlying carpus. The distal end of the radius is now resected by use of a reciprocating saw to the level of Lister's tubercle or slightly more proximally. The resection is made in a plane at right angles to the long axis of the radius. The head of the capitate is amputated at a level with the lesser multangular, and the proximal carpal row and the head of the capitate are removed. If volar and proximal subluxation of the carpus has occurred, as is commonly observed in far-advanced rheumatoid disease, contracture of the volar capsule will have taken place. Volar capsulotomy at the base of the distal radius or a total volar capsulectomy will be necessary if a useful range of extension motion is to be achieved postoperatively. Reaming of the capitate-third metacarpal-medullary canal is next performed by use of a Riordan "Christmas tree" power-driven rasp. This is followed by power rasping of the distal radial canal. A trial fit of prosthetic component parts is now carried out. If extension appears limited, additional bone may need to be resected from the distal radius, or further soft tissue release of the volar capsule may need to be performed. Following copious irrigation of the bony beds to remove fat, blood, and bone debris, methylmethacrylate cement is injected under pressure into the metacarpal, carpal, and radial canals. (However, since 1981, we have elected not to cement the metacarpal component in place if a tight press-fit of the medullary stem can be achieved within the medullary canal of the third metacarpal.) Following curing of the cement, the prosthesis is once again placed through a full range of motion to check for stability. All exposed cement is carefully removed. The dorsal capsule is precisely closed, and if deficient in substance the distal portion of the extensor retinaculum is reflected under the extensor tendons and incorporated into the repair to provide for complete coverage of the prosthetic implant. The extensor pollicis longus is now secured to Lister's tubercle; occasionally a slip of the extensor retinaculum will be utilized to create a pulley sling. A small-diameter drainage tube is placed upon the repaired capsule, and the wound is further closed in layers. Damp pressure dressings are applied to the hand and fingers with the wrist in neutral or slight dorsiflexion.

Because some rheumatoid arthritic patients will show a propensity for small areas of wound separation postoperatively, splinting should be maintained for at least 7 to 10 days or longer until the incision is completely sealed. Once this has been achieved, active and passive range of motion may be begun, generally under the supervision of a hand or occupational therapist. As some patients will have presented with a compromise in active extension of the wrist preoperatively, the use of a part-time day and full-time night splint is essential until adequate volitional control over wrist motion is achieved. This frequently requires 6 or more weeks. Dynamic splinting has also been used on occasion where the regaining of a sufficient arc of motion has been slow.

Case Results

All patients undergoing total wrist arthroplasty have been carefully followed for 6 to 12 weeks postoperatively, when maximum recovery generally has been observed. Patients were then requested to return on a yearly basis for routine evaluation of their condition. A computer analysis form documenting the range of motion, relief of pain, performance of activities of daily living, and any evidence of clinical loosening has been tabulated for each patient.

As with other types of total joint arthroplasty, the most predictable outcome of this type of reconstructive surgery was the observed relief of pain. Using a scale of 1 to 5, with 1 representing absence of pain and 5 incapacitating pain, patients reported postoperative pain scores averaging 1.2, compared with an average preoperative score of 3.7.

An assessment of the range of motion noted postoperatively in comparison with that recorded preoperatively is recorded in Table 11-2. The average arc of flexion and extension noted for all patients preoperatively measured 55.5°, whereas the average postoperative arc of motion equalled 67.3°. Five patients exhibited a loss of motion postoperatively which averaged 21°, three such patients presenting with 90° of flexion-extension preoperatively. Although the design of the prosthetic interface allows for only 90° of flexion-extension, it has been our experience that patients rarely regain this degree of motion postoperatively. Essentially, no change was noted postoperatively in the arc of pronation and supination when compared with the mean preoperative arc of rotation. Similarly, only a slight increase in the arc of radioulnar deviation was observed postoperatively (32.9°) compared with a preoperative arc of 24.5°. Most importantly, none of the 25 patients undergoing total wrist arthroplasty exhibited any degree of radioulnar imbalance postoperatively. One patient who presented with a 10° fixed flexion deformity preoperatively failed to regain any arc of extension postoperatively.

Table 11-2. Range of Motion Before and After Total Wrist Arthroplasty

Type of Motion	*Preoperative Range (Degrees)*	*Postoperative Range (Degrees)*
Flexion	28.4	30.9
Extension	27.1	36.4
Flexion-extension arc	55.5	67.3[a]
Pronation	81.5	79.4
Supination	70.4	70.3
Pronation-supination arc	151.9	149.7[b]
Radial deviation	5.4	9.6
Ulnar deviation	19.1	23.3
Radial-ulnar arc	24.5	32.9[c]

[a]Five patients exhibited a postoperative decrease averaging 21°.
[b]Eight patients exhibited a postoperative decrease averaging 20°.
[c]Three patients exhibited a postoperative decrease averaging 15°.

In reviewing the postoperative complications in this series of patients, it is to be noted that no infections, dislocations, or cases of clinical loosening have occurred. Whereas the initial prosthetic design, which placed the instant center of motion too far radialward, gave rise to a postoperative deformity of ulnar deviation, no case of radial-ulnar imbalance has been observed in this patient group. One patient with far-advanced rheumatoid carpal and metacarpophalangeal joint destruction did fail to regain a useful arc of wrist extension, presumably because of deficient wrist extensors. The prosthesis in this case was removed in favor of an arthrodesis.

Discussion

Our experience with total wrist arthroplasty now spans over 10 years. During that time, refinements in technique and prosthetic design have led us to conclude that the procedure is dependable, predictably giving rise to pain relief consistent with that observed with other types of total joint replacement. The procedure also provides for a useful range of motion postoperatively. Yet the question remains, Why an artificial arthroplasty of the wrist when arthrodesis offers similar advantages?

Bunnell aptly described the wrist as the "keystone" of the hand, a joint that provides for the augmentation of fine motor control of the fingers and hand in addition to aiding with power grasping activities. To this observation we would also add the wrist's ability to place the hand in a variety of postures of flexion and extension with associated degrees of radial and ulnar deviation as might be required because of vocational or avocational needs. Additionally, and perhaps most importantly, patients who have undergone arthrodesis of one wrist and replacement arthroplasty of the other have stated that the mobile wrist is much to be preferred.[9] This has particularly been our observation and philosophy in the treatment of patients with rheumatoid arthritis who exhibit not only wrist involvement but also associated metacarpophalangeal and interphalangeal joint problems. In this patient group, the preservation of even a small arc of wrist motion goes far in assisting with activities that the compromised hand is capable of performing.

Our approach, however, to traumatic or osteoarthritic conditions of the wrist is to recommend arthrodesis, provided the patient's specific needs are not contrary to a permanent loss of wrist motion. Certain occupations such as that of a professional musician or work of a highly technical nature frequently demand preservation of motion.

Much concern has been expressed regarding the use of methylmethacrylate cement in the hand. This concern has arisen over the possibility for the need of revision of an infected or clinically painful, aseptically loosened prosthesis. It has been our observation that whereas a significant reconstructive problem arises when a revision of a failed cemented prosthesis occurs in the metacarpophalangeal joint, such problems do not prevail with failure of a cemented prosthesis at the wrist, because of the greater potential for a salvage arthrodesis should prosthetic removal become necessary.

In a review of the first 100 total wrists performed by the author and 14 other collaborating surgeons employing the originally designed prosthesis from 1974 to 1976, only three cases of loosening requiring revision arose. Similarly, the infection rate among this initial series of patients has been 2 cases in 100. Thus, the likelihood of failure due to infection or aseptic loosening appears to be slight. A logical explanation for the low incidence of clinical loosening may be the low levels of stress to which most wrist prostheses are subjected, especially in patients with rheumatoid arthritis in whom significant associated hand and finger problems exist.

The decided advantage that we feel an articulated metal-and-plastic prosthesis offers is the ability to carry out a more extensive reconstruction of the carpus by reconstitution of the carpometacarpal ratio. Many far-advanced cases of rheumatoid arthritis of the wrist exhibit considerable carpal collapse with fixed deformity and a marked compromise in grip strength. With a metallic prosthesis, the carpal height can be restored, contracted soft tissues released or excised, and early motion begun to facilitate an improvement in wrist function postoperatively.

Cases of recurring dislocation of the prosthesis have not occurred, although three single, isolated episodes of dislocation did arise in the original 100-case series. All three dislocations occurred during the immediate postoperative period as the patients were beginning to awaken from the anesthetic. In each situation, an inadequate release of a contracted volar capsule was felt to be the cause. Thus, as motor tone returned to the wrist flexors with the wrist immobilized in the desired position of a few degrees of dorsiflexion, the metacarpal component dislocated dorsally as a result of the tethering effect of a tight volar capsule. Routine release of the volar capsule has eliminated this problem as was demonstrated in this series of 25 cases in which no acute or late dislocations have been observed.

Our experience with total wrist arthroplasty has further led to the observation that the key to success lies with the problem of soft-tissue closure and the postoperative musculotendinous balance. Frequently, the preoperative examination does not readily permit recognition of an imbalance or absence of one or more wrist extensors. Only when the inhibition of pain has been removed postoperatively and an active range of motion has begun does this problem surface. In some cases, patients will exhibit intact wrist extensors at the time of the operation but postoperatively will show a loss of volitional control over wrist extension with grasping activities. This situation is believed to be due to chronic pain inhibition. Electromyographic studies of wrist extensor activity will in some patients show no electrical activity and thus aid in the identification of this problem. In such situations an intensive muscle retraining should be undertaken.

Certainly it cannot be overemphasized that a successful arc of painfree wrist extension is the most important goal of wrist arthroplasty, for it is this activity that augments hand function to the maximum. Because wrist motors function at a subconscious level, augmenting finger activity, their return to a normal pattern and level of activity may require weeks of postoperative therapy often supplemented by day- and nighttime splinting. Therefore, the role of a hand therapist in the attainment of the maximum result is absolutely critical.

Although the use of methylmethacrylate cement has been the key in providing for a microlock of artificial prosthetic devices, we share the concern and hope of others that a more physiologic method of prosthetic attachment to the skeleton will be found. Thus, since 1981, no cement has been used in securing the metacarpal component to its skeletal bed, for in all cases a sufficiently tight press-fit was achieved. No compromise in the degree of pain relief or functional result has been observed in this very small group of patients compared with the larger initial series of patients. It is hoped that a porous surface prosthesis will prove feasible for the biological attachment of these devices to the skeleton. Work is currently under way on the design and fabrication of a radial stem employing these features.

Lastly, mention should be made of the situation of prosthetic revision or removal and the subsequent arthrodesis of a failed cemented wrist prosthesis. The author has now had experience with seven cases that have required revision or removal of a cemented prosthesis. Four of the seven patients were among the initial 100 patients undergoing total wrist arthroplasty who received the originally designed prosthesis. Two other patients had undergone initial implantation elsewhere, and one had been treated by the author with the modified design.

Four of the seven cases required prosthetic removal because of a fixed deformity that had developed postoperatively because of motor imbalance. Two other patients presented with clinical and radiographic evidence of loosening, and in one patient with rheumatoid arthritis the incision had failed to heal adequately, subsequently developing a dehiscence that could not be managed by secondary skin closure.

In the two patients presenting with clinical evidence of loosening, arthrodesis was refused and a prosthetic exchange carried out. The remaining five patients underwent prosthetic removal and an attempted fusion, three eventually developing a solid fusion. Two were left with a painfree fibrous union, which from their point of view was felt to be satisfactory. In all seven cases, prosthetic removal was facilitated by the creation of a longitudinal saw cut through the dorsal cortex of the metacarpal and the distal radius. This allowed for the expansion of the medullary canal as the prosthesis was tapped free, thereby eliminating the potential for comminution of the cortical bone, which in some patients was quite thin. In the five patients in whom arthrodesis was performed a precisely shaped segment of autogenous iliac bone graft was inserted within the carpal space. (Fig 11-5) The graft was of sufficient dimension to provide

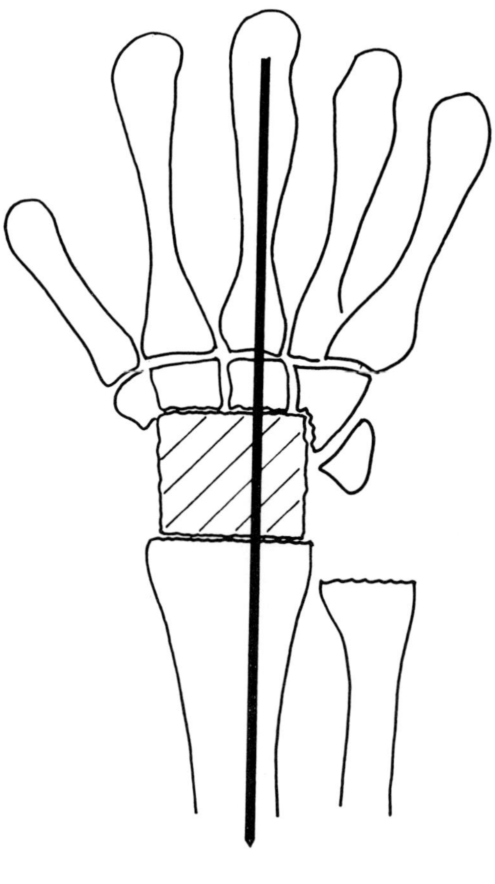

Fig 11-5. Salvage of a failed cemented total wrist prosthesis involves the incorporation of a free segment of iliac bone graft inserted between the freshened bone surfaces of the distal radius and the remaining carpal bed. The graft is then positioned and secured with intramedullary wire fixation.

stability by creating tension within the surrounding soft tissues. Additional stability was achieved by the use of single or multiple skeletal pins. Immobilization was continued for 6 to 12 weeks postoperatively until a satisfactory degree of bony or fibrous stability had been achieved.

Our experience with total wrist arthroplasty dating from its initial use in 1974 leads us to conclude that the procedure is predictable and provides for a useful and painfree arc of motion in patients who exhibit the need for preservation of wrist function. Use of the procedure in monoarticular types of arthritis is generally not recommended at this time. Revision of a failed total wrist prosthesis carries with it the likelihood of a satisfactory degree of function following the establishment of a bony arthrodesis or a fibrous nonunion.

References

1. Volz RG: The development of a total wrist joint. *Clin Orthop Rel Res* 1976;116:209–214.
2. Volz RG: Clinical experiences with a new total wrist prosthesis. *Arch Orthop Unfallchir* 1976;8:205–209.
3. Youm Y, Flatt AE: Kinematics of the wrist. *Clin Orthop* 1980;149:21.
4. Youm Y, McMurtry RY, Flatt AE, et al.: Kinematics of the wrist. *J Bone Joint Surg Am* 1978;60A:423.
5. Boyes JH: *Bunnell's Surgery of the Hand,* ed 4. Philadelphia, JB Lippincott Co, 1964.
6. Volz RG: Total wrist arthroplasty: A clinical and biomechanical analysis in A Inglis (ed): *Symposium: Upper Extremity Total Joint Replacement.* St. Louis, CV Mosby Co, 1982, pp 273–288.
7. Volz RG, Lieb M, Benjamin J: Biomechanics of the wrist. *Clin Orthop Rel Res* 1980;149:112.
8. Werner FW, Palmer AK, Glesson RR: Forearm load transmission: The effect of ulnar lengthening and shortening. Transactions of the 28th Annual Meeting of the ORS, New Orleans, Jan 1982, p 273.
9. Goodman MJ, Millender LH, Nalebuff EA, et al.: Arthroplasty of the rheumatoid wrist with silicone rubber: An early evaluation. *J Hand Surg* 1980;5:114–121.

12

Soft-Tissue Reconstruction of the Hand in Early Rheumatoid Deformity

D. C. R. Ireland

Rheumatoid hand surgery can be broadly classified as early preventive soft-tissue reconstruction or late salvage surgery. The term *preventive* is used perhaps euphemistically, but it refers to prevention of rheumatoid deformity rather than of the rheumatoid disease process. If we accept the premise that untreated early deformity progresses to the late salvage stage, then early surgical intervention, which is able to halt or significantly slow this progressive process, is desirable. The results of early preventive surgery are superior to those of late salvage surgery because the patients are younger, the disease is less advanced, and the joints are preserved, producing a more physiologically functional hand.

Discussion in this chapter is confined to early soft-tissue preventive surgery at the metacarpophalangeal (MP) joint to prevent ulnar drift and at the proximal interphalangeal (PIP) joint to correct swan-neck deformity. The more obvious, equally rewarding, and less controversial procedures of flexor and extensor tenosynovectomy are not considered.

Metacarpophalangeal Joint Ulnar Drift

Ulnar drift of the fingers compromises hand function because radial support for the MP joint is lost, making difficult many of the activities of daily living in which the forearm is held in the neutral rotation position (eg, holding a cup) vis-a-vis. Associated extension lag at the MP joint diminishes wide prehensile gripping function. Gripping strength is diminished as a result of dissipation of longitudinal flexion and extension tendon forces to the ulnar-directed vector force, as these translocated tendons require a moment arm. Whether many of the features (Table 12-1) associated with ulnar drift are causes or effects is debatable; however, experience shows that these features should be corrected if surgical correction of ulnar drift is to be maintained.

Table 12-1. Associated Features of MP Joint-Ulnar Drift

MP joint synovitis
Ulnar translocation of extensor tendons
Ulnar translocation of flexor tendons
Attenuation of dorsal hood radial transverse laminae
Attenuation of radial collateral ligament
Contracture of ulnar intrinsics
Contracture of radial intrinsics
Radial deviation of the "carpometacarpus" at wrist
Excessive fourth and fifth metacarpal descent (carpometacarpal joint flexion)

The indication (Table 12-2) for soft tissue reconstruction for ulnar drift at the MP joints is progressive ulnar drift in the presence of uncontrolled MP joint synovitis in a symptomatic, motivated, cooperative patient with radiologically intact MP joints. The contraindications (Table 12-2) are significant radiological MP joint change, clinical volar subluxation of the proximal phalanx, and incorrigible deformity.

Surgical Technique

The surgical technique, in addition to correcting the associated features (Table 12-1) mentioned above, centers on Flatt's[1] modification of Straub's[2] crossed intrinsic transfer, whereby the deforming ulnar intrinsic force is converted to a correcting radially directed force by transfer of the ulnar intrinsic wing tendon to the radial side of the adjacent finger.

The MP joints are exposed through a transverse incision. The ulnar-translocated tendons are noted, and through a radial hood incision a thorough synovectomy is performed. Especially elusive areas are the volar pouch and the deep surface of the radial collateral ligament. The abductor digiti minimi is tenotomized, leaving the flexor digiti minimi intact. The juncturae tendinum of the extensor tendons between the third, fourth, and fifth metacarpals are

Table 12-2 Early Soft-Tissue Reconstruction for MP Joint Ulnar Drift

Indications	*Contraindications*
Progressive ulnar drift	Clinical volar subluxation of the proximal phalanx
Uncontrollable MP joint synovitis	Incorrigible deformity
Deteriorating hand function in a symptomatic, motivated patient with radiologically normal MP joints	Significant MP joint radiographic change

divided[3] to prevent transfer of the ulnar pull to the more radial extensor tendons caused by descent into flexion deformity of the fourth and fifth carpometacarpal joints. The ulnar intrinsics are incised at the wing tendon attachment to the dorsal hoods and then dissected proximally to ensure that all bony attachments are divided. This dissection should be carried to the musculotendinous junction, proximal to the transverse metacarpal ligament. At least 1 cm of tendon excursion is possible. The tendon is then crossed to the radial side of the adjacent digit under the interdigital veins and attached at the base of the proximal phalanx to the collateral ligament under full excursion of the transfer with the ulnar deviation of the finger corrected. If the Bunnell test for intrinsic tightness remains positive, then radial intrinsic release is necessary.

Ulnar hood-releasing incisions are then made where necessary to enable relocation of the central tendons just radial to the midline by reefing the initial radial hood incision.

At the index finger, if the first dorsal interosseous attachment has subluxated volar to the axis of the MP joint, it is divided and relocated into the dorsal hood beside the central tendon, after the hood has been closed. Too much tension here can produce unwanted overcorrection of the index finger into radial deviation.

The skin incision is then carefully closed over a suction drain.

Attention must now be directed to the wrist, where radial deviation at the carpometacarpal joint (the intercalated segment of this zigzag collapse deformity) must be corrected. This is effected by transfer of the extensor carpi radialis longus to the relocated extensor carpi ulnaris, as described by Clayton.[4] This transfer is indicated when passive ulnar deviation exceeds active ulnar deviation of the wrist.

A bulky, compressive dressing with a volar and ulnar plaster splint is applied to splint the hand statically for 1 week with the MP joints in extension and radial deviation, before mobilizing the MP joints in a dynamic extension-radial deviation assist splint for a further 3 weeks. This splint is worn 24 hours a day. The PIP joints are held in extension during active exercising to further mobilize the MP joints. After discontinuing the dynamic splint, a static night splint is worn indefinitely.

These patients lose the intrinsic ability to spread the fingers, but this is more than compensated for by the improved extrinsic gripping power and prehensile function. The tension developed by a muscle is inversely proportional to fiber length and directly proportional to the cross-sectional area of all the muscle fibers. As these intrinsics have relatively large muscle mass and short fibers, they are capable of developing tension sufficient to withstand any residual deforming forces, including externally applied force.

Fig 12-1 demonstrates an 8 year follow-up of a patient who underwent crossed intrinsic transfer on the right side. Correction of ulnar drift and active MP joint extension has been maintained, whereas the nonoperated left side has deteriorated to the salvage surgery stage. Preservation of the MP joints (Fig 12-2) can be seen in the radiographs on the right, whereas deterioration has

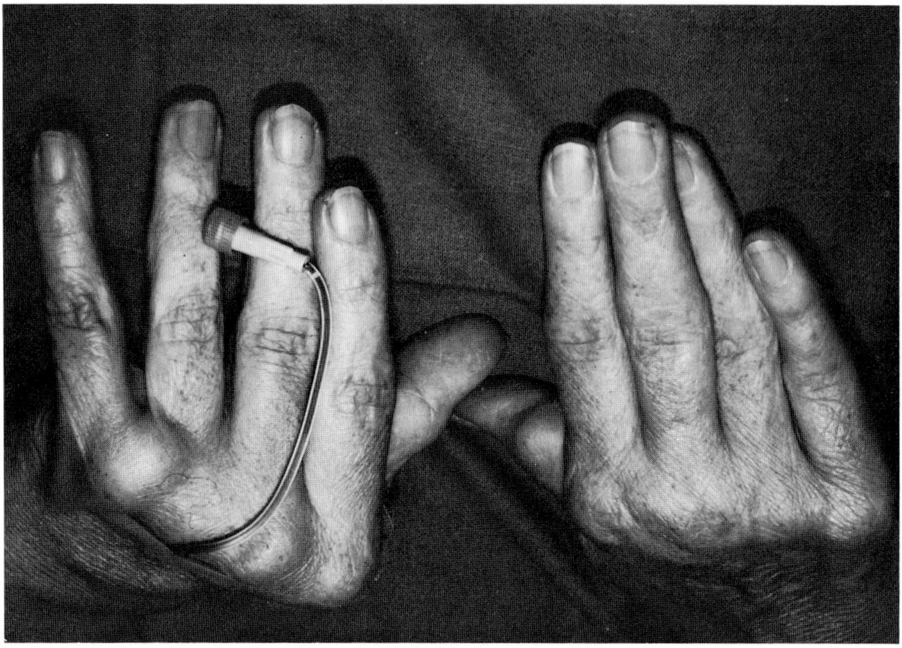

Fig 12-1. Eight-year follow-up of correction of ulnar drift by crossed intrinsic transfer on the right. The left side was not operated upon. Correction of ulnar drift has been maintained, together with active MP joint extension, whereas the nonoperated left side has deteriorated to the salvage surgery stage.

occurred on the left (the patient re-presented for stabilization of the right thumb interphalangeal joint).

Swan-Neck Deformity

Fixed swan-neck deformity can be functionally devastating, because of loss of the ability to grasp objects of any size between the fingers and the palm, leaving only key pinch and double-handed opposition. In spite of severe, long-standing hyperextension contractures at the PIP joints, their articular surfaces remain remarkably well preserved, leaving the potential for joint movement if balanced forces are provided. As with ulnar drift at the MP joint level, the etiology of swan-neck deformity at the PIP joint level is multifactorial. Which is cause and which is effect is arguable; however, the pathology (Table 12-3) associated with swan-neck deformity must be treated if one is to maintain correction of the deformity itself.

The treatment of swan-neck deformity exemplifies the ideal procedure in hand surgery, for it is simple, fundamental, mechanical, and effective. Proximal joint deformity first must be corrected, often as a series of staged proce-

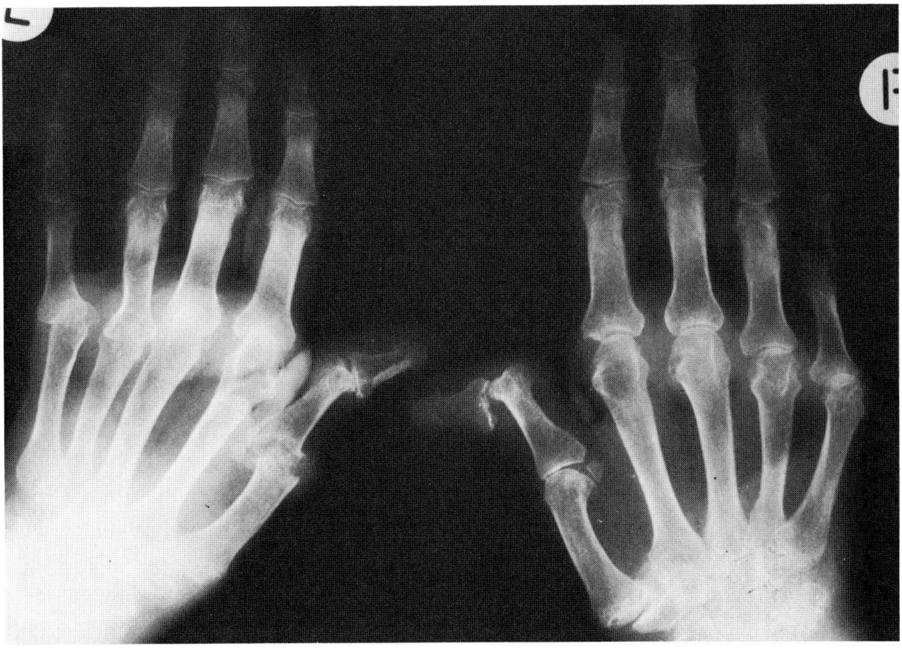

Fig 12-2. Posteroanterior radiographs taken at eight-year follow-up of correction of ulnar drift by crossed intrinsic transfer. On the right (operated) side, correction of deformity is seen and joint surfaces have been preserved at the MP joint level, whereas on the left (unoperated) side, dislocation and deterioration have progressed.

dures, before the hyperextended PIP joint can be actively mobilized. At the wrist, volar subluxation or dislocation is corrected by implant arthroplasty or arthrodesis to restore correct flexor/extensor balance with respect to length and tension. At the MP joint, fixed flexion contracture with destroyed or dislocated joint surfaces requires implant arthroplasty. If the joint surface is preserved, a volar release, intrinsic releases, and extensor tenotomy and tenodesis to the

Table 12-3. Swan-Neck Deformity: Associated Pathology

Intrinsic contracture
MP joint fixed flexion/subluxation/dislocation
Flexor digitorum sublimis rupture
Flexor tendon adhesions
Central slip contracture
Wrist volar subluxation/dislocation
Landsmeer's oblique retinacular ligament rupture
PIP joint collateral ligament contracture

base of the proximal phalanx[5] may be necessary to restore MP joint extension. When the long extensor is tenodesed in this way, the radial wing tendon must be preserved to extend the interphalangeal joints.

Once the proximal influencing deformities have been corrected, attention can next be directed to the target PIP joint intrinsic causes of hyperextension and their secondary effects. Swan-neck deformity, which is amenable to soft tissue reconstruction, requires radiologically intact joint surfaces. It can be divided into three stages.

Stage 1

Mild but progressive cases, where the Bunnell test reveals tight intrinsics in the presence of a full range of passive PIP joint flexion, with the MP joints flexed, are treated by Littler[6] radial and ulnar intrinsic releases.

Stage 2

When the PIP joint has been preserved but passive flexion is restricted to 30°, then, in addition to intrinsic releases, the PIP joints are manipulated closed into 100° of flexion. This must be followed by flexor tenolysosynovectomy. Flexor tendons that have not moved for even a few months adhere to each other and to the deep surface of the fibro-osseous tunnel. Intratendinous rheumatoid nodules and inflammatory synovium must be removed so that passive tension on the flexor tendons produces 90° of PIP joint flexion. This procedure can be performed through a single transverse incision in the palm at the level of the A.1 pulley. Postoperative splinting maintains the MP joints fully extended and the PIP joints flexed at 90°. This static splint is replaced at 2 days postoperatively with a dynamic flexion-assist splint to hold the PIP joints at 90° of flexion, allowing full active extension against resistance. This splint is worn 23 hours a day for 5 weeks. A static night splint, which maintains the MP joints in neutral extension and the PIP joints flexed to 60°, is worn indefinitely.

Stage 3

When the PIP joints cannot be passively flexed beyond the neutral position, but are radiologically preserved, an open procedure is indicated. Landsmeer's oblique retinacular ligament is reconstructed by the Littler[7] method. The wing tendon is incised proximally and dissected distally off the extensor apparatus, preserving its distal attachment. This is passed volar to the axis of the PIP joint under Cleland's ligament for later attachment to the flexor tendon sheath at the A.2 pulley. The other intrinsic is now released, and the PIP joint is manipulated into 100° of flexion. Flexor tenolysosynovectomy, as described above, follows. The reconstructed Landsmeer's oblique retinacular ligament is now attached to the flexor tendon sheath at the A.2 pulley, under tension, at 45° of PIP joint flexion. The joints are now pinned in 90° of flexion for 10 days. Postoperatively, the MP joints are statically splinted in neutral extension, and the distal interphalangeal joints are actively mobilized at day 1 to move the lysed flexor tendons on each other. At 10 days, the pins are removed and the PIP joints actively mobilized. Slow movers require dynamic flexion-assist splinting through nail hooks. Patients with more mobile tendons are fitted with a 45° dorsal extension-block splint and allowed to flex actively.

This treatment regime for the three phases of swan-neck deformity with radiologically intact PIP joints amenable to soft-tissue reconstruction is summarized in Table 12-4.

The improvement in hand function following mobilization of fixed, extended finger joints can be dramatic. The PIP joint must be radiologically intact, and flexor tenolysosynovectomy is essential. Unless dynamic and static splinting is continued for a prolonged period postoperatively, there is a tendency for extension deformity to recur over a 6-month period. From a functional point of view, it is far preferable to develop some fixed flexion contracture at the PIP joint and to maintain flexion.

Conclusion

Early "preventive" soft-tissue surgery for rheumatoid hand deformity is extremely rewarding provided the indications and contraindications are observed. By correcting deformity at an early phase and rebalancing joint

Table 12-4. Swan-Neck Deformity: Soft-Tissue Reconstructive Treatment

P.I.P. Joint Stage	*Problem*	*Treatment*
Stage 1: Almost-full flexion with MP flexed	Intrinsic contractures	Intrinsic releases
Stage 2: 30° flexion	Intrinsic contractures Joint contracture Flexor adhesions	Intrinsic releases Closed manipulation of PIP joint Flexor Tenolysosynovectomy Dynamic splinting
Stage 3: 0° flexion	Intrinsic contractures Joint contracture Flexor adhesions Ruptured LORL	Intrinsic release Open manipulation of PIP joint Flexor tenolysosynovectomy Littler LORL reconstruction Dynamic splinting

LORL, Landsmeer's oblique retinocular ligament.

forces, progression of deformity to the late salvage surgery stage can be significantly delayed or halted. The postoperative dynamic and static splinting regime, together with the hand therapy regime that follows the treatment of ulnar drift and swan-neck deformity, is as essential to maintaining the correction and achieving the desired result as is the surgical technique.

References

1. Ellison MR, Flatt AE, Kelly KJ: Ulnar drift of the fingers in rheumatoid disease. *J Bone Joint Surg Am* 1971;53A:1061–1082.
2. Straub LR: The intrinsic muscles in disease with particular reference to the rheumatoid hand, in *Dixième Congrès International de Chirurgie Orthopédique et de Traumatologie, Paris, 4–9 Septembre 1966.* Brussels, Les Publications Acta Medica Belgica, 1967, pp 863-872.
3. Zancolli EA: *Structural and Dynamic Bases of Hand Surgery,* ed 2. Philadelphia, JB Lippincott Co, 1979.
4. Clayton ML, Ferlic DC: Tendon transfer for radial rotation of the wrist in rheumatoid arthritis. *Clin Orthop* 1974;100:176–185.
5. Nalebuff EA, Millender LH: Surgical treatment of swan-neck deformity in rheumatoid arthritis. *Orthop Clin North Am* 1975;6:733–752.
6. Littler JW, cited by Riordan DC, Harris C: Intrinsic contracture in the hand and its surgical treatment, *J Bone Joint Surg Am* 1954;36A:10–20.
7. Littler JW: Restoration of the oblique retinacular ligament for correcting hyperextension deformity of the proximal interphalangeal joint. In *La main rhumatismale.* Paris, L'Expansion Scientifique Francaise, 1966, pp 39–41.

13

Early Care of the Burned Hand

Raymond L. Warpeha and
Juan Angelats

The treatment goal in acute burns of the hand is to attain wound closure while maintaining motion in the fingers. The burn wound must be closed by epithelialization or graft. To prevent secondary scar deformity, the resulting skin surface must be of good quality so that it can withstand the shearing "trauma" of a pressure garment worn for 6 to 12 months. Burn wounds that epithelialize by 3 weeks will have a sound and abrasion-resistant surface. Each increment of time beyond this period increases the chances of having an epithelial cover of poor quality while dermal fibrosis and scar hypertrophy are on the rise. This combination of factors may preclude the use of the all-important pressure glove or garment, which even if well fitted places shearing forces upon the skin during hand and finger motion. With a skin cover of poor quality, the painful ulceration caused by pressure garment abrasion and active motion may not heal with the garment in place. Without the garment, the deleterious forces of scar act freely upon the soft tissues and secondarily upon the joints by reducing their range of motion.

Geography of Hand Burns

Hand burns may occur as an isolated injury, but over half occur with burns involving other body parts in addition to the upper extremities (Table 13-1). The majority of hand burns occur on the dorsal surface. Many of these burns extend to the thin skin of the palmar surface of the thenar eminence and along the ulnar border of the fifth digit (Fig 13-1). Although the remaining palmar skin might be subject to a similar degree of thermal insult, the insulative properties of the thick stratum corneum minimizes dermal damage in most hand burns. Other factors that favor palmar skin protection are reflex fist

Table 13-1. Burns of the Hands Among 300 Consecutive Admissions to Loyola University Burn Center, 1982–1984

Burn Locations	*No. of Cases*	*% of Total Admissions*
One hand only	14	5
Both hands only	7	2
One hand and upper extremity	3	1
One hand and other body parts	49	16
Both hands and other body parts	87	29
Total	160	53

clenching and facial protection by the hands with the dorsal surfaces facing the thermal insult.

Depth of Injury

Depending upon heat intensity and duration of exposure burns of the hands will vary in depth and can be categorized as dermal and subdermal. Dermal burns can be further divided into superficial and deep, based solely upon clinical examination, as no presently available apparatus or test can define the depth of injury.

Superficial burns range from erythema to blistered skin having a pink and often wet base with good capillary refill. Deep dermal burns appear opaque and relatively dry and represent a range of injuries from one that may only be slightly deeper than a blistered wound to one that approaches the dermal-subcutaneous junction. Although clinical examination cannot distinguish the depth of injury in dermal burns, laminar excision of the eschar with a calibrated dermatome will help make this distinction (see "Technical Aspects of Excision and Grafting" below).

Subdermal burns involve the superficial fascia beyond the dermal injury and may involve the deep fascia and structures such as tendons and joints. Although subdermal burns may not be distinguishable from deep dermal burns, except by laminar excision to bleeding tissue, the parchment-like appearance and feel with loss of subcutaneous mobility point to this level of injury.

Care of the Acute Wound

Acute hand burns should be cleansed and the loose, dead tissues excised; this is followed by the application of a topical antibacterial agent in a closed dressing. Active finger motion is started immediately, and during periods of rest the hand

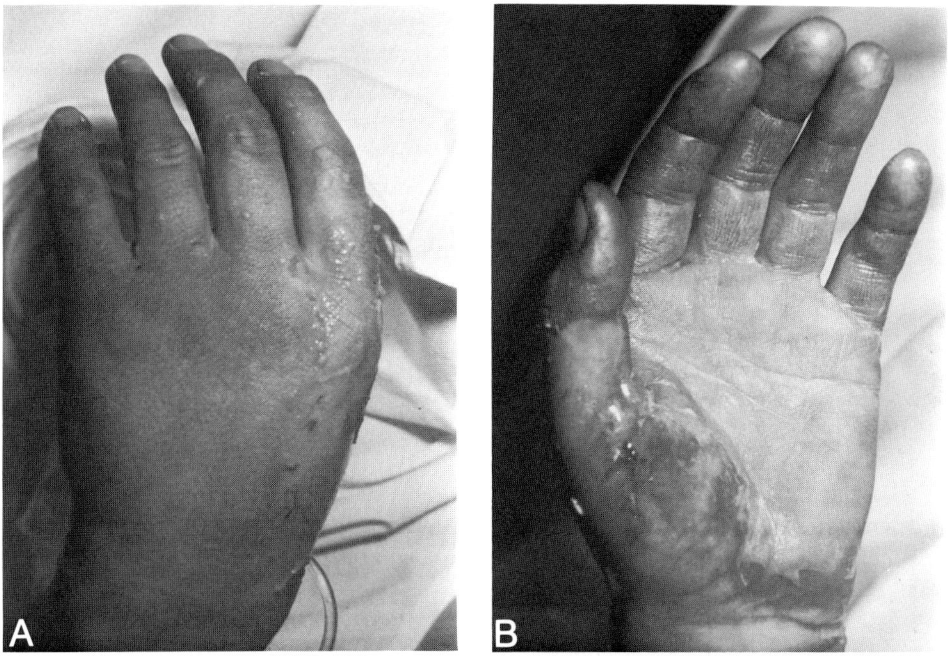

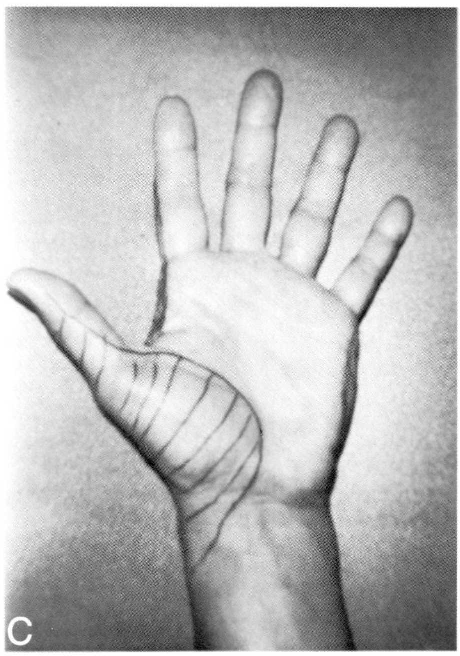

Fig 13-1. *A*, Typical burn of dorsum of the hand extending to the thin skin over the thenar eminence. *B*, *C*, Outline of common palmar component of "dorsal" hand burn.

is placed in a splint with the metacarpophalangeal (MP) joints in flexion. The burned hand is kept elevated above the level of the heart.

Evaluation of Circulation

In circumferential burns of the upper extremity, the arterial circulation is monitored by palpation or, where this is not possible, by Doppler study. If the Doppler radial pulse is lost to the compressive forces of burn edema, an escharotomy is performed along the lateral border of the forearm or arm, proximally from the unburned skin across the wrist onto the dorsum of the hand. To prevent linear contracture resulting from the healing dermal injury, the incision across joints should be zig-zagged, particularly when crossing dermal burns of the wrist. In severe subdermal injury, which may extend to the fascia and affect deeper structures, or in electrical injuries with sensory or motor deficit, fasciotomy of the forearm and/or dorsal interosseous compartments is indicated. Wang[1] has shown that early débridement and vascular reconstruction of extensive electrical injuries of the hand and wrist can salvage much motor and sensory function.

Because the stratum corneum of the palmar skin of the fingers often protects this skin from dermal damage, escharotomy in the midlateral line of the finger is not often needed, but is of value in promoting distal circulation when circumferential dermal burns of the fingers occur.

Excision of the Burn Wound

The pink, translucent, superficial burns are allowed to epithelialize, as this is expected to be complete by 3 weeks, resulting in a good surface that is resistant to the shearing forces within a pressure glove. If for any reason epithelialization is not imminent at 2 weeks, excision and grafting are carried out at that time. Active motion and splinting are faithfully maintained.

Opaque dermal or subdermal wounds are excised in the operating room when the patient's general condition warrants. Inhalation injury and large burns often delay such wound coverage and militate against patient cooperation in physical therapy. Hand coverage has a high priority over most other areas of the body because of the severe functional losses that accompany long delay in wound closure. Fortunately, graft failure on prepared hand wounds is rare because of the good vascularization of the tissues at all levels of excision.

Laminar excision of the burn wound within the first few days is usually accompanied by less blood loss, presumably due to less hyperemia in the dermis. However, excision of the dermal burns and successful closure with grafts at any point within the first 3 weeks of injury are readily accomplished. If joint motion is maintained prior to wound closure, there is less urgency to excise and close the hand burn. Conversely, lack of cooperation, voluntary or involuntary, increases the need to obtain wound closure in the adult. Frequently, young children find it difficult to cooperate fully with the physical therapist. Nevertheless, children rarely experience permanent contractures if their wounds are closed and placed in pressure garments within a reasonable period of time.

Technical Aspects of Excision and Grafting

To facilitate uniform excision, the Brown dermatome is used to excise burn eschar whenever technically feasible. Subeschar injections of saline are used in areas of concavity or over bony prominences. A guarded dermatome blade is used where the oscillating dermatome cannot be applied. A blade opening of 0.015 to 0.020 inch is used in a small test area and increased or decreased as judged necessary from the dermal bleeding or lack of it. Occasionally an opaque burn is quite superficial, with bleeding occurring at a thickness of about 0.010 inch. One may choose to discontinue excision and allow for spontaneous epithelialization, which would be expected to occur within 3 weeks, or one might choose at this time to dermabrade the surface and apply a thin (0.008 to 0.010 inch) split-thickness skin graft. At about 0.030 inch, the full thickness of the dorsal hand dermis is approached, and excision must then include the subdermal areolar tissues. These tissues are laminated usually with a limited amount of subcutaneous fat and a loose, deep layer of well-vascularized areolar tissues which lie in apposition to the dorsal tendons and their expansion in the fingers. If the depth of the injury requires excision to this point, the excision is better carried out by careful knife dissection with magnification, preserving the peritenon. Dermal hand burns can have a mixture of depths, and the dermatome settings and other techniques of wound excision must be varied as each region of the burn is approached. It is particularly important that the margins of the burn wounds be properly excised and closed, particularly along the thenar eminence and the little finger. It is the scar hypertrophy and linear shortening along these margins that are responsible for many of the secondary hand deformities (see Chapter 14).

If during the course of excision of eschar one is unable to separate satisfactorily the dead tissue from the underlying tendon and joint, excision is discontinued and these areas are left to separate spontaneously. The dorsal surfaces of the proximal interphalangeal (PIP) joints and, less commonly, of the MP joints are the most frequently involved in this fashion. Those adjacent tissues with a good vascular bed are closed with grafts, despite the remaining attached eschar. Open joints are fixed with Kirschner wires in a position of function and allowed to granulate and are then grafted. With open joint wounds, the extensor apparatus is invariably destroyed, thus preventing future mobilization.

Enzymatic débridement has been used, but the result is an incomplete separation of eschar. This is said to reduce the need for escharotomy because of its softening effect upon the eschar. As a preliminary to mechanical débridement, the present author finds enzymatic preparation of the wound a mechanical impediment to sharp excision, which depends upon firm eschar to be successful.

Grafting

If the eschar is excised to healthy, viable tissue, only hematoma formation will prevent graft take. Therefore absolute hemostatis is essential. This can be accomplished by compression of the wound with moist sponges for several minutes to attain clotting in the capillary vessels followed by coagulation of small-arterial bleeding under a thin veil of saline applied to the wound by syringe.

Dermal wounds are covered with skin grafts 0.008 to 0.012 inch thick taken with the Brown dermatome. Skin grafts are only meshed when being applied to dermal burns, and the deeper the burn, the less efficacious is meshing. Meshed skin produces a permanent, less desirable cosmetic result, and we apply meshed skin to excised dermal burns only when there is a shortage of skin. When the burn wound has been excised beyond the dermis, thicker grafts of 0.012 to 0.016 inch are used to enhance the long-term mobility of the dermal tissues. The skin is rapidly affixed to the wound with skin staples, and the hand is placed in bivalve 5-inch plastic splints with the MP joints in full flexion. Little bulk is used in the dressing so that the MP joints can be properly positioned as the plaster sets. The dressings are removed at 4 days and active motion is reinstated. Pin fixation of the MP joints is not used as it appears to delay the onset of joint motion.

Pressure garments are made and applied within a week to 10 days after grafting. These garments are worn for about 6 to 12 months, depending upon the rate of resolution of hypertrophic scar. Burn syndactyly can be eliminated or reduced by the application of pressure to the web spaces by means of special elastic devices made to apply continuous pressure in these areas.

Special attention is paid to possible early flexion contracture of the little finger occurring at the junction of the burned dermal skin and unburned palmar skin. At the first sign of this contracture, which cannot be corrected by active motion alone, a passive extension splint is applied at all times when active motion is not being carried out.

Early care of the burned hand begins with proper wound management and closure and ends with a hand with good function only after many months of controlling hypertrophic scar and preserving joint motion.

14

Reconstruction of the Burned Hand

Raymond L. Warpeha and Juan Angelats

The most efficient management of burn deformity of the hand is to prevent it by appropriate measures of wound closure and joint mobilization. When preventive measures have failed or the burn produces loss of substance, reconstructive surgical procedures often help restore lost function and appearance. The following classification of hand burn deformity is given to pinpoint the physical factors causing the deformity and suggesting logical treatment:

- I. Primary
  - A. Skin shortage
    - 1. Dorsal
    - 2. Palmar
  - B. Linear shortening
    - 1. At wound margin
    - 2. Within wound
- II. Secondary (joint position)
- III. Structural loss
- IV. Combination of the above

Primary Deformity

Skin shortage is three-dimensional and is indistinguishably locked in with dermal scarring. Because most hand burns occur on the dorsum, most shortage deformities limit metacarpophalangeal MP joint flexion (Fig 14-1). In the first 4 to 6 months following injury the healing skin becomes plaquelike, and its elastic pull may overpower the ability of the joints to complete their range of motion. During this early period, these forces are best treated by a pressure glove and active motion of all joints of the hand. If the hypertrophic shortening

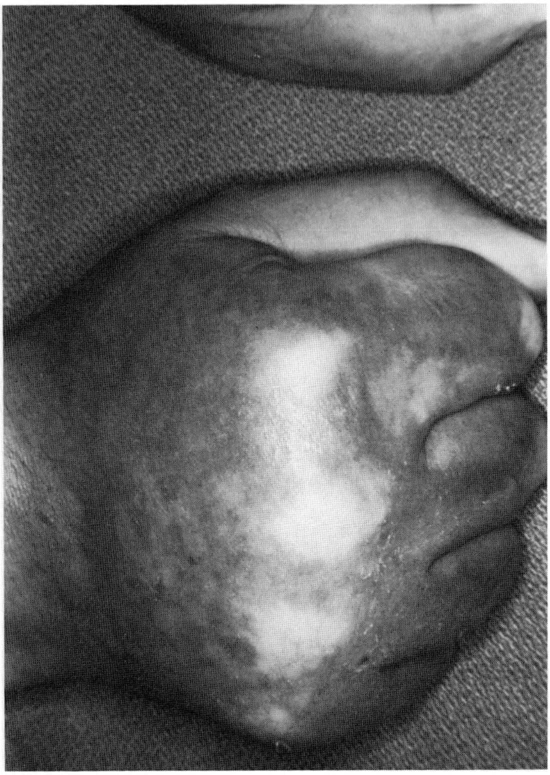

Fig 14-1. Dorsal hand burn at 3 months postburn. Although full MP joint flexion is attained, this is done only with difficulty as is obvious from the tight, white skin over the knuckles.

forces are overwhelming and there is poor skin cover, excision of all scar, often to fascia, is indicated. Intermediate split-thickness grafts in the range of 0.014 to 0.016 inch should be used for cover and pressure garments and physical therapy immediately reinstated.

If one encounters a fixed shortage of skin that shows mature scar, usually toward the end of the first year following injury, excision and grafting of the shortened tissues are required. Excision of all burn scar on the plane bordering normal tissues will release the soft tissue contracture and present a surface with easily controllable small-vessel bleeding (Fig 14-2). This is an ideal bed for a skin graft of sufficient thickness, 0.014 to 0.016 inch, to add permanent mobility to the previously restrained parts. Once this dorsal scar is excised, mobility of the affected joints is tested and release of contracture of the capsular and pericapsular structures may be necessary. Obviously, postoperative physical therapy is necessary and proceeds more effectively after these measures.

Many of the deformities in the burned hand occur at the borders of the burn with normal skin. The dermal scar hypertrophy along these lines shortens and

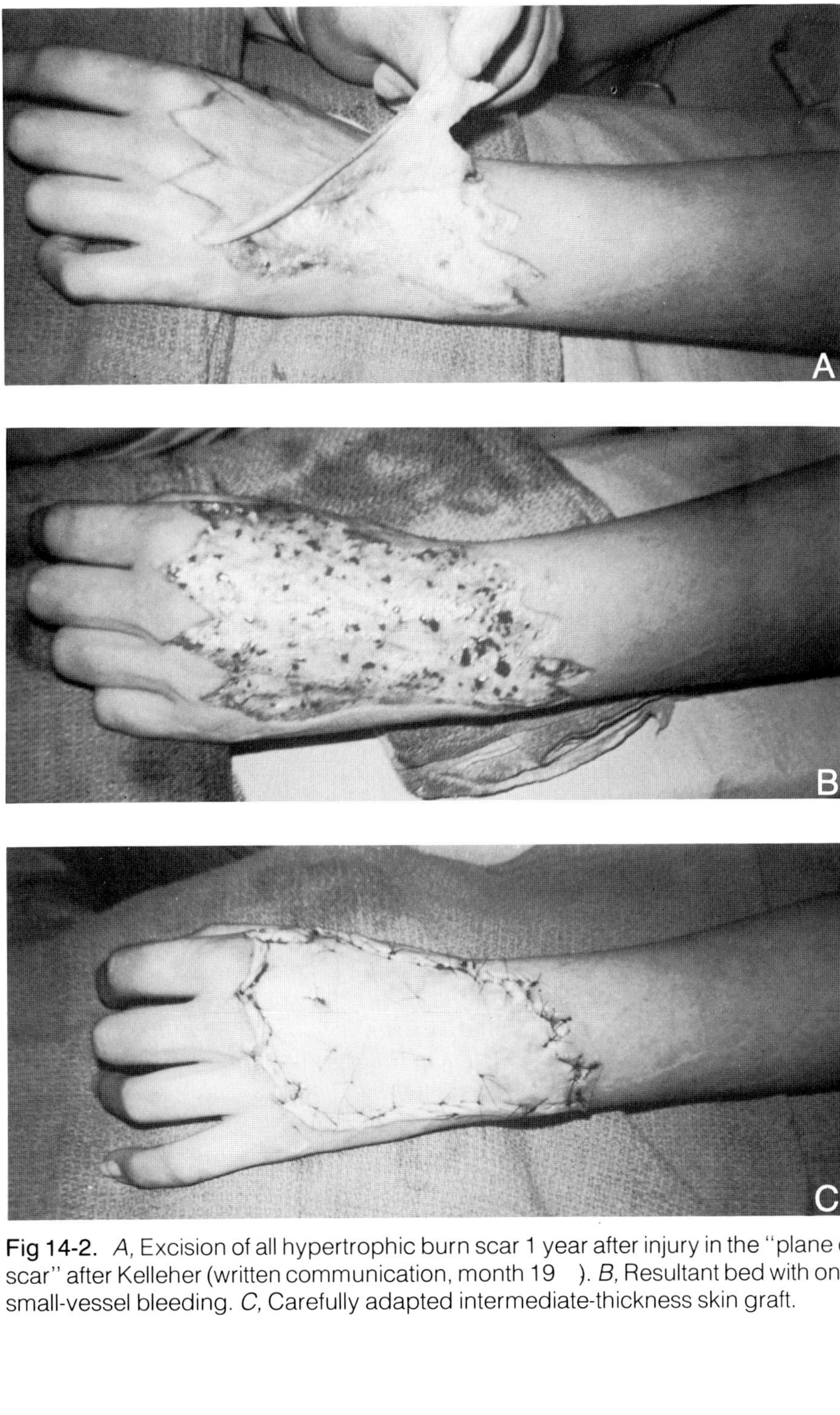

Fig 14-2. *A*, Excision of all hypertrophic burn scar 1 year after injury in the "plane of scar" after Kelleher (written communication, month 19). *B*, Resultant bed with only small-vessel bleeding. *C*, Carefully adapted intermediate-thickness skin graft.

forms the characteristic burn syndactyly of the second to fourth web spaces, contracture of the first web space, and limitation of abduction of the thumb and flexion contracture of the little finger (Figs 14-3, Fig 14-4).

Release of these linear contractures is readily achieved by transecting these bands, thus forming open gaps. The gap must then be filled with supple tissue and so placed as not to reshorten and reproduce the original deformity. In marginal scarring, the Z-plasty flap procedure, which supplies complementary flaps across the line of shortening, results in one healthy tissue side and one scar tissue side, which, when transposed effectively, lengthens the shortened band and repositions the healing incision over a longer and more angulated course. This works well for linear scars of modest dimension, such as a mild to moderate degree of syndactyly. However, in more marked degrees of deformity, interdigital advancement flaps create a more effective correction (Fig 14-5).

Z-plasty flaps in burn scar are subject to necrosis from decreased blood supply of the scar and perhaps vascular compression in the twisted flap base. For this reason, small, multiple Z-plasty flaps with limbs of 1 to 2 cm are preferred. These flaps, therefore, should be atraumatically elevated, leaving as much underlying attached subcutaneous tissue as one is able to mobilize without tension. Minor flap tip loss is common and will not defeat the purpose of the procedure, as it is the bases of the transposed flaps that elongate the linear contracture, and these remain viable.

Where marginal scar is not linear but broadly involves the marginal tissues, the scar should be totally excised and grafted with skin of good quality.

Palmar burn deformity, which usually results in loss of extension and flexion contracture, is treated by excision of scar and grafting. The recurrent nature of these deformities in the face of a good skin graft frequently requires adding of thick graft or the introduction of distant flap tissue.

Secondary Deformity

Secondary joint deformities such as boutonnière or swan-neck deformity are common with hand burns and take the same form as when produced by other causes. They are treated by similar release procedures plus the correction, where possible, of the foreshortened skin or linear contractures as previously discussed. Fortunately, children with secondary joint deformity caused by burn scar contracture regain joint motion rapidly after the primary scar restraint is successfully removed and replaced with supple skin and physical therapy is applied.

With fixed joint deformities secondary to open joints and extensor tendon destruction on the dorsum of the finger, little can be accomplished if the extensor mechanism cannot be reconstructed. Arthrodesis and ray amputation contribute much to improving hand function when these deformities are isolated.

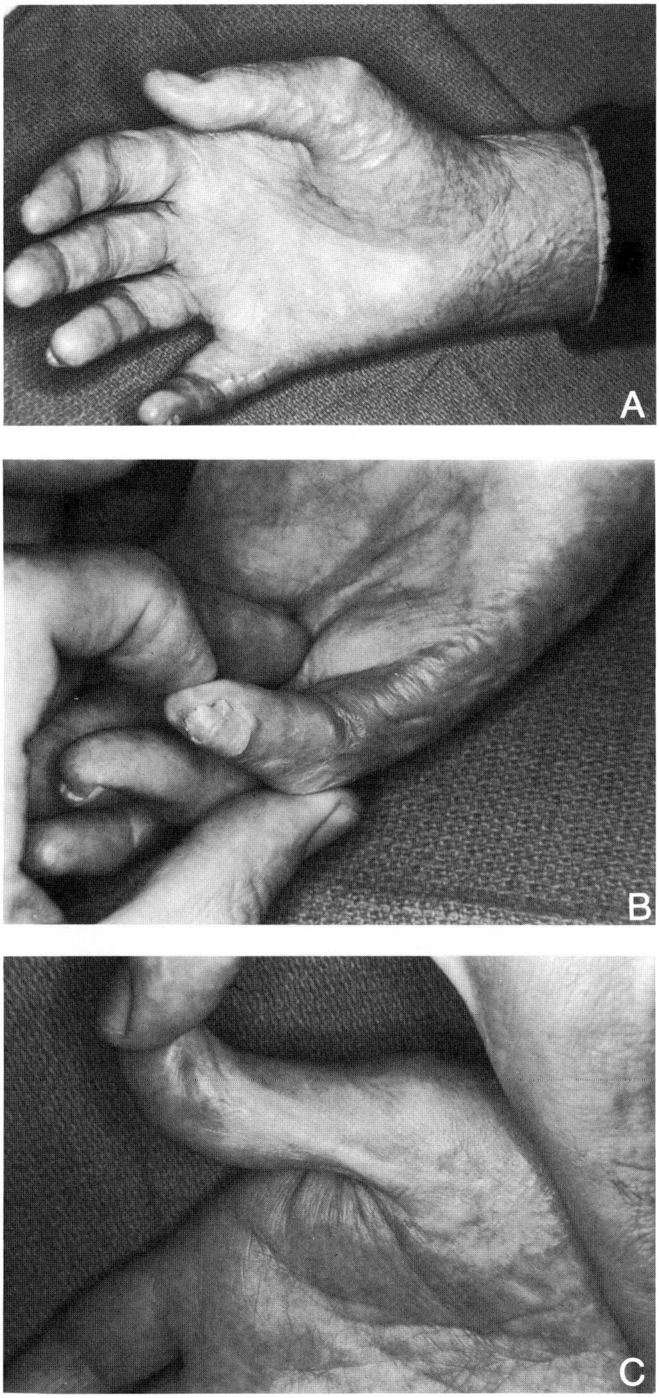

Fig 14-3. *A*, Linear contracture of skin along the margins of the burn on the palmar surface, causing flexion contracture of the little finger (*B*) and limitation of abduction extension of the thumb (*C*).

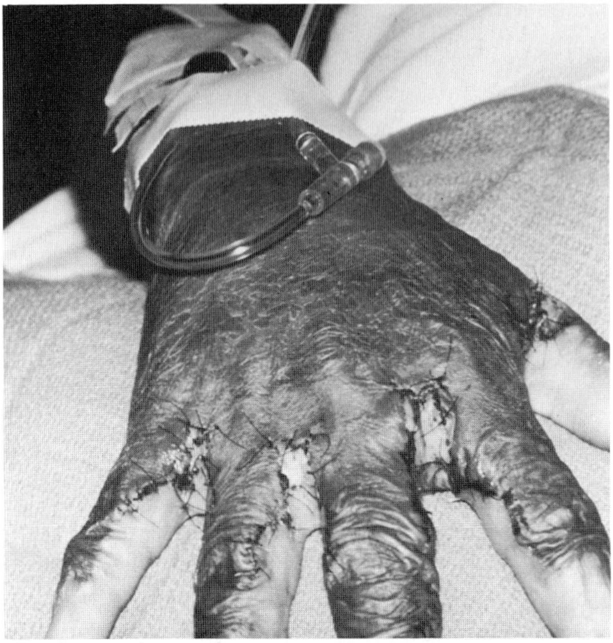

Fig 14-4. Advancement flap correction of burn syndactyly after incising the linear contractures at the second through the fourth web spaces, plus multiple short-limb Z-plasty of the first web space contracture.

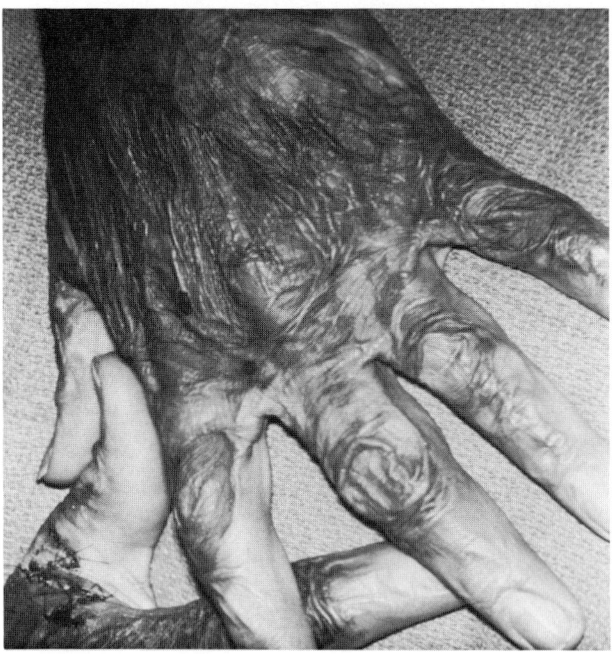

Fig 14-5. Burn syndactyly due to linear shortening at the margin of the dorsal burn and normal web space skin.

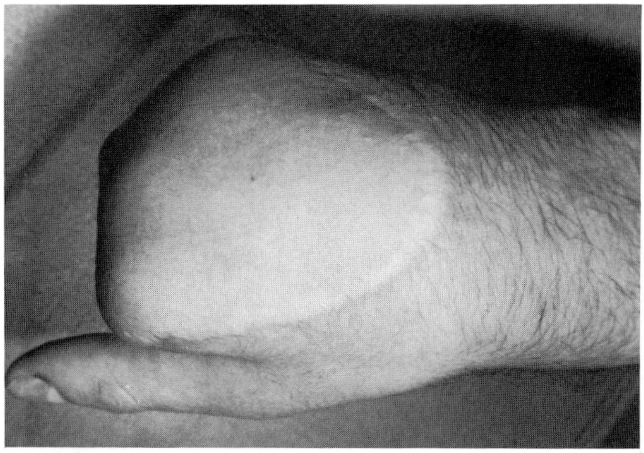

Fig 14-6. Hot press injury of the hand with total loss of all fingers beyond the MP joints. Exposed dermal tendons required a groin flap for wound closure.

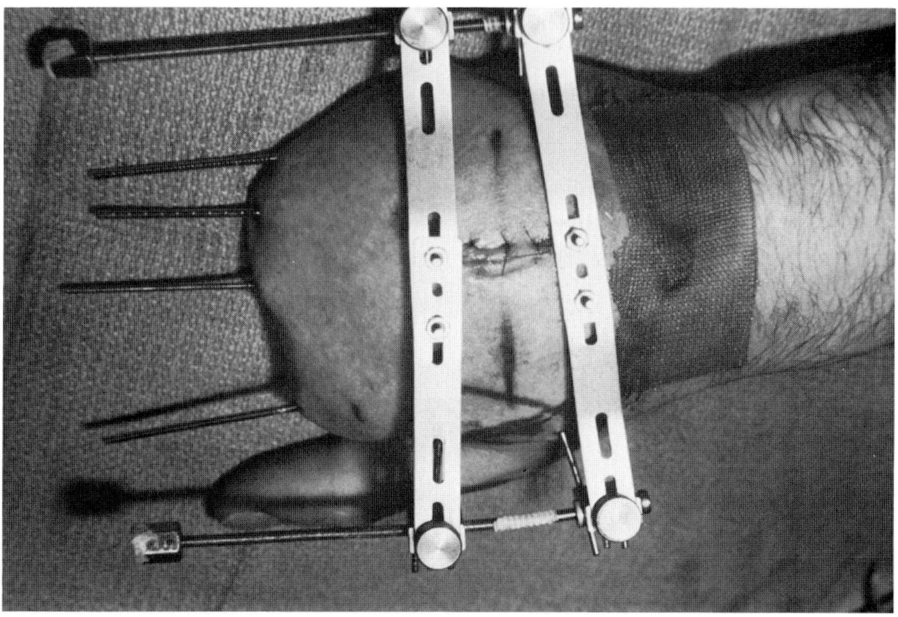

Fig 14-7. Postoperative appearance of the hand after transection of the second, third, and fourth metacarpals and application of a mini-Hoffman appliance.

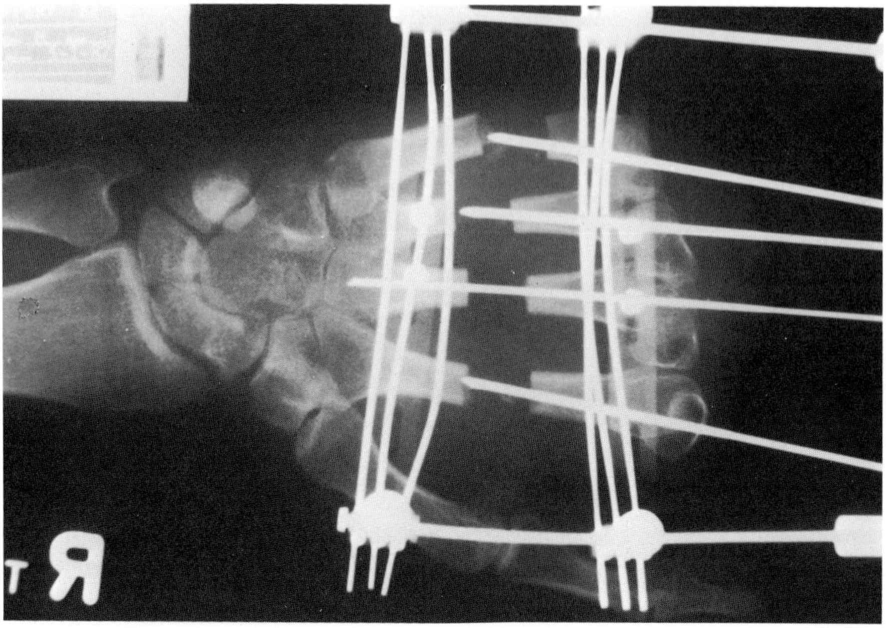

Fig 14-8. Postoperative radiograph showing initial distraction of the transected metacarpals.

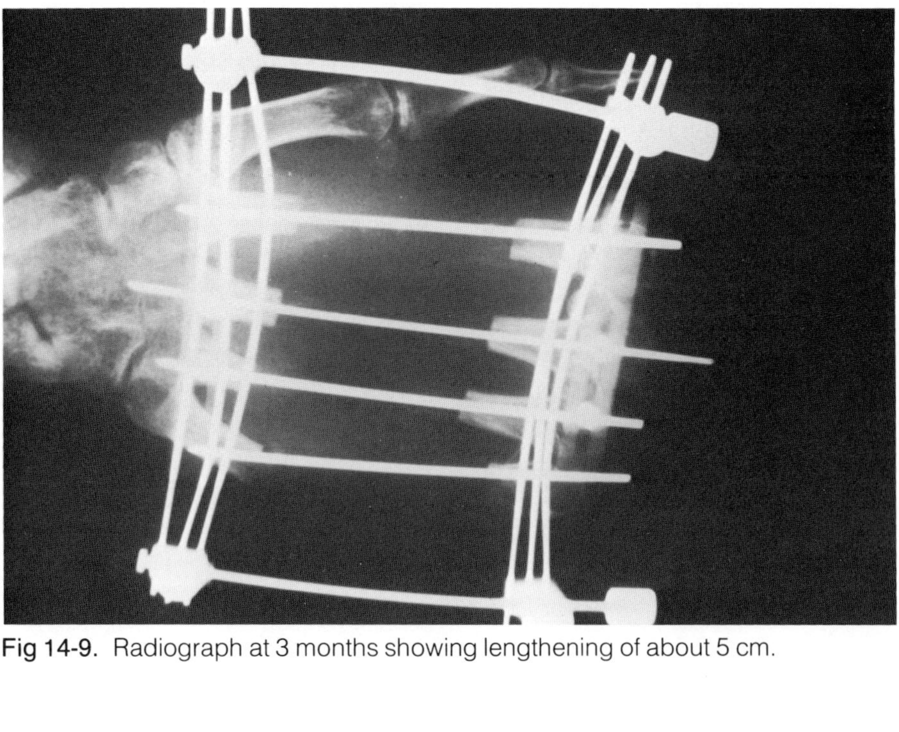

Fig 14-9. Radiograph at 3 months showing lengthening of about 5 cm.

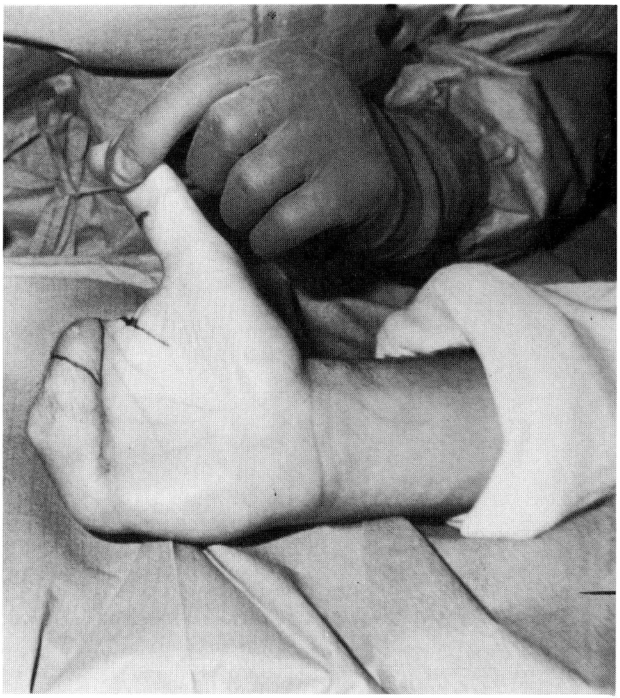

Fig 14-10. Palmar view with Z-plasty markings before transposition. The proximal, more sensitive flap will be transposed to the insensitive tissues at the distal-radial point of the index stump.

Loss of Substance

Occasionally, hand burns are of such depth as to cause full-thickness loss of all finger and/or thumb substance. Although flap tissue may be necessary and able to cover the remaining proximal structures, individual finger structure is difficult and often impossible to restore. Reconstructive efforts are directed at maximizing the oppositional or grasp function of the thumb and fingers. This may be as simple as deepening the first web space by Z-plasty. It may mean lengthening the thumb by various methods of thumb reconstruction. Figs 14-6 through 14-11 show a novel approach to mitt lengthening in a 22-year-old male who sustained the loss of all his fingers near the MP joints following a hot press injury, which required a groin flap to cover the exposed extensor tendon on the dorsum of the hand. With the use of a mini-Hoffman appliance, the osteotomized metacarpals were distracted over a period of 3 months, then bone grafted to give a 5-cm increase in length of the mitt. A palmar Z-plasty was used to transpose sensitive palmar skin to the previously insensitive distal-radial border of the mitt.

Microsurgery and free flaps will expand the reconstructive possibilities in treatment of the burned hand, and perhaps these procedures might be entertained in the acute period before secondary deformity is allowed to occur.

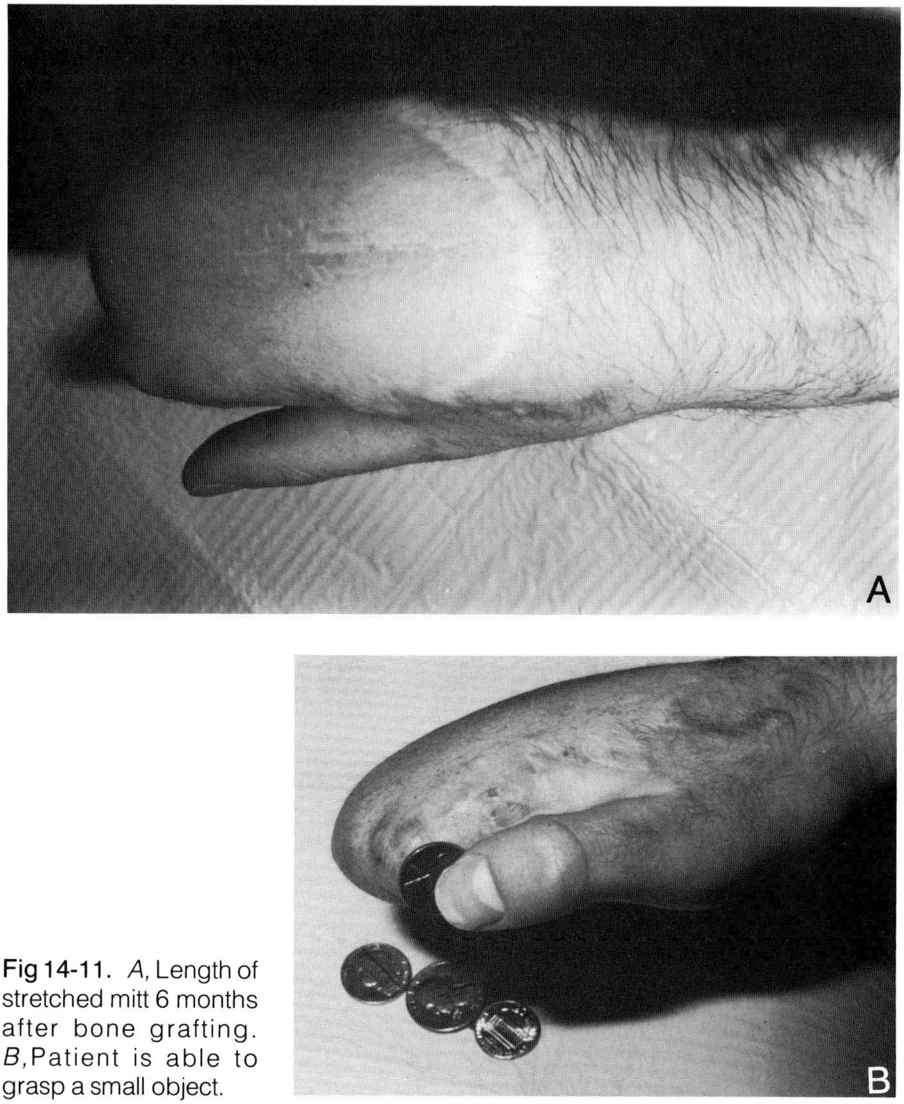

Fig 14-11. *A,* Length of stretched mitt 6 months after bone grafting. *B,* Patient is able to grasp a small object.

15

Flap Skin Cover on the Hand: Three New Additions

Ravin L. Thatte and
Uddhav A. Patil

The SEPA Flap

The SEPA flap is a new axial pattern flap based on the superficial external pudendal arteriovenous system.[1,2]

Anatomy

The superficial external pudendal artery (SEPA) arises from the medial side of the femoral artery and after supplying the labial or the scrotal skin courses from the pubic tubercle to the umbilicus to supply the skin in that area (Fig 15-1). The lower two thirds of its course lies in the superficial fascia, and the upper third lies subdermally.[1,2] Cadaveric dissection[2] reveals that the SEPA cross-anastomoses with its opposite member (Fig 15-2) and sends communicating branches to the superficial inferior epigastric artery (SIEA) on the same side. The venous drainage of the SEPA flap is more than adequate, consisting of the superficial external pudendal vein and its two venae comitantes, which drain into the great saphenous vein. The superficial external pudendal vein is usually larger than the artery.

Clinical Considerations

An inferiorly based skin flap between the pubic symphysis and the umbilicus is feasible on either side of the midline (Fig 15-3). When a combined flap is planned on both sides of the midline (bilateral combined SEPA flap; see Fig 15-4), it has the advantage of the cross-anastomosis between the two SEPAs (Fig 15-2). A SEPA flap based on one side of the midline can be extended laterally to

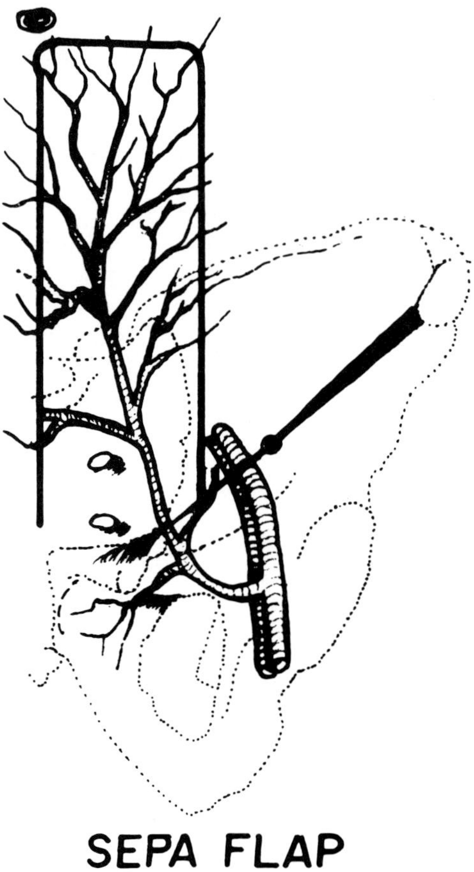

Fig 15-1. The hemipelvis is outlined, and the territory of the external pudendal artery is marked. Its origin is from the medial side of the femoral artery.

include the anastomosis between the SEPA and the SIEA. In the standing, sitting, or supine position the human hand most naturally lies either by the side of the body or is placed across the lower abdomen. By its location, therefore, the SEPA flap is ideal for skin cover of the hand. The flap drapes extremely well over the dorsum of the hand (Fig 15-4), fits snugly in the first web space (Fig 15-5), and can be used quite conveniently to make a thumb by the osteoplastic method (Fig 15-6). For small defects on the dorsum of the fingers, a narrow, unilateral flap can be used with safety.

Case 1

Nine days prior to hospital admission, this male patient suffered an electrical burn injury to the dorsum of the left middle and ring fingers, resulting in loss of skin, subcutaneous tissue, and part of the extensor tendon. The proximal interphalangeal (PIP) joint of the middle finger was exposed and dislocated,

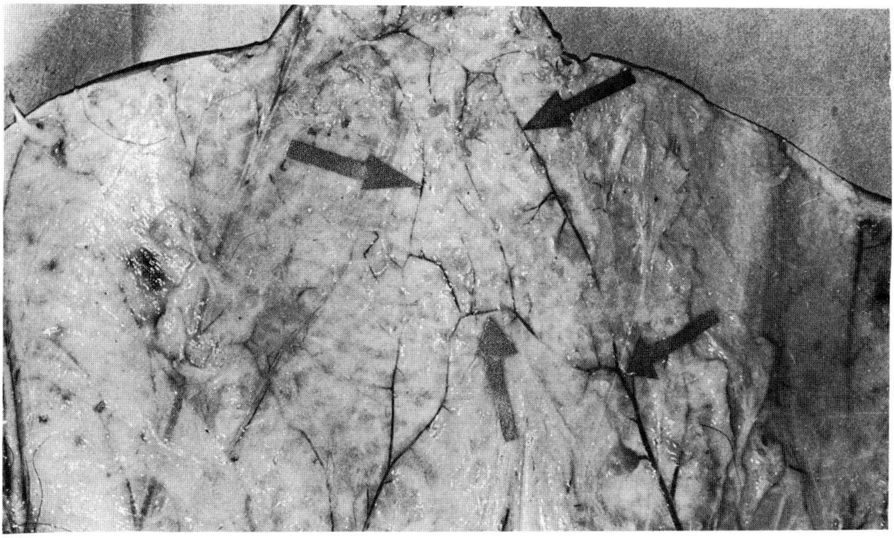

Fig 15-2. Cadaveric dissection of the superficial external pudendal arteries (*horizontal arrows*). The *vertical arrow* shows cross-anastomosis between the arteries.

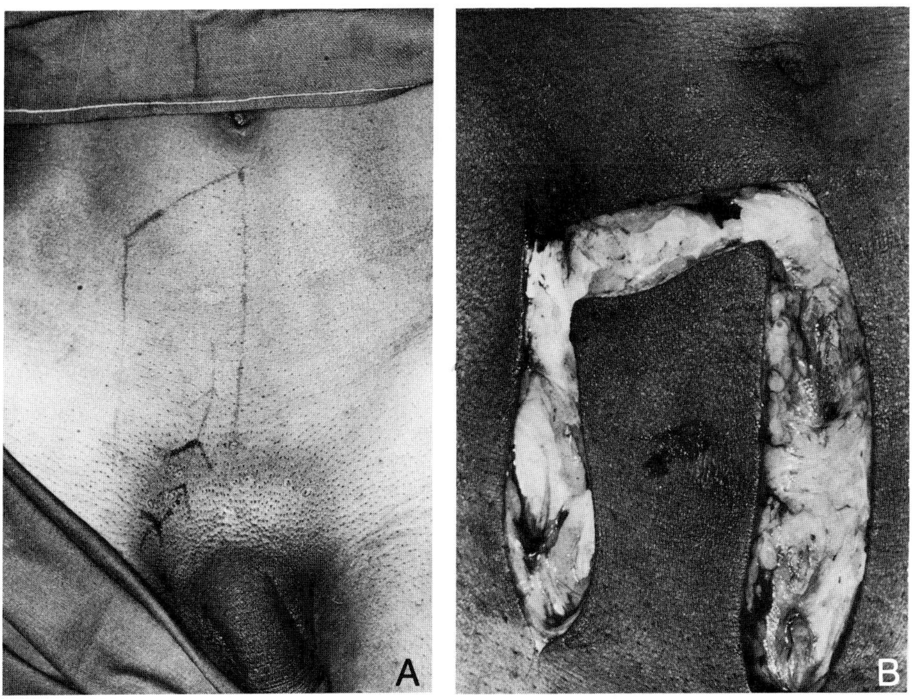

Fig 15-3. A narrow, unilateral SEPA flap is marked (*A*) and cut (*B*).

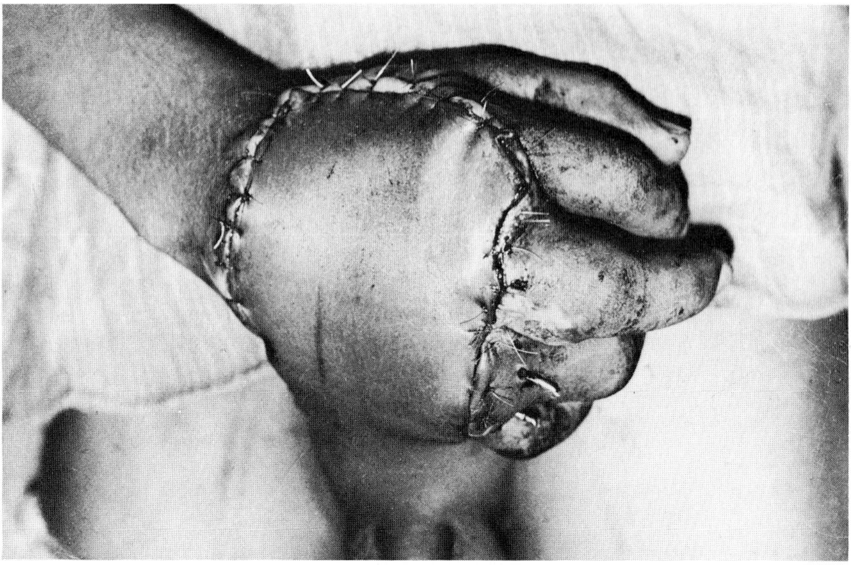

Fig 15-4. Avulsion crush of the dorsum of the right hand repaired with a bilateral SEPA flap. Note the comfortable lie of the hand. No immobilization was used from the 4th postoperative day.

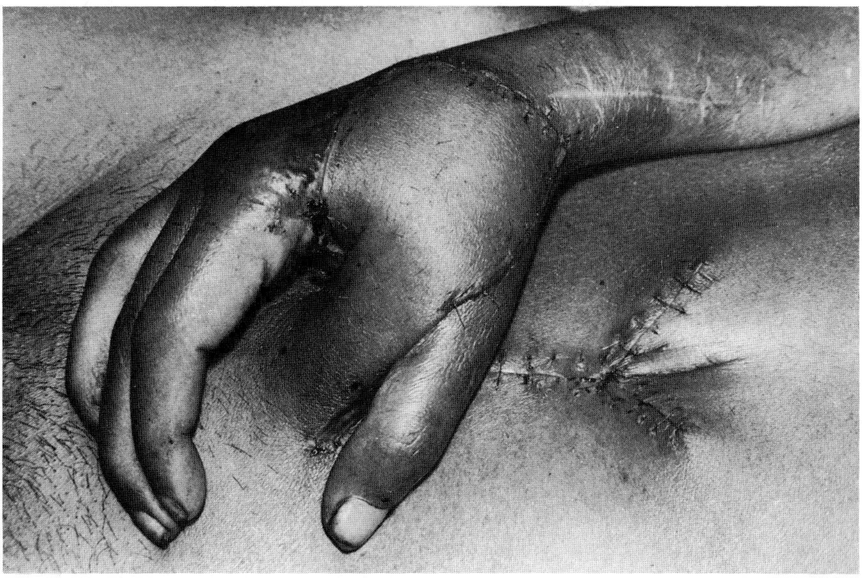

Fig 15-5. Repair of a traumatic adduction contracture in the first web space of the right hand. A local transposition flap has proved inadequate. Photograph shows a bilateral SEPA flap in place on the 10th postoperative day. The donor area has been closed primarily.

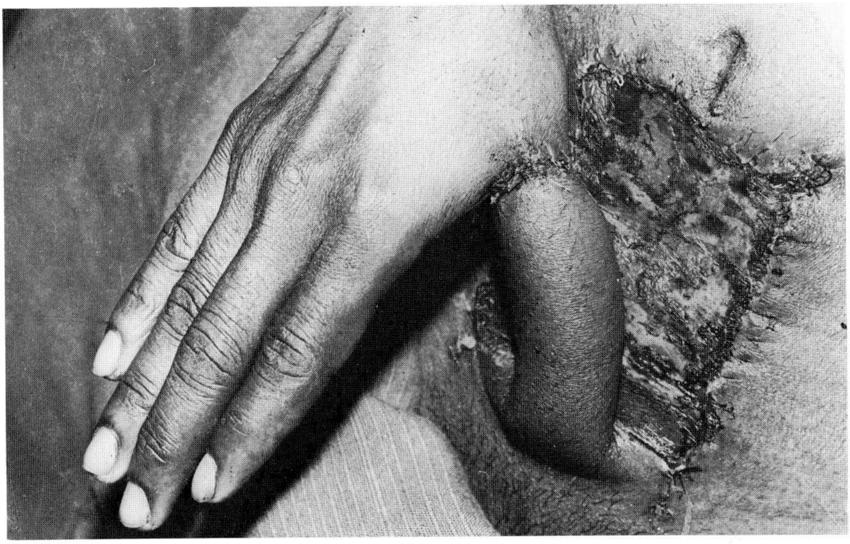

Fig 15-6. Reconstruction of a traumatically amputated thumb by the osteoplastic method (first stage). The defect left by the flap will be covered by a skin graft.

then reduced and fixed with a metal wire after the wound was thoroughly cleaned and débrided (Fig 15-7A). The areas over the fingers needing skin flap cover were unequal, but this difficulty was well taken care of by designing an unequal bilateral SEPA flap which fit quite well over the defect (Fig 15-7, B and C). A recent examination reveals that the flap is bulky, but it can be cut quite thin in its upper one third. In this case, because the injury was due to an electrical current, the risk involved in cutting the flap thin was avoided.

Interposition of Anterior Rectus Sheath to Prevent Dorsal Adhesions

Injuries to the skin of the dorsum of the hand are frequently accompanied by lacerations of the extensor tendons. In some cases the tendons are not actually cut but are mangled in continuity, with loss of paratenon, and there may be gross contamination of the bed on which the tendons move. This situation is an invitation for scar formation and contractures, restriction of mobility, and secondary stiffness at the metacarpophalangeal joints. The problem is not remedied by achieving skin cover alone on the dorsum of the hand, particularly when a staged skin flap transfer is contemplated, because mobilization of the fingers cannot be fully attempted before the flap is divided. It appears logical to assume that tendon adhesions will be considerably less if a one-stage restoration of skin cover is achieved by small-vessel anastomosis with the help of a microscope, with physiotherapy begun almost immediately thereafter.

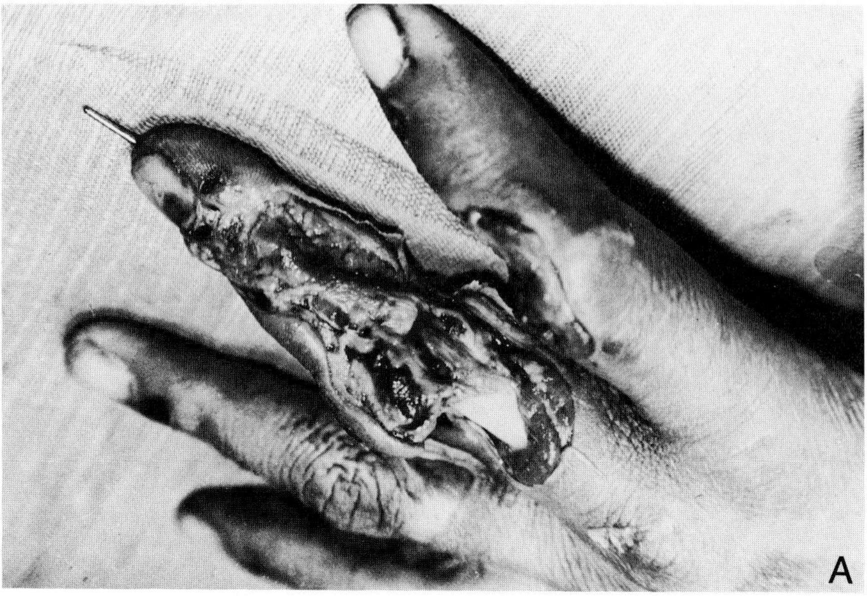

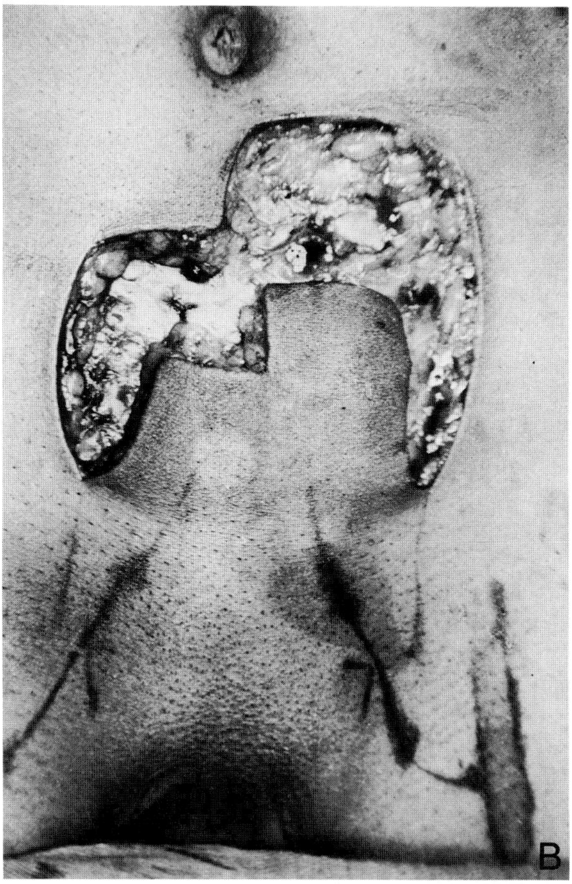

Fig 15-7. *A*, Injury to the dorsum of the middle and index fingers by an electric current. The area needing flap skin cover over the two fingers is unequal. *B*, An unequal bilateral SEPA flap is raised. *C*, The flap covers both fingers adequately and conveniently.

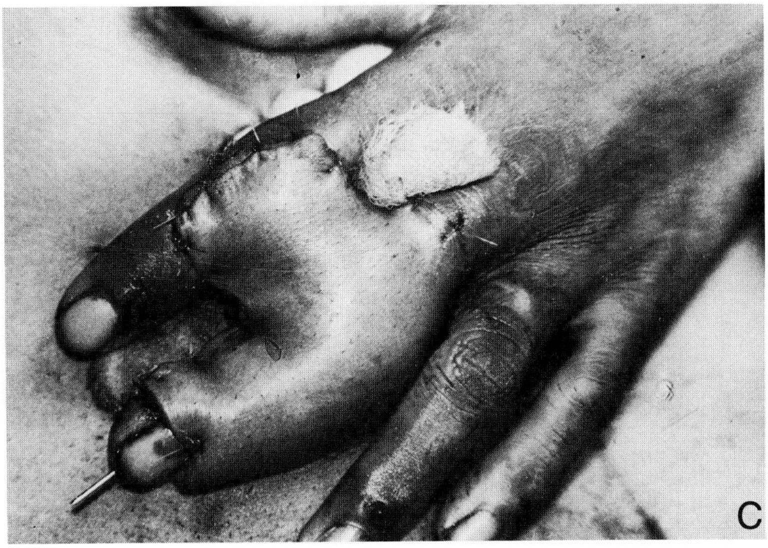

Fig 15-7. Continued

However, transfer of tissue by microvascular anastomosis is not a universally available procedure, and even where available there are constraints on its use; for example, microsurgery of the hand might be contraindicated when other parts of the body are grievously injured as well.

With this background, while achieving skin flap cover in two stages over the dorsum of a hand in which extensor tendons are bereft of their gliding and protective mechanism, we have interposed underneath the tendons a part of the anterior rectus sheath with or without external oblique aponeurosis.

Case 2

This male patient was seen with a severe dorsal contracture of the ulnar half of the right hand a year following a deep chemical burn injury (Fig 15-8). An x-ray revealed that the metacarpophalangeal joint of the little finger was damaged at the articular surface of the fifth metacarpal.

At surgery the scar was completely excised, revealing frayed extensor tendons of the ring and middle fingers. The extensor tendon to the little finger was missing. A right SEPA flap, with a skin territory extending into the area of anastomosis with the SIEA, was raised to cover the defect (Fig 15-9), and in addition a sheet of the anterior rectus sheath was raised from underneath. This sheath was passed under the tendons and then turned over on itself to enclose both sides of the tendons (Fig 15-10). The flap was sutured over this newly created sheath (Fig 15-11). Eight weeks later the ulnar deviation of the hand was further corrected by transposing the available flap skin after creating a fresh defect in the area of the metacarpophalangeal joints. Twelve weeks from

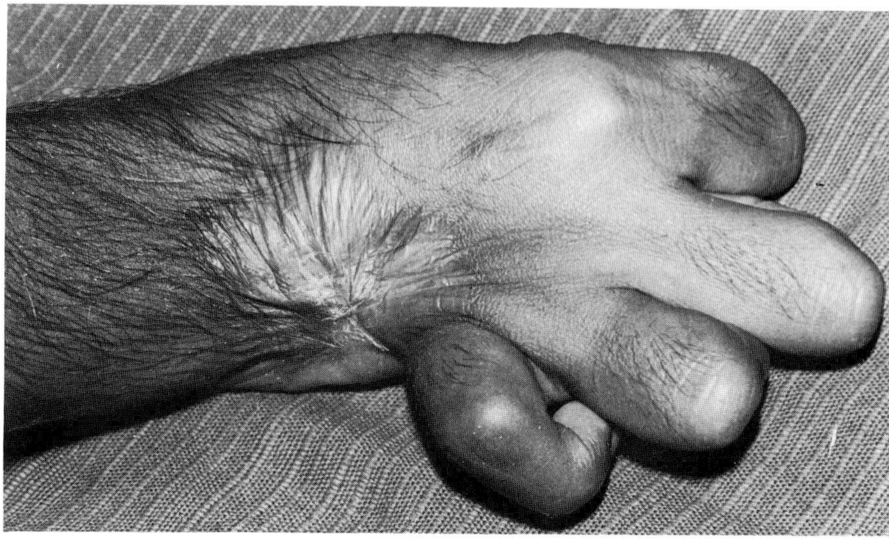

Fig 15-8. Dorsal contracture of the hand following a deep chemical burn. Note the position of fingers while an attempt is made to form a fist.

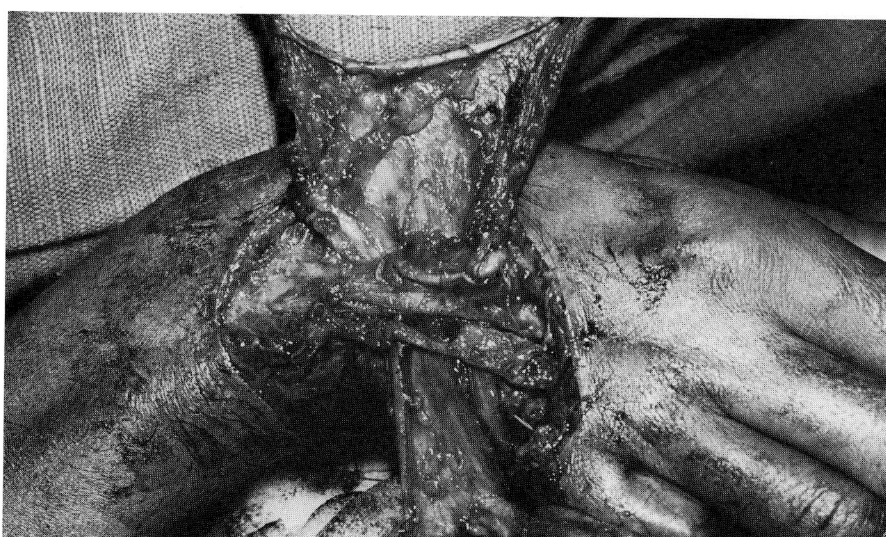

Fig 15-9. A part of the anterior rectus sheath under the flap is raised with an inferior base.

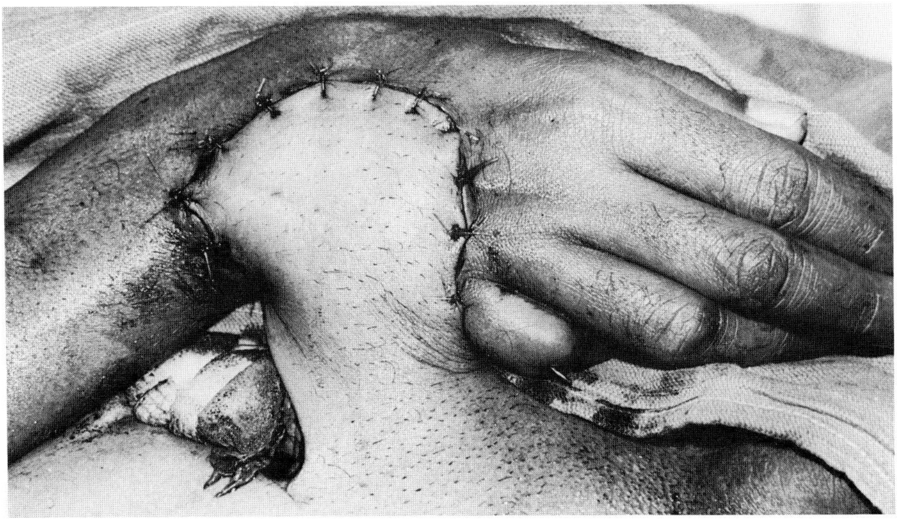

Fig 15-10. A SEPA flap with additional territory of the SIEA is raised and sutured over the defect.

the time of the first surgery the hand was restored to near-normal function with the help of active and passive physiotherapy and splinting (Fig 15-12).

Case 3

This adult male patient suffered a severe friction avulsion injury to the dorsum of the right hand when he was dragged on an oil-smeared road after falling out of a skidding open jeep. The wound was débrided and cleansed under anesthesia to reveal laceration of the extensor tendon of the little finger and severe fraying of the other extensor tendons (Fig 15-11). A large, inferiorly based skin flap from the lower abdomen was raised to achieve cover over the injured hand, and a segment of anterior rectus sheath of a corresponding size

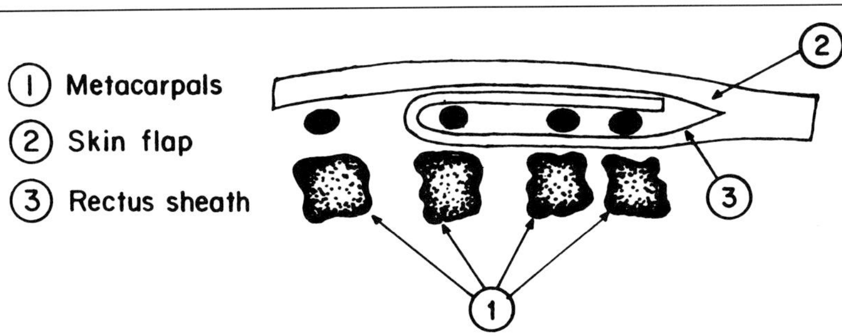

Fig 15-11. Schematic representation showing how the sheath is passed under the tendons and rolled over to make a protective cover for the tendons, after which the flap is sutured to the defect.

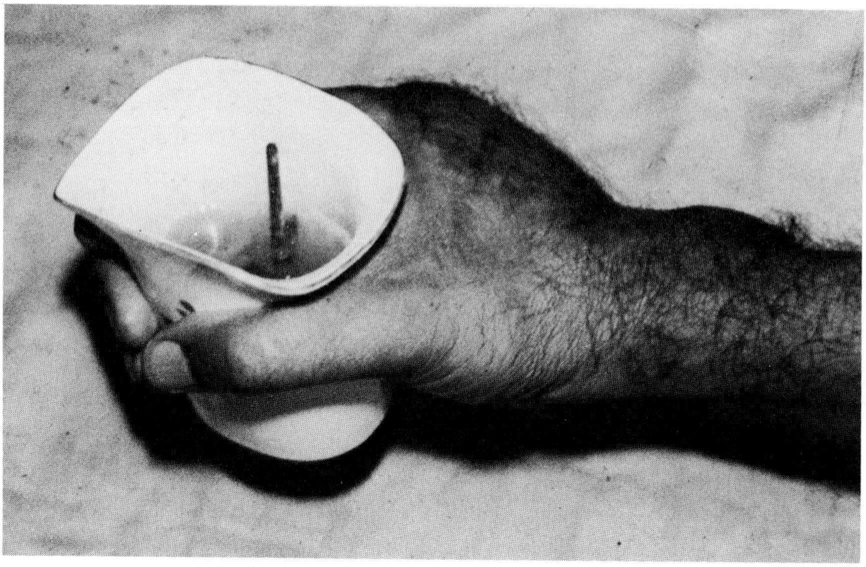

Fig 15-12. The result 3 months later.

was interposed under the tendons by the method described to prevent adhesions. The hand had excellent function when last seen, a year after surgery.

Discussion

These clinical examples cannot resolve whether the interposition of rectus sheath underneath or around the tendons prevents adhesions, or even whether the anterior rectus sheath survives as live tissue under the circumstances described here.

Our own observations, however, have been quite encouraging. At the time of division of the skin flap, when the fascial bridges were detached, the rectus sheath appeared unaltered. It also had the leash of small vessels which were observed when the sheath was initially raised. The experience of the senior author[3] in raising flaps of fascia alone in the lower extremity also lends weight to the feeling that the rectus sheath might survive in the clinical circumstances described above. Recent work on flaps consisting of the whole of the lower abdominal skin based on only one rectus muscle for reconstruction of the breast has revealed, through some interesting angiographic studies, that there is profuse cross-anastomosis between the cartwheel of six superficial and two deep vessels in the region of the lower abdomen.[4] It appears likely, therefore, that a 4-inch-long and equally broad part of the anterior rectus sheath, with or without the external oblique aponeurosis, with its lower abdominal attachment and cover intact, will be able to survive and subserve the function of preventing adhesions, particularly because fascial structures are known to have a very low metabolic rate.

Deepithelialized "Turnover" Skin Flaps

Volar skin losses in the proximal two thirds of a finger are conventionally treated by a cross-finger flap. The method involves two stages and requires immobilization (albeit partial) of the affected finger as well as of the adjacent normal finger. A local "turnover" flap[5] overcomes these problems.

Case 4

This 22-year-old, right-handed manual worker was referred with a skin defect over the volar surface of the middle phalanx of the right middle finger (Fig 15-13A). The defect was the result of an abscess in the same area that had been incised 1 week earlier. A bare profundus tendon was seen in the floor of the defect, and skin flap cover was considered essential to heal the area and restore function. The metacarpophalangeal and interphalangeal joints of the finger

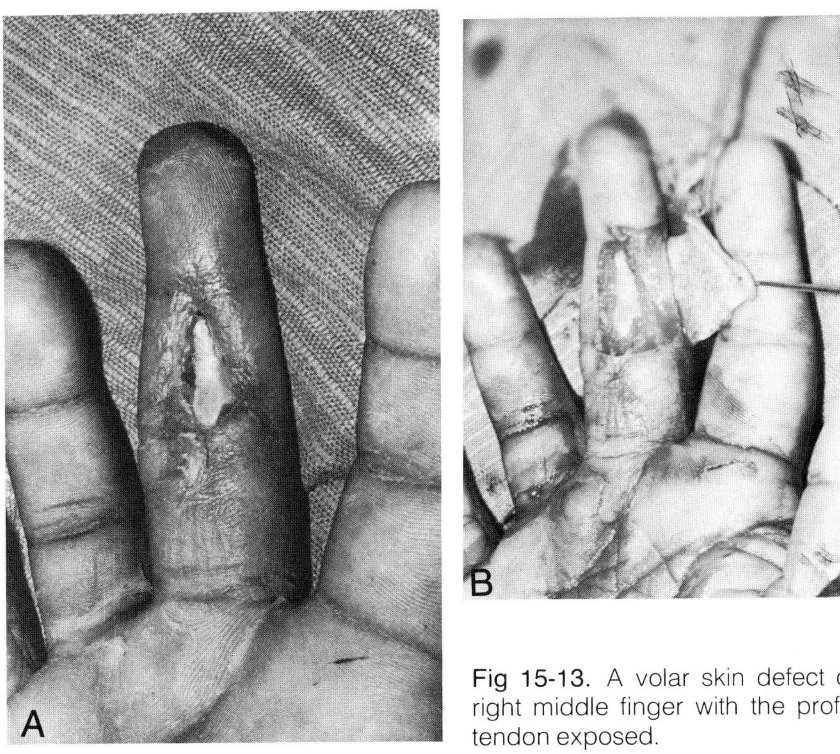

Fig 15-13. A volar skin defect on the right middle finger with the profundus tendon exposed.

were stiff and painful. Surgery was performed under a digital block with 2% Xylocaine. The scar surrounding the wound was excised, leaving a final defect measuring 2 × 1 cm needing flap skin cover. An area measuring 2 cm along the finger and 3 cm across the finger was marked out on the radial and dorsal surfaces of the same finger for deepithelialization (Fig 15-14). After deepithelialization, a flap was raised from this area on the dorsum (Fig 15-13B), leaving the crosshatched area as the base of the flap, which was then turned over to cover the volar defect and sutured in place. The turnover flap and the secondary defect were both covered with a splitthickness skin graft. The graft took completely, mobilization was started on the 3rd postoperative day, and the finger showed excellent function 4 weeks later (Fig 15-15, A and B).

Case 5

A patient presented with an infected wound on the volar surface of the little finger, with osteomyelitis of the proximal and middle phalanges and destruction of the PIP joint (Fig 15-16, A and B). The lesion required excision of affected bone and flap skin cover. A local turnover flap was quite adequate to heal the wound after the bone ends were excised (Fig 15-16C). There is little expectation of PIP joint motion, however. A functional position with an arthrodesis at the level of the PIP joint is contemplated at a future date.

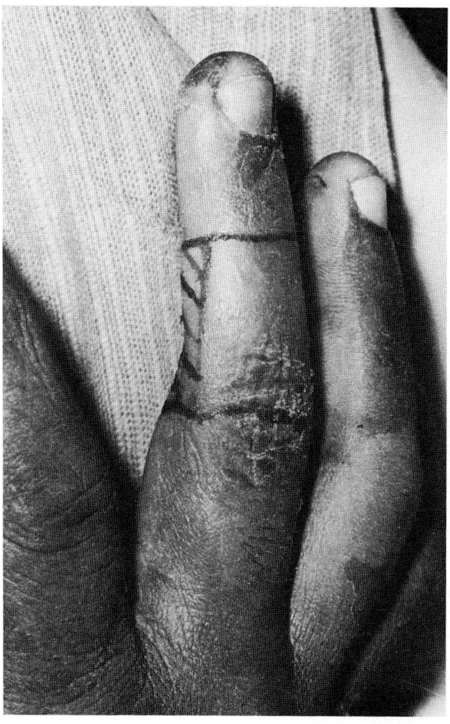

Fig 15-14. An area on the dorsal aspect of the digit is marked for deepithelialization.

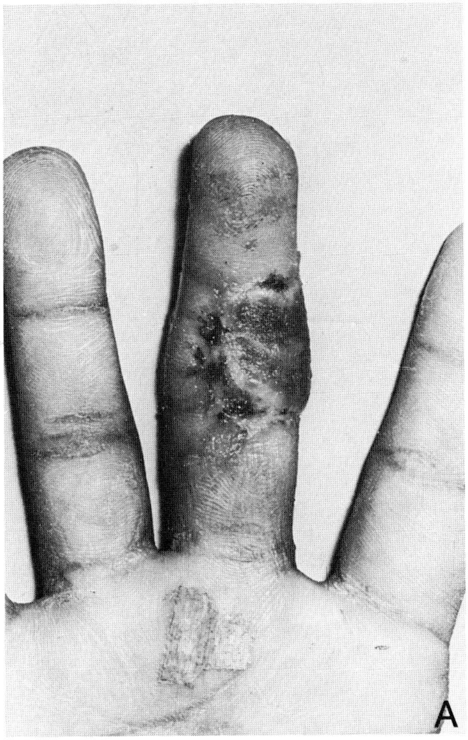

Fig 15-15. Range of movement 4 weeks later.

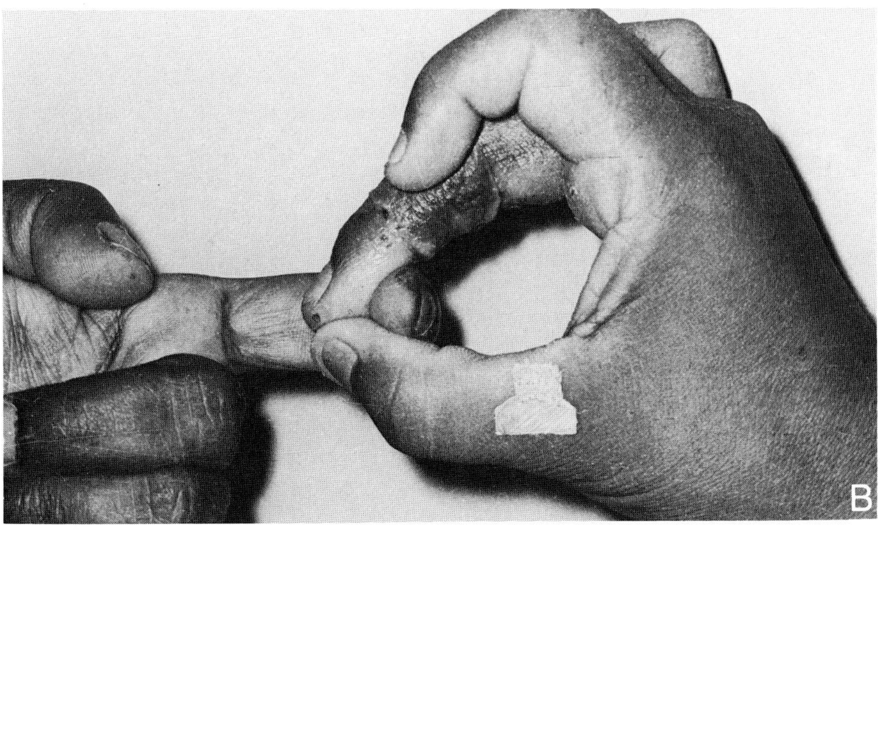

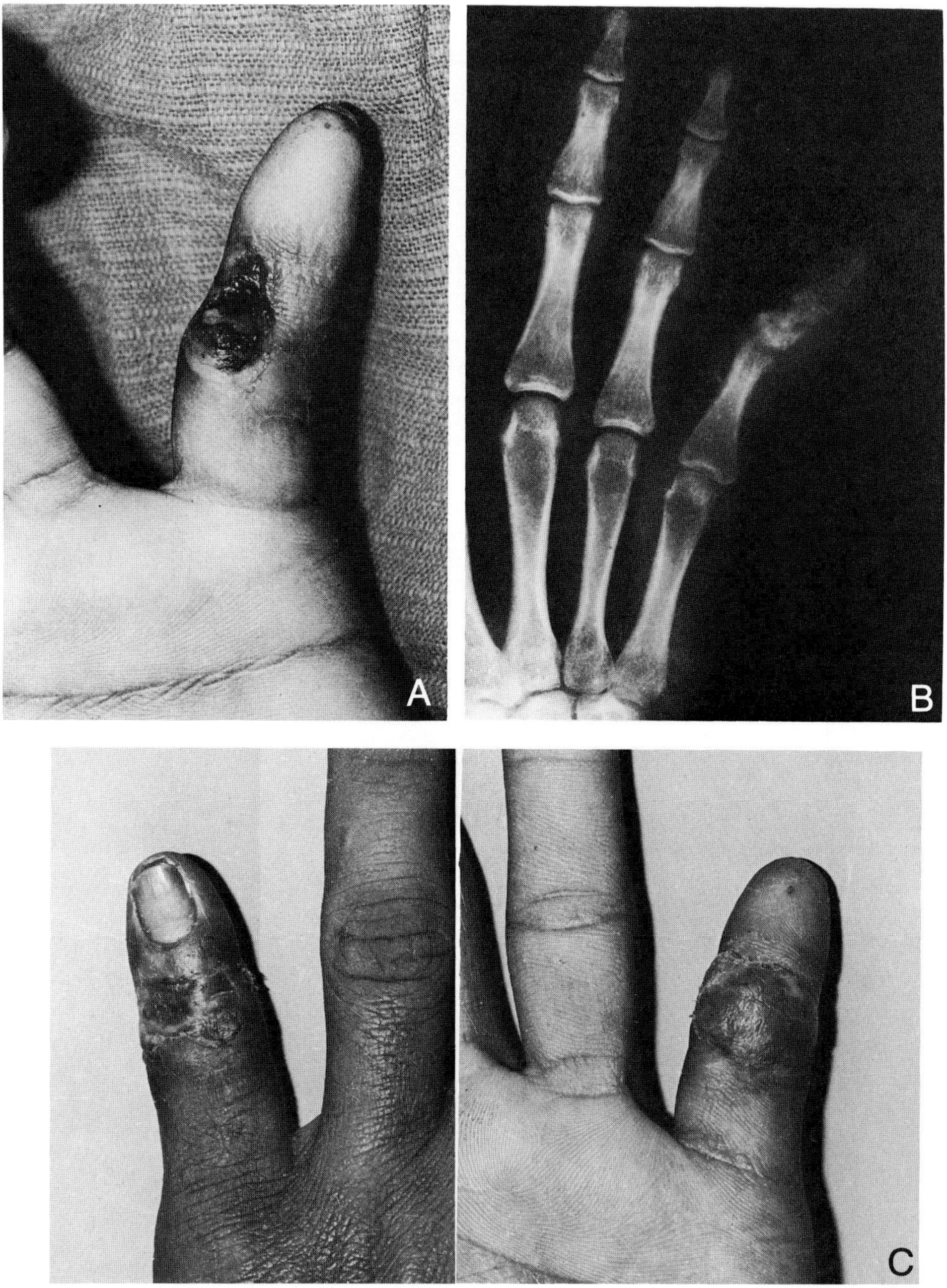

Fig 15-16. An area of skin loss on the left little finger. *B*, Osteomyelitis of the middle and proximal phalanges. *C*, Healed area after a local turnover flap and excision of pathological bone (*left*, dorsal view; *right*, volar view). Surgery for better positioning of finger will be undergone later.

Acknowledgment

The authors would like to thank the British Journal of Plastic Surgery for kindly supplying some of the material contained within this chapter.

References

1. Dias AD: The superficial external pudendal artery (SEPA) axial-pattern flap. *Br J Plast Surg,* 1984;37:256.
2. Patil UA: *The SEPA Flap,* thesis. University of Bombay, Bombay, 1983.
3. Thatte RL, Laud NS: The use of the fascia of the lower leg as a roll over flap. Its possible clinical application in reconstructive surgery. *Br J Plast Surg* 1984;37:88–94.
4. Scheflan M, Dinner MI: The transverse abdominal island flap. Part I: Indications, contraindications, results and complications. *Ann Plast Surg* 1983;10:24.
5. Thatte RL, Gopalakrishna A, Prasad SA: The use of de-epithelialised 'turn-over' flaps in the hand. *Br J Plast Surg* 1982; 35:293–299.

16

The Management of Acute Upper Extremity Nerve Injuries

C.A. Luekens, Jr.

Surgeons who are called upon to treat acute peripheral nerve injuries face a considerable challenge in reaching their goal of reestablishing function. Overall management of the wound, the timing and technical performance of nerve suture, and the supervision of postsurgical rehabilitation are the only means by which the surgeon can influence the outcome. Many other presently uncontrollable factors, including age, type of injury, and physiological mechanisms, will also be determinants in the final result.

Nerve Microanatomy

To understand the physiology of injury and regeneration, as well as modern methods of nerve suture, one must review the internal anatomy of a nerve (Fig 16-1). Each axon is covered by myelin and closely enmeshed in the collagen fibers that form the endoneurium. A group of axons is, in turn, surrounded by a consolidation of the connective tissue fibers, the perineurium, which defines a fascicle within its boundaries. Each peripheral nerve consists of a few to several dozen fascicles, some containing sensory and some motor nerve fibers, and some even containing both (mixed fascicle). The epineurium encases the nerve as a sheath, protecting it from stretching and kinking.

Types of Injury

The nerve and its epineural sheath may have been completely transected (neurotmesis), or the sheath may be left intact but the nerve fibers separated by crush or stretch (axonotmesis). These injuries are followed by degeneration of

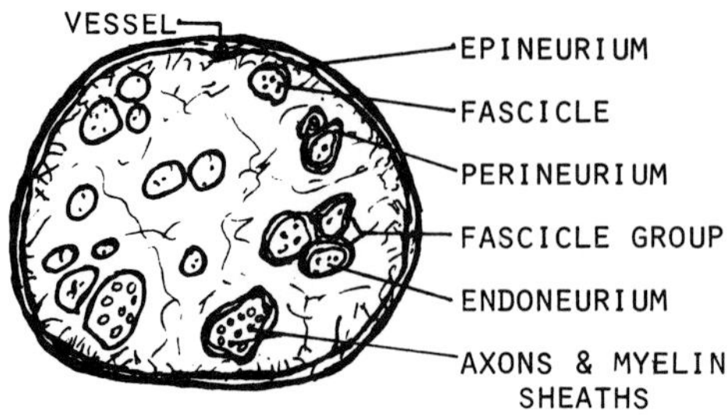

Fig 16-1. Nerve microanatomy.

the distal axons and some proximal degeneration and marked physiological reaction in the cell body near the spinal cord.

The term neurapraxia refers to injury in which electrical conduction is temporarily, and for variable lengths of time, interrupted across the injury site, but all anatomical structures remain intact.

Injuries are also classified as either (1) sharp, clean, noncontaminated wounds; (2) crush or explosive wounds; or (3) contaminated or infected wounds. The timing and method of nerve repair are dependent on the condition of the wound itself. Basic principles of wound débridement, delayed closure, and sepsis prevention and control always take precedence over nerve repair.

Clinical Diagnosis

The health practitioner examining a patient with a suspected nerve injury must be knowledgeable as to the course of the nerves and their cutaneous sensory distribution and muscle innervation. Therefore, to confirm a nerve injury, the anatomical position of the nerves in relation to the injury site must be assessed.

Although the radial nerve provides only a small area of skin sensibility over the dorsum of the radial aspect of the hand and thumb, it innervates all the extensor muscles of the hand and wrist, as well as the brachioradialis and the triceps.

Injury to the median nerve results in a devastating loss of hand sensibility involving the thumb, index, and long fingers, as well as important loss of thumb dexterity because of thenar muscle paralysis. If the injury is near the elbow, the thumb, index, and long finger flexors are also denervated along with the pronators and the radial wrist flexor.

The muscles innervated by the ulnar nerve provide power grip to the hand, and when lost compromise strong flexion of the wrist and the ring and little fingers, as well as pinch and ability to abduct and adduct the fingers. The loss of interosseous muscle function may also cause finger clawing. Sensibility loss is to the little finger and the ulnar half of the ring finger.

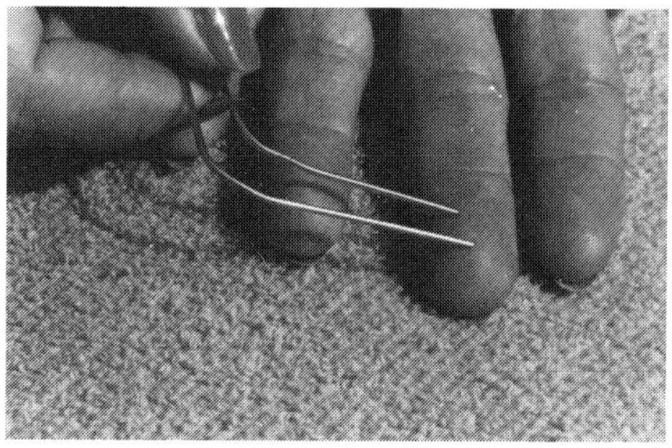

Fig 16-2. Sensory examination by Weber two-point discrimination method using a reshaped ordinary paper clip. Source: Reprinted from *Current Concepts in Hand Surgery* by Boswick JA Jr (ed) with permission of Lea & Febiger Inc, Copyright © 1983.

Detection of sensory loss requires careful examination. The common practice of using a sharp pin should be avoided, because one not only intimidates the patient, especially a child, but may miss significant defects. Subtle and early sensory loss is more accurately determined by light touch or two-point discrimination techniques (Fig 16-2).

The "wrinkle test" (Fig 16-3) employs a phenomenon that may be useful in detecting sensory denervation in the fingers, especially in unconscious or uncooperative patients and in small children. It is based on the fact that water is absorbed into the epidermis osmotically in normally innervated skin, but not into denervated skin. The test is performed by placing all the digits of both hands in a container of warm water for at least 15 minutes. Denervated skin should remain smooth, whereas the control areas of normally innervated skin should absorb water and become wrinkled. Some patients show less wrinkling than others. Mild neurapraxia does not affect the process. As reinnervation occurs, so does the wrinkling. The loss of wrinkling has been noted to occur as early as 5 hours after complete laceration of an ulnar nerve. Therefore, this test not only may be helpful soon after injury, but is easy to perform and requires no sophisticated equipment.

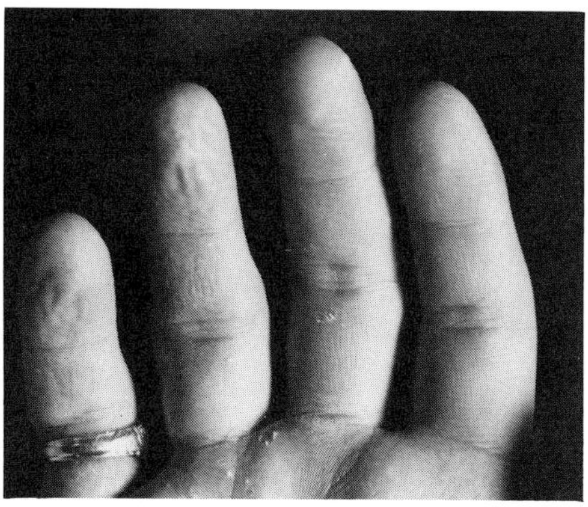

Fig 16-3. Wrinkle test. Median nerve laceration has denervated the skin, which then fails to wrinkle after immersion in warm water for 15 minutes. Compare with wrinkled digits innervated by normal ulnar nerve. Source: Reprinted from *Current Concepts in Hand Surgery* by Boswick JA Jr (ed) with permission of Lea & Febiger Inc, Copyright © 1983.

To determine muscle weakness due to denervation, one should palpate the muscle or tendon while asking the patient to actively contract it. This method decreases the likelihood that the patient can substitute other muscles to perform the requested motion (Fig 16-4).

Electrical Studies

Electrical techniques can be helpful in determining the degree of injury to a nerve.[1] There is, however, a variable time lapse following injury before the abnormalities appear. A nerve distal to a complete laceration may conduct normally up to 20 hours postinjury. Therefore, nerve conduction velocity (NCV) examination may be helpful 2 or more days after injury. If there is a decrease in conduction across the lesion site *and* distally, there is probably a complete axonotmesis or neurotmesis. If one finds decreased NCV across the lesion but normal conduction distally, a neurapraxia is probable. The electromyogram (EMG) will not show evidence of muscle denervation until approximately 10 to 14 days postinjury, and not at all if the injury is a neurapraxia.

The strength duration (SD) curve is a measure of a muscle's ability to respond to an electrical stimulus applied to the motor point of the muscle.[2] A current strength is determined to be just high enough to cause a palpable muscle contraction. As the current is applied over decreasing time intervals, a typical curve will be plotted. As the duration is decreased, strength must eventually be increased in order for the muscle to contract. When the duration of current necessary (the chronaxie) becomes greatly prolonged (more than one millisec), it is evident that there is denervation. This technique may be the only early means to differentiate between a patient with true denervation and one who cannot move the muscles (as in unconsciousness or conversion hysteria) or will not move them (eg, in malingering).

Timing of Repair

The issue of primary versus secondary repair has been debated for years. Those who favor secondary repair cite the advantages that the operation can be performed under elective conditions, and that the extent of nerve scarring will be more apparent. Theoretically, the nerve has been thought to be physiologically better prepared to grow across the repair sites because at approximately 2 weeks postinjury the nerve cell activity reaches a peak.

However, more recent evidence, as shown by VanBeek et al[3] and Cabaud et al,[4] is that axons cross the repair site within 48 hours and move into new neural tubes being formed by Schwann cells, even while previous axons, endoneurium, and myelin are degenerating and being removed. It is evident that repair response begins within a few hours at the injury site and that there is little reason to delay suturing for physiological reasons. Primary repair makes dis-

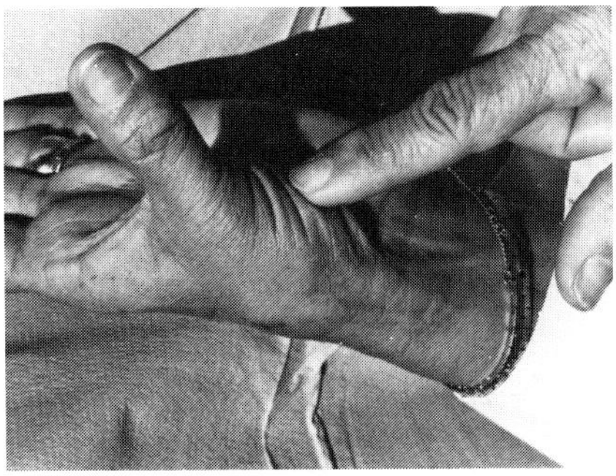

Fig 16-4. Muscle strength examination. Examiner not only tests power but palpates contraction of the muscle in question. Source: Reprinted from *Current Concepts in Hand Surgery* by Boswick JA Jr (ed) with permission of Lea & Febiger Inc, Copyright © 1983.

section easier and safer, because there will be essentially no scar tissue, less nerve tension will ensue, only one operation is required, and muscle denervation time will be less.

However, the nature of the wounding agent and the wound condition must ultimately determine the timing of nerve repair. Delayed primary or secondary repair is safer and will give better results than attempts at primary repair in an unsatisfactory wound.[5]

Types of Repair

The ideal method of repair would be to use no suture, have no tension on the nerve, and obtain accurate reapproximation of each axon, or at least each fascicle, to its distal segment. Unfortunately, we have not reached that perfect state of the art. Work with lasers and plasma "glue" has started, but at present one must attempt to reach the goal as nearly as possible with fine, nonreactive suture and bring together epineurium and/or groups of fascicles, or if identifiable, individual motor fascicles in a mixed nerve.[6,7] Although Sunderland's cross-sectional diagrams of major nerves are useful in finding motor fascicles,[8] other techniques such as electrical stimulation,[9] staining of a nerve biopsy, and choline acetyltransferase assay[10] are also available, but cumbersome. Whichever technique is elected, adequate magnification, gentle nerve handling, prevention of epineurial interposition, preservation of blood supply to the nerve, avoidance of any tension, and as accurate an approximation of fascicles as possible, are all mandatory.

Postoperative Management

Since Millesi[11] and others have stressed that no tension at the site of repair can be accepted, it follows that postoperative immobilization of adjacent joints in extremes of position is contraindicated. One should determine at the time of repair what joint motion will place zero tension on the nerve and then immobilize the joint accordingly for 3 weeks. Active motion can then be started, protecting the nerve from sudden or extreme stretching for a second 3 weeks. Muscle strengthening measures should ideally be started soon after injury and be continued during and after immobilization.

Sensory reeducation[12] is a valuable technique to enhance the quality of sensibility return and should be started as soon as the first evidence of regained sensation is detected.

Results

Type of injury, type of repair, timing, site of the lesion, age of the patient, criteria used, and rehabilitation and motivation of the patient are all factors influencing results. Reports of large, standardized series with adequate follow-up since the use of routine magnification and newer techniques are not yet available. A report by Omer[13] on 140 epineurial repairs of upper extremity nerve lacerations in the Vietnam War revealed that 45% had "functional" motor and sensory return in below-the-elbow lacerations. No patient with an above-the-elbow neurorrhaphy experienced recovery of the intrinsic muscles of the hand.

Epineural and fascicular or interfascicular repairs have not yet been shown to have statistically different results when evaluated from a functional standpoint. Kloss and Lister,[14] however, have reported using interfascicular grafts in complete lesions, thereby relieving all tension at the suture line and providing 60% of the patients with significant motor return and 95% with sensory return, as measured by 6 to 10 mm of two-point discrimination. It is evident that the results of nerve repairs in the past have been disappointing, especially when one considers that for most surgical procedures a failure rate of 10% to 15% is considered high.

In a recent editorial, Sir Sidney Sunderland[15] has pointed out that new research in controlling collagen formation, stimulating neurotrophic substances, and perhaps developing nerve homografts may be necessary to allow additional significant improvement in neurorrhaphy results. In the interim, surgeons and therapists must strive to use and develop the principles and techniques presently known in their attempt to reach the goal of functional recovery following a peripheral nerve injury.

References

1. Delagi EF: Electrodiagnosis in peripheral nerve lesions, in Omer G, Spinner M (eds): *Management of Peripheral Nerve Problems.* Philadelphia, WB Saunders Co, 1980, p 30.

2. Luekens CA, Jr: Nerve injuries in the upper extremity, in Boswick J, (ed): *Current Concepts in Hand Surgery.* Philadelphia, Lea & Febiger, 1983, p 88.
3. VanBeek AL, Eder M, Zook EG: Nerve regeneration: Evidence for immediate sprout formation. *J Hand Surg* 1982;7:79.
4. Cabaud HE, Rodkey WG, Nameth TJ: Progressive ultra structural changes after peripheral nerve transection and repair. *J Hand Surg* 1982;7:353.
5. Jabaley M: Technical aspects of peripheral nerve repair. *J Hand Surg* 1984;9B:14–19.
6. Snyder CC: Epineural repair. *Orthop Clin North Am* 1981;12:267–276.
7. Kutz J, Shealy G, Lubbers L: Interfascicular nerve repair. *Orthop Clin North Am* 1981;12:277–285.
8. Sunderland S: *Nerves and Nerve Injuries,* ed 2. Edinburgh, Churchill Livingstone, 1978.
9. Gaul JS Jr: Electrical fascicle identification as an adjunct to nerve repair. *J Hand Surg* 1983;8:289–296.
10. Engel J, Ganel A, Melamed R, et al: Choline acetyltransferase for differentiation between motor and sensory nerve fibers. *Ann Plast Surg* 1979;4:376–380.
11. Millesi H: Nerve grafts, indications, techniques and prognosis, in Omer G, Spinner M (eds): *Management of Peripheral Nerve Problems.* Philadelphia, WB Saunders Co, 1980, p 410.
12. Dellon AL, Curtis RM, Edgerton MT: Re-education of sensation in the hand following nerve injury and repair. *Plast Reconstr Surg* 1974;53:297–305.
13. Omer GE: The evaluation of clinical results following peripheral nerve suture, in Omer G, Spinner M (eds): *Management of Peripheral Nerve Problems.* Philadelphia, WB Saunders Co, 1980, p 431.
14. Kloss JG, Lister G: Results of interfascicular nerve grafting for secondary repair of segmental defects in the upper extremity. Read before the Annual Meeting of The American Society for Surgery of the Hand, Las Vegas, NV, Feb 1981.
15. Sunderland S: Editorial: Nerve repair. *J Hand Surg* 1984;9A:1–3.

17

The Palmar Branch of the Median Nerve and Its Surgical Importance

L. Mannerfelt and
R. Oetker

Research has been conducted during the last 20 years on the anatomical variations of the motor branch of the median nerve.[1-6] Only a few publications on variations of the palmar branch of the median nerve (PBMN) are available. In 1973 Taleisnik[7] reported his discovery of branches running in an ulnar and distal direction from the PBMN. This chapter surveys the different variations of the PBMN at the wrist and at the ulnar aspect of the palm. The relations between the PBMN and the tendon of the palmaris longus are discussed as well.

Normal Anatomy of the PBMN and Its Variations

The PBMN branches from the median nerve on its radial aspect at a relatively constant distance (40 to 60 mm) proximal to the rasceta[8] (Fig 17-1A). Hirasawa[9] reported that the PBMN could emerge from the median nerve even at the level of the pronator teres muscle. There are numerous variations to this arrangement as well; for example, there can be two or three PBMN emerging from the median nerve.

The PBMN maintains close contact with the ulnar aspect of the sheath of the flexor carpi radialis tendon. The nerve sometimes runs in its own channel, which is closely attached to the ulnar aspect of the flexor carpi radialis tendon sheath (Fig 17-1B).

The PBMN divides into three principal branches (Fig 17-2):

1. a radial branch innervating the thenar area
2. a median branch
3. the branch or branches described by Taleisnik[7], which run in a distal-ulnar direction.

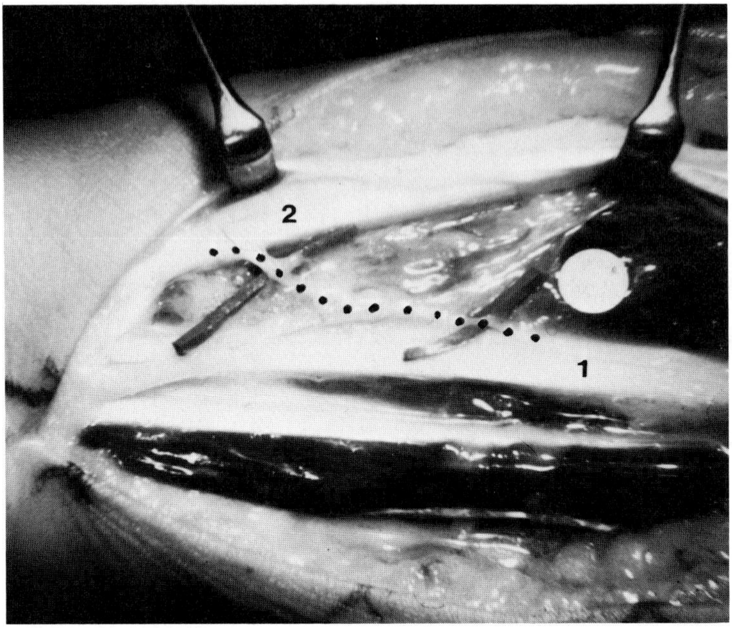

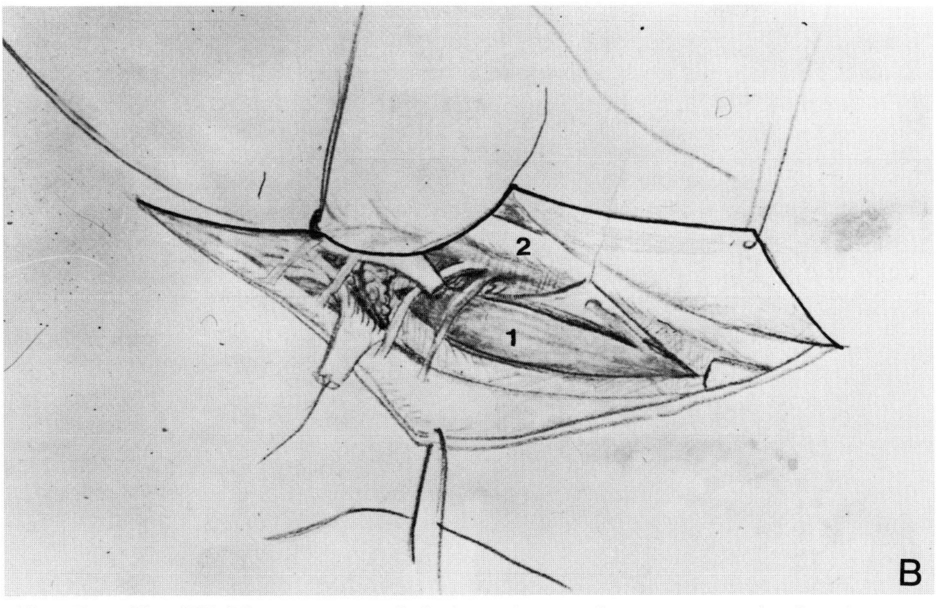

Fig 17-1. The PBMN emerges radially from the median nerve proximal to the rasceta and runs in a distal direction on the ulnar aspect of the flexor carpi radialis tendon sheath, sometimes in its own channel. The palmaris longus tendon is divided 1 cm proximally from its ulnar and radial shank. *A*, Intraoperative photograph; *B*, schematic diagram; *1*, median nerve; *2*, flexor carpi radialis tendon. (All figures in this article show the right hand from the ulnar side as seen by the surgeon.)

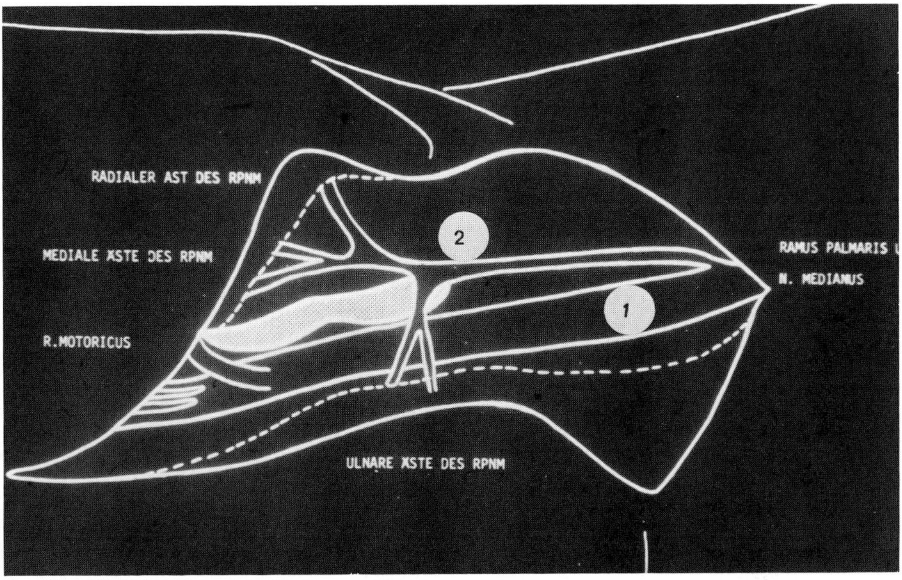

Fig 17-2. The three branches of the PBMN: radial, median, and ulnar. *1,* Median nerve; *2,* PBMN.

As early as 1931 Hirasawa[9] demonstrated that some of the branches of the PBMN could anastomose with the palmar branch of the ulnar nerve (PBUN). Nerve anastomoses of this kind are well known, for instance, the Martin-Gruber anastomosis and the Riche-Cannieu anastomosis.[10] These nerve connections between the median and the ulnar nerve are regarded as a motoric ansa connection. It is doubtless possible that the connection between the PBMN and the PBUN could be regarded as a sensory ansa connection.

Normal Anatomy of the Palmaris Longus Tendon and Its Variations

The tendon of the palmaris longus muscle lies between the skin and the fascia. The insertion is distal to the rasceta and has two branches, one radial and one ulnar, both inserting into the fascia of the thenar and hypothenar. The tendon continues in the median line with the palmar aponeurosis (Fig 17-3). According to Reimann et al[11], in an American population the palmaris longus tendon is absent in 12.9% of the population.

Present Investigation

In our outpatient department more and more patients are referred with pain in the scar of the proximal palm after release of the carpal ligament. The reason for

Table 17-1. Frequency of Absence of the Palmaris Longus Tendon

Author	*Race*	n	*Tendon Absent (%)*
Reimann (1944)[11]	American	1,600	12.9
Adachi (1909)[11]	Japanese	884	3.4
Nakano (1923)[11]	Chinese	95	2.2

this postoperative pain, in our opinion, is the presence of microneuromas of the PBMN, which crosses the line of incision.

Materials and Methods

The purpose of this study was to find out intraoperatively whether the distal-ulnar-running branches described by Taleisnik[7] are normal or variations, and if the latter, how often one could observe such branches.

Two prospective studies were performed. In the first series[12] we studied the anatomy of the PBMN in 103 consecutive cases of carpal tunnel release. The second series was an in-depth study of the PBMN during 50 operations of carpal tunnel release. In this study the correlation between the PBMN and the presence or absence of the palmaris longus was studied as well.

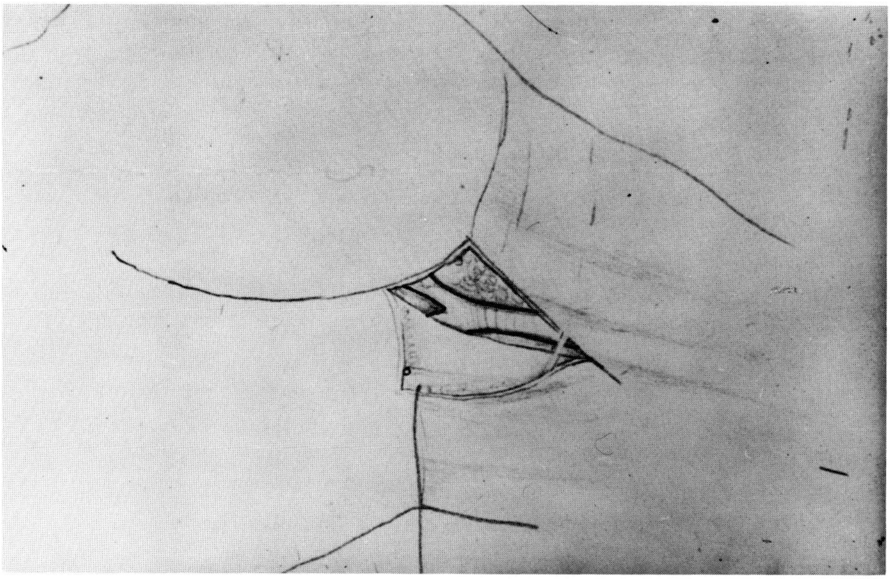

Fig 17-3. The palmaris longus tendon inserts distal to the rasceta with one radial and one ulnar shank at the base of the thenar and hypothenar muscles.

Operative Technique

The skin incision runs parallel with the thenar base skin crease, continuing obliquely over the rasceta and thence in a proximal-ulnar direction. The palmaris longus tendon is divided at a point 1½ cm proximal from its insertion, according to the method of Kopell and Thompson.[13] The fascia is divided in the median line, and the PBMN is identified at the radial aspect of the median nerve and is isolated and held to the side with the aid of a fine rubber band (Fig 17-4). In the beginning of our first study we followed the PBMN thoroughly in a distal direction. This technique is no longer deemed necessary, as there is a risk of traumatization.

Under the microscope the branches of the PBMN were followed in a distal direction. Very often we found several branches running in a distal-ulnar direction. Before releasing the carpal ligament all the branches running in the distal-ulnar direction are secured by rubber bands (Fig 17-5).

Results

Frequency of PBMN Branches Running in a Distal-Ulnar Direction

In the first series (103 cases) we found PBMN branches in 65% of cases, and in the second, more detailed study (50 cases) we found them in 96% (Table 17-1).

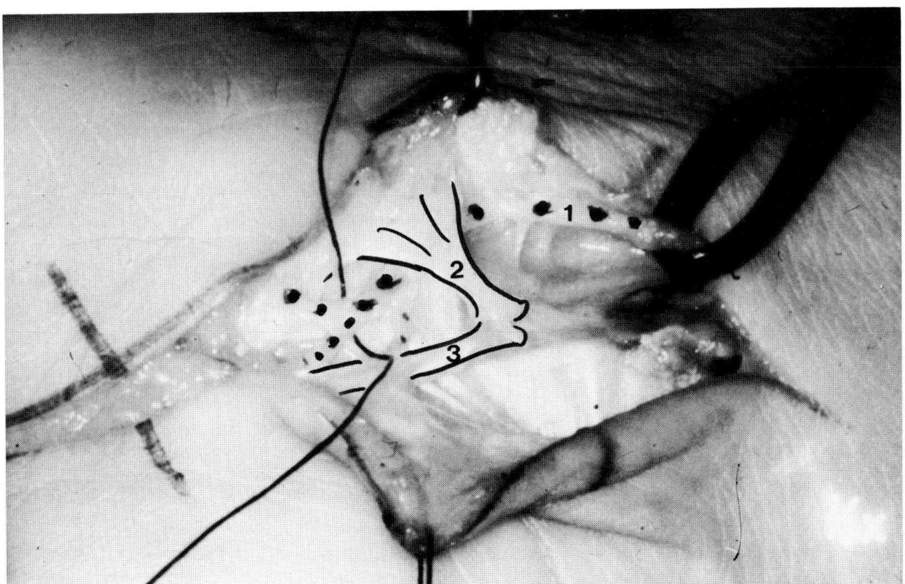

Fig 17-4. The PBMN (*1*) is isolated and secured with a rubber band. The nerve runs in this case deep to the radial shank (*2*) of the palmaris longus tendon; *3*, ulnar shank.

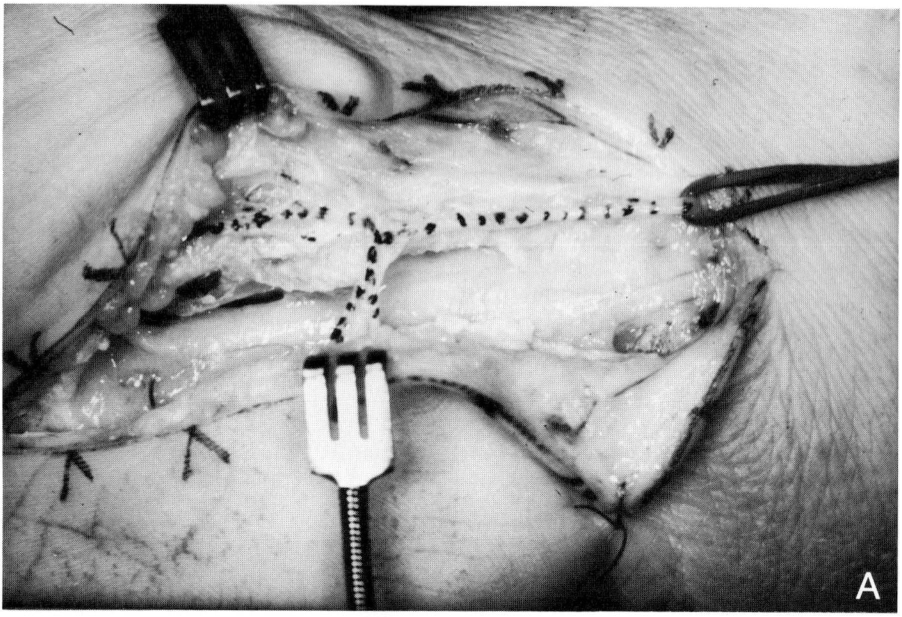

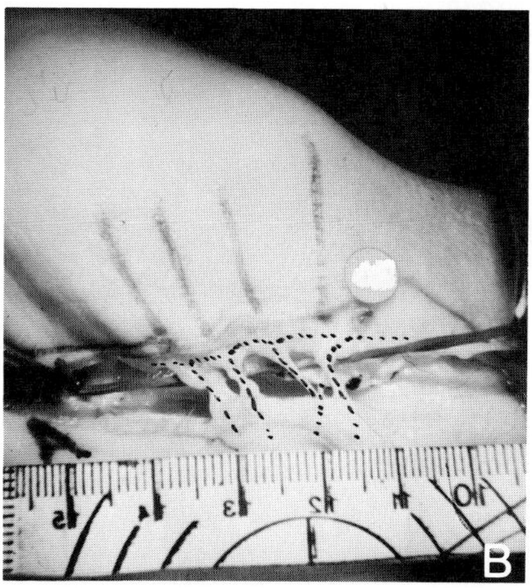

Fig 17-5. Branches of the PBMN run in a distal-ulnar direction crossing the line of incision. The nerves are secured with the aid of a rubber band. After this procedure the carpal ligament will be divided in a proximal-to-distal direction. *A* Here one branch of the PBMN running in ulnar direction divides into two smaller branches as it crosses the incision. *B* There can be up to four branches emerging from the PBMN succesively (at different levels) and running to the hypothenar. All the four of them cross the incision and should be secured before dividing the carpal ligament.

In the second study we tested the hypothesis that distal-ulnar-running branches from the PBMN could emerge from the median nerve at a level proximal to the rasceta. In fact we found that branches could leave the median nerve as far as 3 mm proximal to the rasceta (Fig 17-6).

In the first series we found distal-ulnar-running branches of the PBMN in an area from 9 to 26 mm distal from the rasceta. In the second series we found ulnar-distal-running branches emerging from the median nerve as far as 3 mm proximal and 39 mm distal to the rasceta (Fig 17-7).

Table 17-2. Number of Distal-Ulnar-Running PBMN Branches (Series 2)

No. of Branches	*No. of Cases*
1	20
2	13
3	9
4	6
	48(96%)

Diameter of the Distal-Ulnar-Running Branches of the PBMN

From 3 mm proximal to 9 mm distal to the rasceta the branches showed diameters of around 0.9 mm, and distal to this area the diameters averaged 0.6 mm. The most important and thickest ulnar-running branches therefore are located in the area around the rasceta.

Relationship Between the PBMN and the Palmaris Longus Tendon

In the first series we found an absence of the palmaris longus tendon in 13% of cases, and in the second series this tendon was absent in 18%. When the palmaris longus tendon was present, it divided into one radial and one ulnar branch before the insertion. In the second study we found that ulnar-running branches of the PBMN went under the radial shank and after that over (superficial to) the ulnar shank (Fig 17-8).

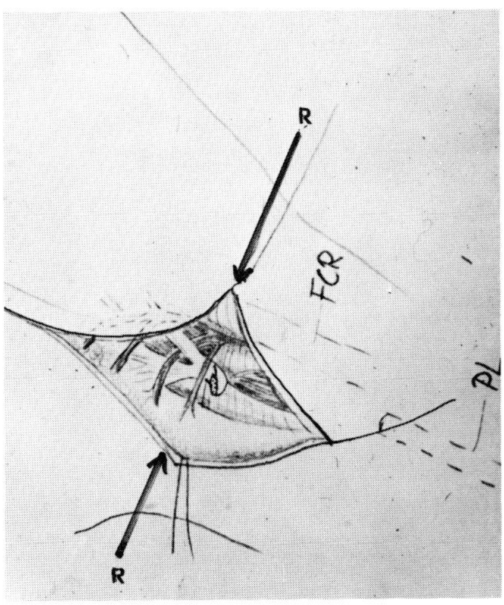

Fig 17-6. Branches from the PBMN run in an ulnar direction over and under the radial shank of the palmaris longus tendon. One branch is seen 3 mm proximal to the rasceta (*R*).

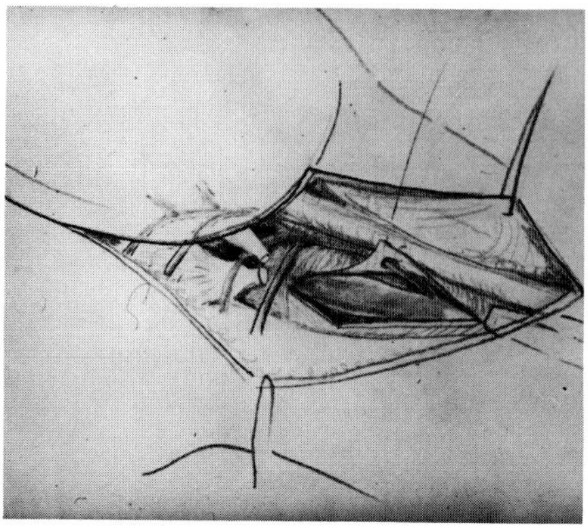

Fig 17-7. In this case, a branch of the PBMN emerges from the median nerve proximal to the rasceta.

Communications Between the PBMN and the PBUN and the Incision Proposed by Taleisnik

As already mentioned, Hirasawa[9] in 1931 demonstrated communications between the PBMN and the PBUN in the proximal volar part of the hand. Nevertheless, we tried the incision proposed by Taleisnik[7] for release of the carpal tunnel. In some cases we found branches from the PBMN running in an ulnar direction transverse to the incision proposed by Taleisnik[7]. We also found

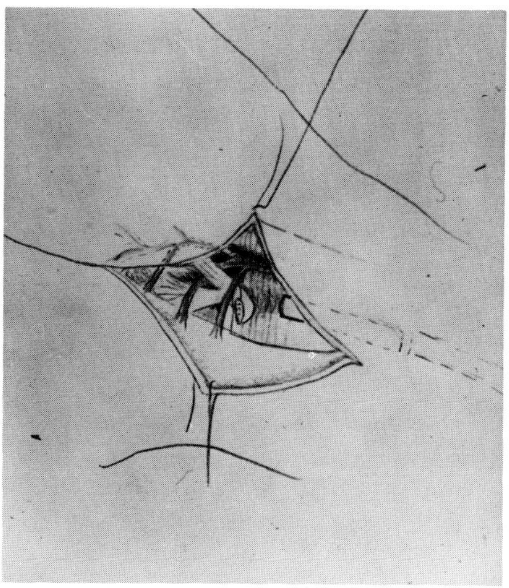

Fig 17-8. One ulnar-running branch of the PBMN is situated under the radial shank of the palmaris longus tendon and thereafter runs superficial to the ulnar shank.

that these branches connected with branches from the PBUN (Figs 17-9, 17-10, A and B).

Engber and Gmeiner[14] published their investigation on the PBUN in 1980. They also used an incision on the ulnar side of the axis of the fourth ray, as Taleisnik[7] proposed. They noted postoperatively painful neuromas on the radial side of the hypothenar. They dissected 21 bodies and found variations of the PBUN in the radial direction.

Discussion

In patients previously operated on at other hospitals we found cases involving transection of the PBMN. This was most often the case when the surgeon had tried to release the carpal ligament through a transverse incision in the height of the rasceta, a procedure very often performed under local anesthesia (Fig 17-11, A and B). In other cases we found microneuromas in the scar at the thenar base. We diagnosed these microneuromas as resulting from transected branches of the PBMN (Fig 17-12). Not uncommonly we found nerve lesions with neuroma after extirpation of a palmar radial ganglion (Fig 17-13).

The surgical importance of the palmar branch of the median nerve is evident, and when using the incision technique of Taleisnik[7], utmost care should be taken not to damage the connections between the PBMN and the PBUN. This incision is therefore, according to our experience, not without danger.

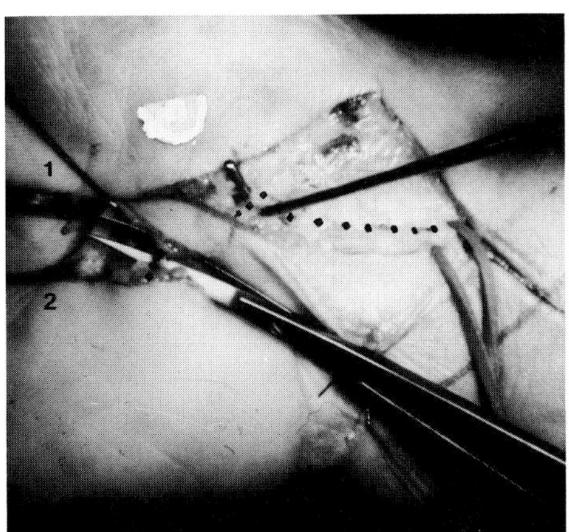

Fig 17-9. Two incisions have been made for release of the carpal ligament. One is our standard incision (*1*) and the other the incision proposed by Taleisnik (*2*). Branches from the PBMN cross the incision proposed by Taleisnik. Over the scissors one can see a prominent branch of the PBMN running in an ulnar direction.

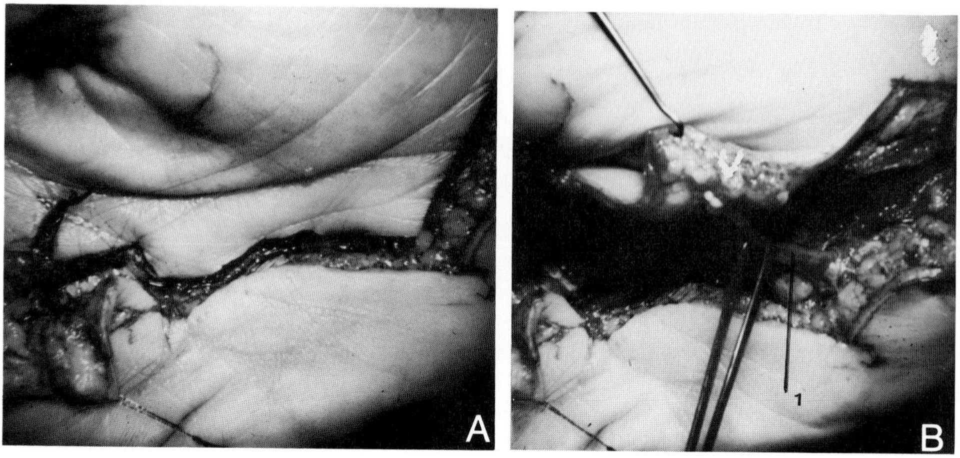

Fig 17-10. *A*. An acute hand injury with a longitudinal cut in the palm, 5 mm in an ulnar direction from the base of the thenar. *B*. During preparation for reconstruction of the transected deep structures, a prominent palmar branch of the ulnar nerve (*1*) was found and secured with a rubber band.

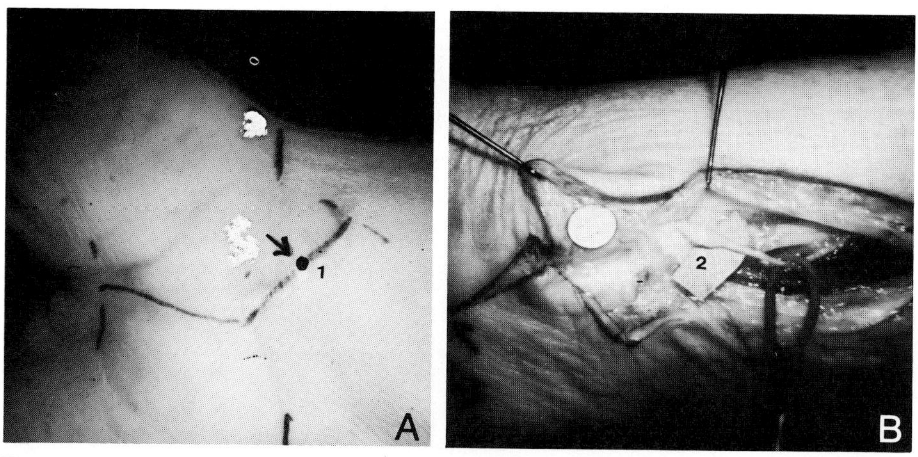

Fig 17-11. A painful neuroma of the PBMN 3 mm proximal to the rasceta after insufficient carpal tunnel release performed under local anesthesia. *A*, Preoperative; *B*, intraoperative photograph.

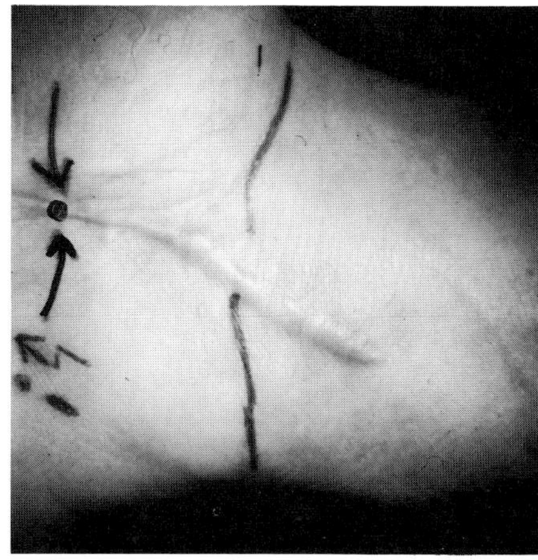

Fig 17-12. Isolated pain is experienced in the operative scar at the thenar base after carpal tunnel release. The cause is a neuroma secondary to transection of a branch of the PBMN.

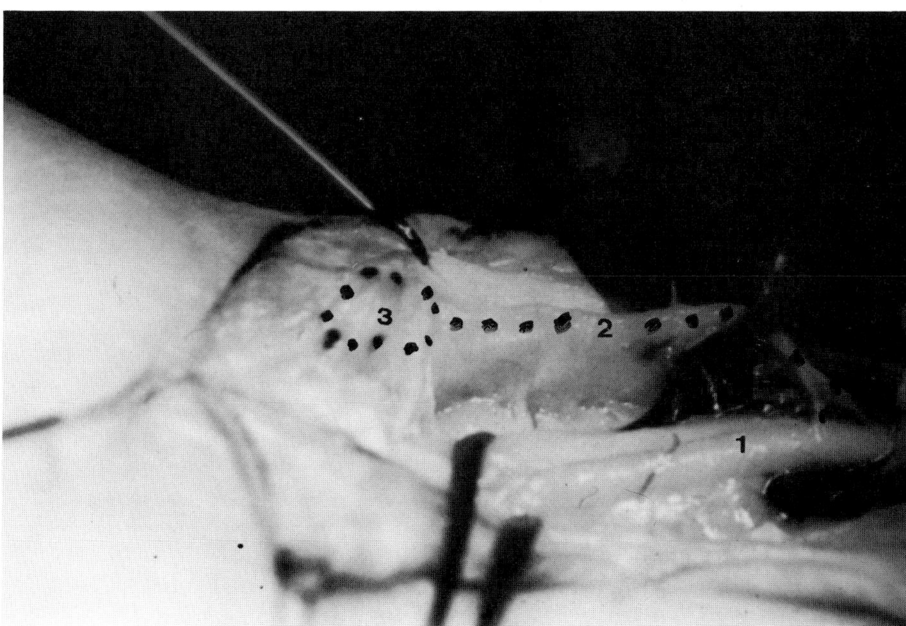

Fig 17-13. Iatrogenic neuroma of the PBMN proximal to the rasceta after extirpation of a radial palmar ganglion. In this case also, the operation was performed under local anesthesia without a bloodless field. *1*, Median nerve; *2*, PBMN; *3*, Neuroma.

Conclusion

On the basis of studies of more than 150 cases of carpal tunnel release with special reference to the PBMN, we are of the opinion that the PBMN must be identified and safely isolated before the carpal ligament is fully divided. We have also found that one must be extremely careful in those cases where the palmaris longus tendon is absent, because there are probably more variations of the PBMN in these cases.

References

1. Kaplan EB: *Functional and Surgical Anatomy of the Hand.* Philadelphia, JB Lippincott Co, 1965.
2. Papathanassiou BT: A variant of the motor branch of the median nerve in the hand. *J Bone Joint Surg* 1968;50B:156–157.
3. Entin MA: Carpal tunnel syndrome and its variants. *Surg Clin North Am* 1968;48:1097–1112.
4. Linburg RM, Albright JA: An anomalous branch of the median nerve. *J Bone Joint Surg* 1970;52A:182–183.
5. Mannerfelt L, Hybbinette CH: Important anomaly of the thenar motor branch of the median nerve. *Bull Hosp J Dis Orthop Inst* 1972;33:15–21.
6. Lanz U: Anatomical variations of the median nerve in the carpal tunnel. *J Hand Surg* 1977;2:44–53.
7. Taleisnik J: The palmar cutaneous branch of the median nerve and the approach to the carpal tunnel. *J Bone Joint Surg* 1973;55A:1212–1217.
8. Sunderland S: *Nerves and Nerve Injuries,* ed 2. Edinburgh, Churchill Livingstone, 1978.
9. Hirasawa K: Der N. medianus—Die Anastomose zwischen dem N. medianus und dem N. ulnaris. *Anat Inst Kyoto* 1931, pp 135–140.
10. Mannerfelt L: Studies on the hand in ulnar nerve paralysis. *Acta Orthop Scand,* 1966 (suppl 87).
11. Reimann AF, Daseler EH, Anson BJ, et al: The palmaris longus muscle and tendon. *Anat Rec* 1944;89:495–505.
12. Albersmeyer R, Goldberg W, Mannerfelt L: Die besondere Bedeutung des R. palmaris n. mediani bei der Operation des Karpaltunnelsyndroms. *Orthop Praxis* 1981;7:574–575.
13. Kopell H, Thompson WAL: *Peripheral Entrapment Neuropathies.* Baltimore, The Williams & Wilkins Co, 1963.
14. Engber WD, Gmeiner JG: Palmar cutaneous branch of the ulnar nerve. *J Hand Surg* 1980;5:26–29.

18

Upper Extremity Surgery in the Spinal Cord Injury Patient

Charles Hamlin

Upper extremity reconstructive surgery in the quadriplegic patient has a short history. Although there is mention in the German literature of a functional brace in the 1920s, relatively little attention was paid to this patient population until hand surgery emerged as a viable specialty after World War II. Certainly, this had to do with what was until then the natural history of this patient group. For although many of these spinal cord injury patients did indeed survive their accidents, they were not long-term survivors. Other major areas of concern such as spine stabilization, bowel and bladder training, and psychological and sexual counseling necessarily took precedence over sophisticated or even primitive hand reconstruction.

Yet hand function was, and is now to perhaps an even greater degree, essential to any quality of life for these patients. As care has improved and long-term survival has become a reality, upper extremity function has become a basic part of the formula equating meaningful life with the concepts of independence, vocational and avocational skills, and self-esteem. In a survey taken from this patient group in 1976,[1] which asked their preference for either normal bowel and bladder function, sexual function, lower extremity function, or upper extremity function, 77% indicated that they would prefer to have their hand function back.

Unfortunately, even after attention from the hand specialists was focused on this group, progress was still slow and problematical. Pioneers such as Bunnell, Lipscomb, Henderson, and Freehafer, often using principles adapted from polio experience, showed that function could be restored. Yet the cost to the patient was often great in terms of time and the number of procedures and necessary revisions, and of course the cost was magnified by the physical and psychological price already paid. Thus, with the development of the functional flexor hinge brace at Rancho Los Amigos Hospital in 1963,[2] surgical hand reconstruction lost favor, and spinal cord physicians and physiatrists rejected hand surgery for their patients as an area too full of problems and lacking predictability.

A number of surgeons working independently can be given credit for overcoming the resistance that existed toward reconstructive hand surgery in the quadriplegic. Erik Moberg in Sweden, Eduardo Zancolli in Argentina, and Douglas Lamb in Scotland should be given special mention for their attention to this group of patients, and their published data demonstrated that the functional gains were not only predictable, but were achieved in large numbers of patients and at little risk of functional loss.[3-5] James House at the University of Minnesota should also be credited for this thoughtful approach to this group.[6] These surgeons earned the respect of spinal cord centers around the world. A national network for care of the spinal cord injury patient was organized in this country in the 1970s, and it is not inaccurate to say that hand surgery should be, and most often is, a part of the team approach essential to the well-being of these patients. The work reviewed in this chapter comes out of the experience of the hand clinic started at Craig Hospital in Denver, Colorado, in 1978.

Important to the development of a proper approach to upper extremity reconstruction in the quadriplegic was the work that came out of an international symposium held in Edinburgh, Scotland, in 1978. A new classification emerged (Table 18-1), based not on a cervical level of injury, which was often asymmetrical and incomplete, but instead on the assessment of the number of available motors in an upper extremity, the quality of sensation, and the facility of hand-eye coordination. This classification has permitted a clearer picture of surgical options as they relate to the postinjury musculoskeletal examination, and more realistic expectations for their success. Based on this classification, four distinct areas of attention have emerged, and it is toward finding solutions in these areas that the focus of the Craig Hospital Hand Clinic is directed.

Table 18-1. Motor Classifications for Sensory Classification OCu Groups

Group	*Characteristics*
OCu0	Weak BR and wrist extensors suitable together to provide wrist extension
OCu1	BR
OCu2	BR, ECRL
OCu3	BR, ECRL, ECRB
OCu4	BR, ECRL, ECRB, PT
OCu5	BR, ECRL, ECRB, PT, FCR
OCu6	BR, ECRL, ECRB, PT, FCR, finger extensors
OCu7	BR, ECRL, ECRB, PT, FCR, finger and thumb extensors
OCu8	Lacks only intrinsics

Source: McDowell CL, Moberg EA, Graham-Smith A: International conference on surgical rehabilitation of the upper limb in tetraplegia. J Hand Surg 1979;4:387.
BR, brachioradialis; ECRL, extensor carpi radialis longus; ECRB, extensor carpi radialis brevis; PT, pronator teres; FCR, flexor carpi radialis.

Elbow Extension

In the OCu2 patient, no active elbow extension is present. As these patients are now wheelchair bound and are relatively shorter with respect to their immediate environment, it becomes even more important that they have active elbow extension. By transferring the posterior one third or one half of the deltoid muscle to the triceps insertion and achieving length with an intercalated graft, the immediate global environment of the patient is significantly enlarged[7] (Fig 18-1). Although toe extensors have been recommended as the donor graft, the anterior tibialis tendon or a piece of defatted fascia lata is a stronger bridge graft (Fig 18-2). Also, by taking some cortical bone off the humerus with the deltoid and inserting the graft into the olecranon, there is less chance of slippage and relative graft lengthening, and a shorter period of immobilization is possible (5 weeks). There appears to be some resistance on the part of the patients or referring doctors to undertake this procedure, perhaps because a long-arm extension cast is required for a long period of immobilization. In fact, the prognosis is better with this procedure, and there are fewer complications and fewer revisions than with the other surgeries that will be described.

Wrist Extension

The natural tenodesis of wrist extension enhancing digital flexion is used by all of us and requires strong, active wrist extension. In the group 1 patient, the brachioradialis is the only active muscle functioning below the elbow. Freehafer proposed the transfer of the brachioradialis for wrist extension[8] but has spoken of attendant problems with this transfer. Perhaps most important among these is unopposed elbow flexion, for if the power of the brachioradialis is dissipated by elbow flexion, the force transmitted to the wrist extensor is similarly weakened. Thus, in a candidate for this procedure, a deltoid-to-triceps transfer should be considered as a first procedure to stabilize the elbow and ensure the effectiveness of the transfer.

The specific goal of this transfer is to drive the flexor hinge brace by active wrist extension (Fig 18-3), but if strong enough wrist extension is achieved, these patients may become candidates for a flexor pollicis longus tenodesis to achieve key grip.

Key Grip

Key grip, or lateral pinch, as proposed by Moberg[7] (Fig 18-4), is a significant functional gain. The thumb interphalangeal (IP) joint is stabilized, and the flexor pollicis longus tendon is secured to the radius. Moberg, working with Brand, has recommended that the thumb flexor be rerouted across the palm

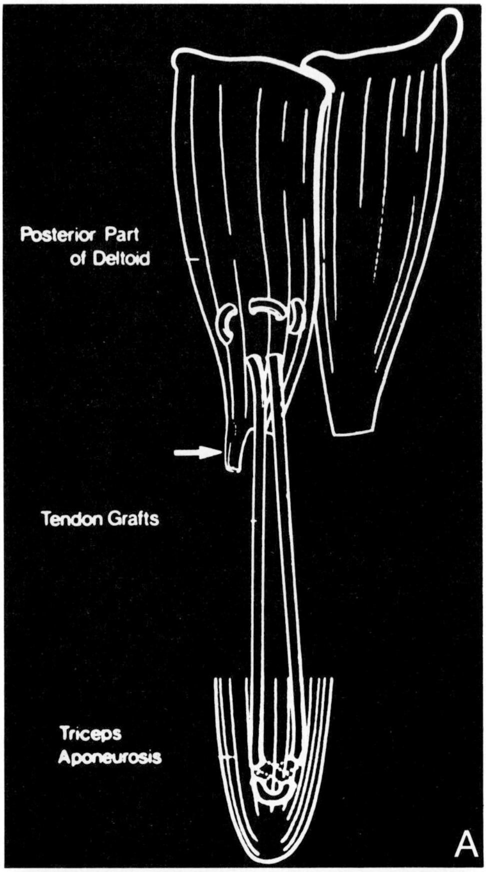

Fig 18-1. *A,* Schematic representation of the deltoid-to-triceps transfer using the intercalated tendon grafts, usually toe extensors, as recommended by Moberg. Source: Reprinted from *The Upper Limb in Tetraplegia* by Moberg E, with permission of Georg Thieme Publishers, Copyright © 1978. *B* and *C,* A patient 6 months after posterior deltoid-to-triceps transfer, demonstrating active elbow extension.

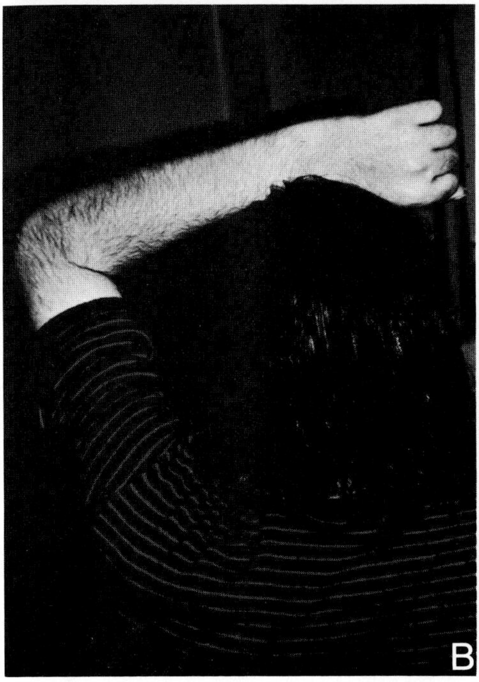

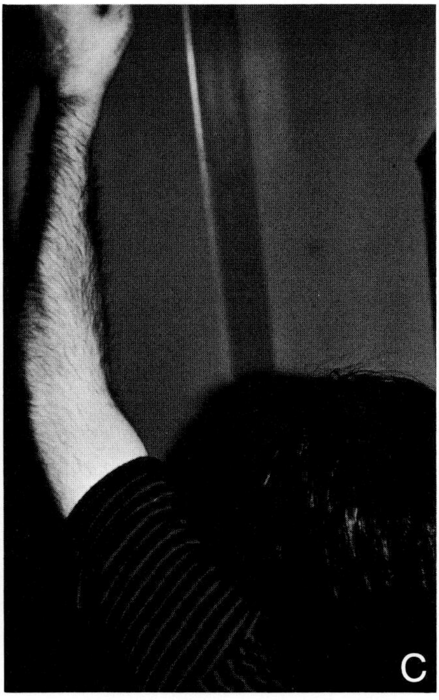

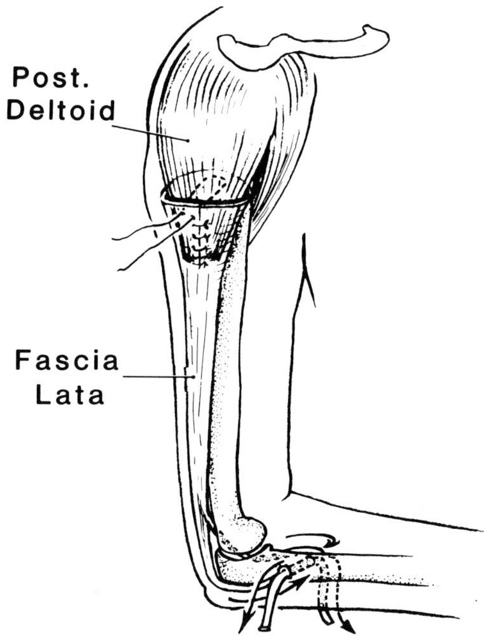

Fig 18-2. The deltoid-to-triceps transfer using a single intercalated piece of fascia lata inserted into the olecranon. This provides greater strength through both the intercalated tendon material and the bony insertion. Source: Courtesy of Vincent R Hentz, Stanford University, Palo Alto, California.

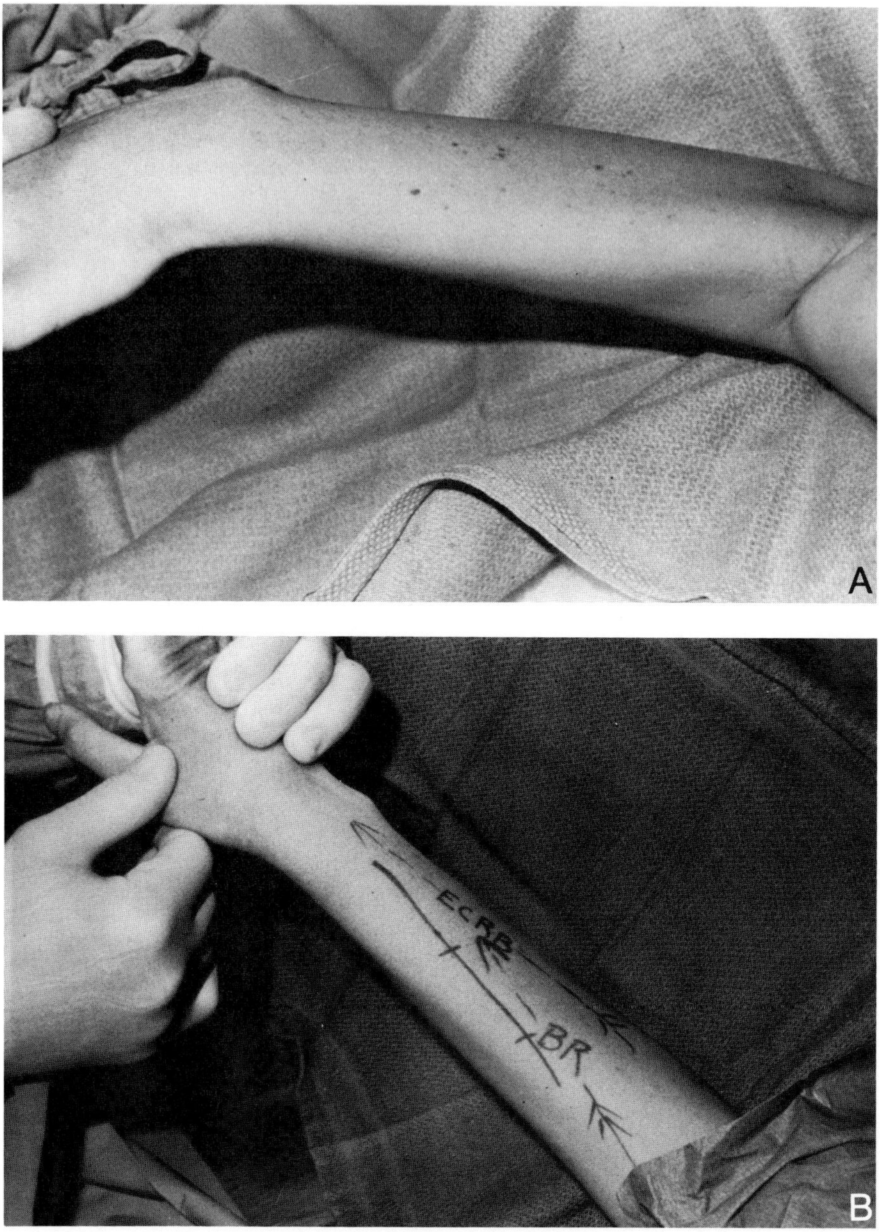

Fig 18-3. *A,* A grade 1 patient demonstrating antigravity flexion of the elbow with the brachioradialis muscle. *B,* Schematic diagram of the brachioradialis to extensor carpi radialis brevis transfer, augmenting or providing wrist extension. *C,* Tenorrhaphy of the brachioradialis to the extensor carpi radialis brevis with tension to permit good wrist extension. The brachioradialis must be freed up throughout its course in the forearm. *D,* The classic flexor hinge brace as developed at Ranchos Los Amigos Hospital. Brachioradialis transfer to augment wrist extension can drive the flexor hinge brace.

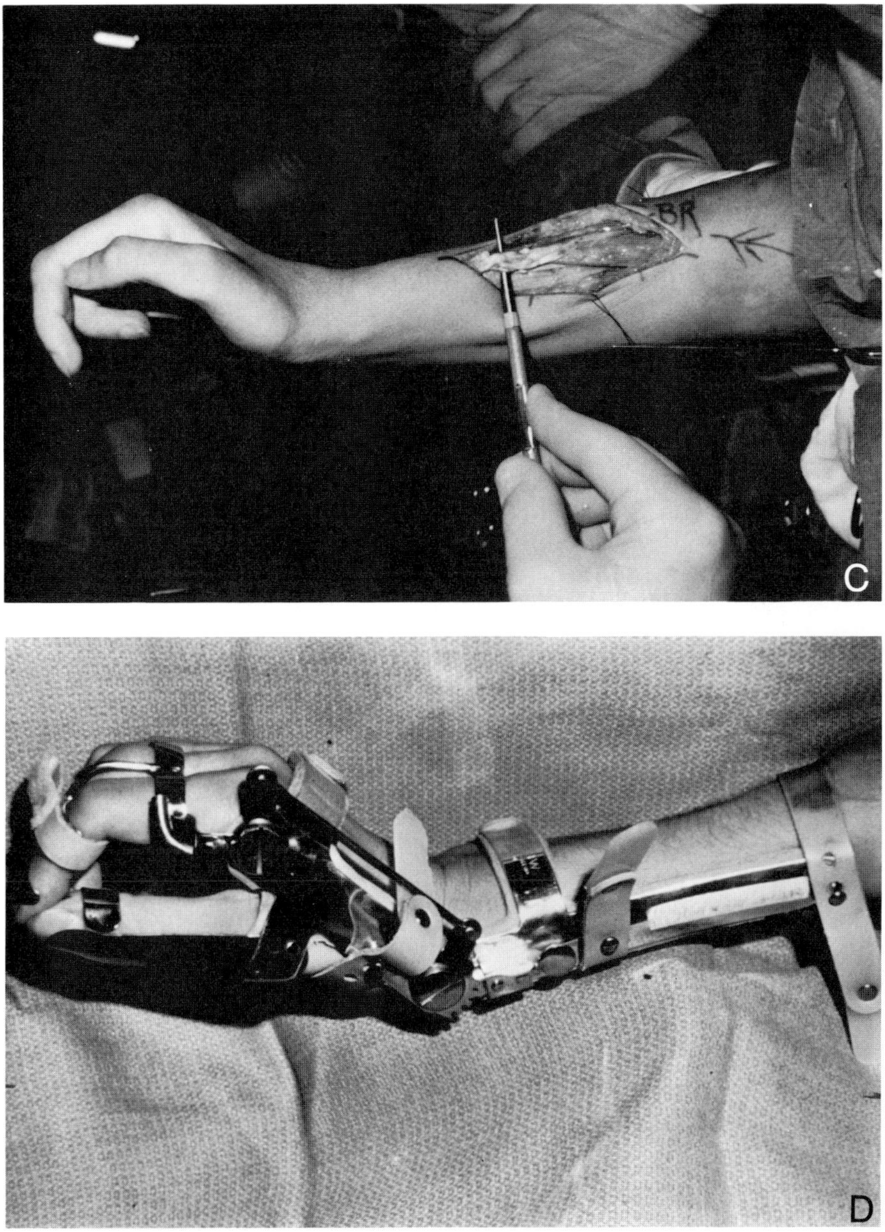
BR
C
D

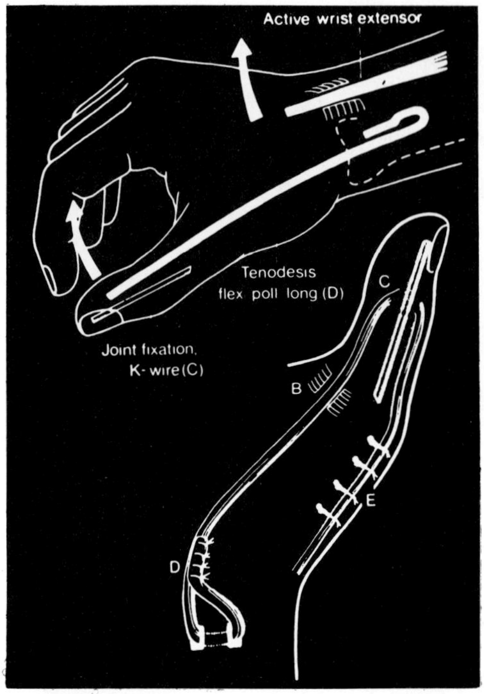

Fig 18-4. The flexor pollicis longus tenodesis with thumb IP joint stabilization, as described by Moberg to provide lateral or key pinch. Source: Reprinted with permission from *The Journal of Bone and Joint Surgery* (1975;57A:196). Copyright © 1975, Journal of Bone and Joint Surgery, Inc.

and through the canal of Guyon to its tenodesis to achieve more power by more closely simulating the major pinch muscle, the adductor pollicis (Fig 18-5). Gravitational wrist flexion opens the pinch, and active wrist extension brings the thumb against the index finger platform (Fig 18-6). This key pinch eliminates the need for a brace, and up to 7 lb of pinch has been recorded.

Five areas of concern have emerged from following the group of 20 patients who have undergone this reconstructive procedure. Thumbtip tenderness and pin migration can be problems associated with IP joint stabilization. A strong, threaded pin, which is less likely to migrate, should be used to stabilize the IP joint, and it should be passed in a proximal-to-distal direction across the joint, leaving the thumbtip and pad undisturbed. This is especially important as this area enjoys the most acute sensibility of all the parts of the hand.

Thumb metacarpophalangeal (MP) and carpometacarpal (CMC) joint stability must be assessed, as there can be attritional loss of ligament support from weight shifts and transfers. Both hyperflexion and hyperextension can be present at the MP joint, dissipating important strength desired at the thumbtip. Formal arthrodesis or local MP joint tenodesis can restore stability and hence improve power delivery to the thumb pad. If the CMC joint is unstable, the abnormal rocking and gliding here can be mirrored distally, resulting in unpredictable placement of the thumb against the index finger platform. Liga-

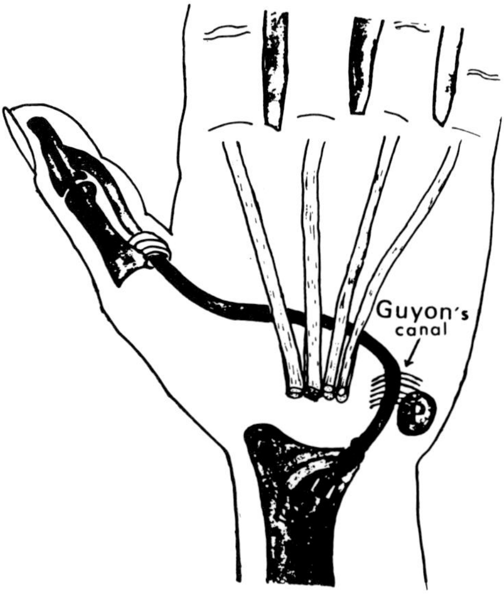

Fig 18-5. The modification of the key grip tenodesis with the flexor pollicis longus passed across the palm, beneath the extrinsic flexor tendons, and proximally to the tenodesis site through Guyon's canal. This better stimulates the powerful adductor pollicis muscle and gives a better force vector of the thumb against the index finger. Source: Courtesy of E Moberg, Göteborg, Sweden.

ment reconstruction (Eaton) or CMC arthrodesis can solve this problem. Obviously, one of the three joints of the thumb must provide good motion to ensure success of this key grip.

Often, through extensor tone or spasm, the index finger maintains an extensor habitus so that it is not properly positioned during key grip (Fig 18-7). The thumb can slide under the platform or miss it altogether, thus weakening or eliminating pinch entirely. By rerouting the extensor indicis proprius tendon palmar to the axis of MP joint motion (Fig 18-8), a "paradoxical" tenodesis is created at the joint, so that MP flexion is maintained during the opening phase that occurs with gravitational wrist flexion. With active wrist extension, the index finger is in position to receive the thumb in pinch.

Finally, hyperflexion of the index proximal interphalangeal (PIP) joint, by either flexor spasm or attritional loss of the extensor mechanism over this joint, can shorten the platform for pinch, permitting the thumb to slide off the index finger, or limiting the size of objects that can be held. Extensor mechanism reconstruction or a formal PIP arthrodesis addresses this problem.

Despite these five problem areas, the Moberg key grip procedure has significant rewards for the properly selected patient. In addition, it is achieved with respect for two of Moberg's precepts: that nothing shall be taken from the patient's existing function, and that the procedure can be reversed if the patient is unhappy with the result.

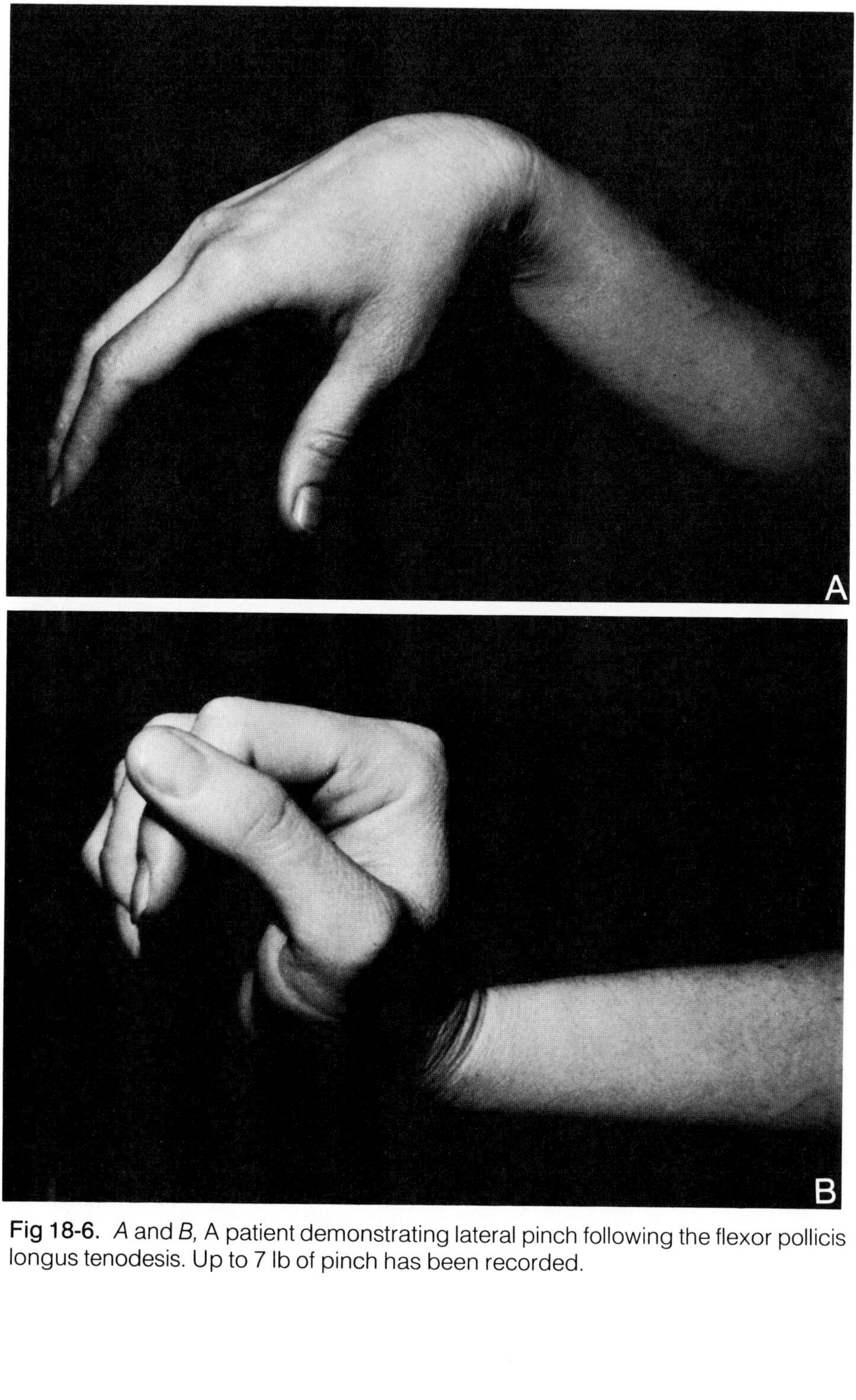

Fig 18-6. *A* and *B*, A patient demonstrating lateral pinch following the flexor pollicis longus tenodesis. Up to 7 lb of pinch has been recorded.

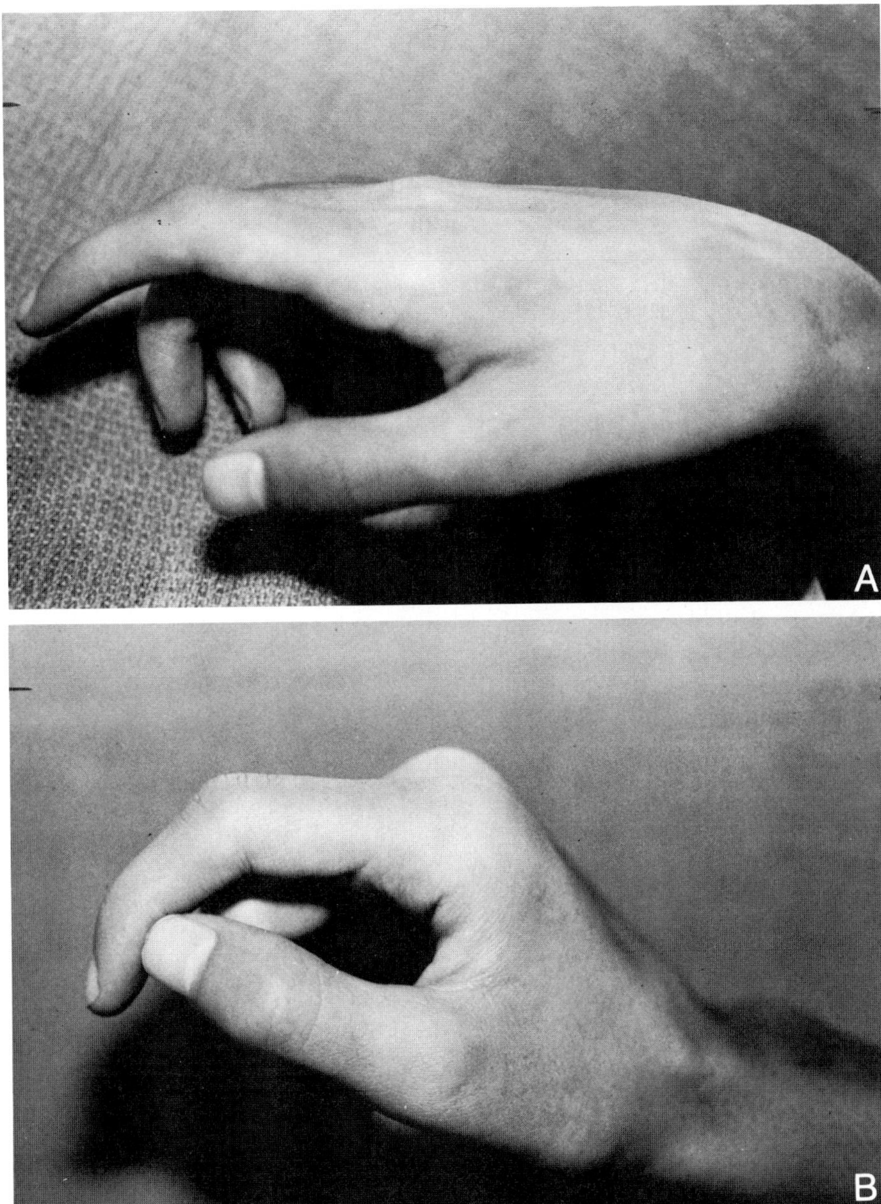

Fig 18-7. *A*, "Extensor habitus" from an overpull of the extensor indicis proprius. *B*, The result of extensor habitus is improper positioning of the thumb against the index finger platform and a dissipation of pinch force.

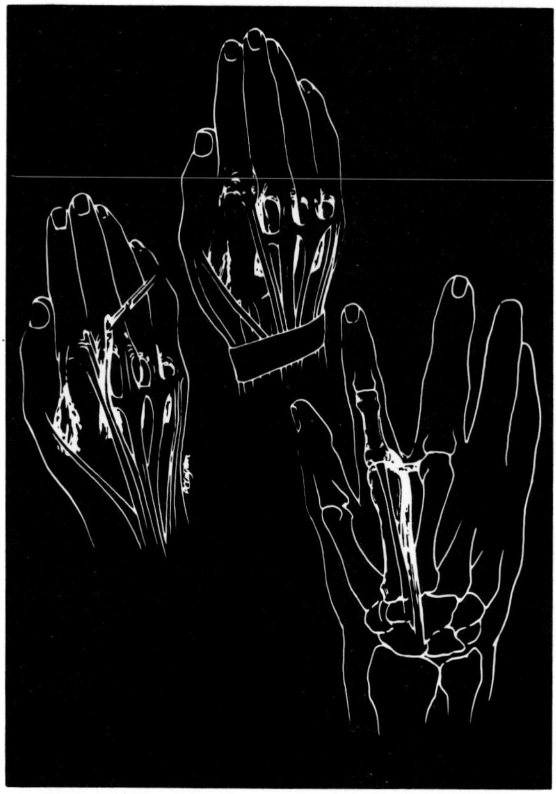

Fig 18-8. Schematic drawing of the tenodesis of the extensor indicis proprius palmar to the axis of index MP joint motion. This eliminates the extensor habitus and ensures a strong platform for the thumb in key grip.

Active Pinch and Grasp

In the patient with more available motors, group 5 or better, Zancolli and House have both advocated a two-stage reconstruction that provides both active pinch and grasp.[4,6] The first stage is an extrinsic and intrinsic extensor tenodesis, permitting the fingers and thumb to open through active wrist flexion (Fig 18-9). The work phase or flexor phase involves tendon transfers for digital flexion and thumb flexion rotation (Fig 18-10). Critical available motors include the extensor carpi radialis longus (ECRL), the pronator teres, and the brachioradialis in the group 5 patient, and more may be available depending on the level of cervical injury. Of critical importance are the preservation of a good wrist extensor and the availability of a good flexor carpi radialis to flex the wrist. If the preoperative motor exam does not clearly define good extensor carpi radialis brevis function, open testing may be indicated. Usually, the presence of a grade 3 or better flexor carpi radialis finds the extensor carpi radialis brevis adequate for wrist extension after transferring the extensor carpi radialis longus.

Four problem areas have been defined in this two-stage procedure. In achieving a firm extensor tenodesis, it is important to have good bone fixation and, ideally, no loss of muscle-tendon unit continuity. By routing the extensor digitorum communis (EDC) tendons of the index, long, and ring fingers under a bridge of bone in the radius, while leaving the extensor pollicis longus and the EDC undisturbed, tendon continuity to all digits is preserved. When the extensor digiti quinti and a slip of the abductor pollicis longus are then cut and sutured to the central tendons, all digits are tenodesed and the balance of the transverse metacarpal arch can be preserved by adjusting the tension of these cut border tendons when they are sutured to the central tendon group (Fig 18-11). Simply to tenodese these border tendons with the central tendons would create a claw in extension because the angle of approach to the tenodesis site makes them relatively tighter.

Often, the PIP extensor mechanism has suffered attritional damage, causing the intrinsic muscles to migrate palmar to the axis of PIP motion. This negates any chance for an intrinsic tenodesis operation to achieve interphalangeal joint extension. In this situation, the lasso tenodesis (Zancolli), using the paralyzed flexor digitorum superficialis muscle tendon unit, can give some MP flexion tone during the wrist extension that accompanies active digital flexion (Fig 18-12).

If the thumb IP and MP joints demonstrate laxity, hyperflexion can use up flexor force desired in the thumb post as a whole. Tenodesis or arthrodesis of one or both of these joints ensures a more predictable power delivery to the thumb pad. Ironically, patients often learn to use the "hook" that results from hyperflexion of the thumb IP joint and do not wish to give it up.

Finally, adhesions are always a statistical possibility with tendon transfers, the more so with multiple transfers done at the same time in a limited area. The extensor carpi radialis longus to flexor digitorum profundus transfer for power grip and the lasso tenodesis for MP flexion probably should not be done at the same time because of the chance of adhesions between the flexor digitorum profundus and the flexor digitorum superficialis at the A1 and A2 pulley level.

Although the two-stage reconstruction "takes away" or "borrows" functioning muscles in the group 5 patient, thereby violating Moberg's precepts, the rewards of the surgery can be great. Our experience finds this group to have a higher level of patient satisfaction than the key grip group in our follow-up evaluations (Fig 18-13).

Conclusion

Presently, the spinal cord injury patient is very likely to be a young survivor and a long-term survivor. It is very important to be able to provide for these young men and women some realistic functional gains through upper extremity surgical reconstruction. Although hard, measurable data such as pinch and grasp strength measurements are an important record of these gains, there are other intangibles such as efficiency, dexterity, and self-esteem, which are perhaps equally important. When one considers that these patients may require 1 to 2

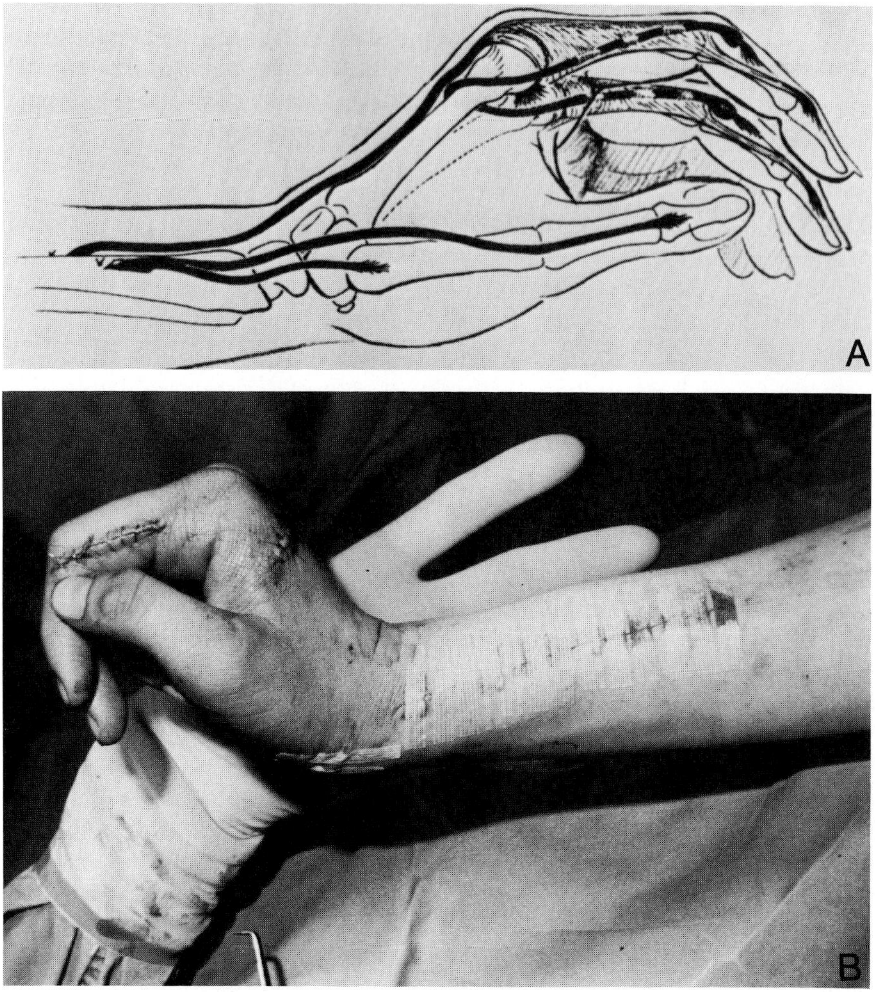

Fig 18-9. *A,* Schematic drawing demonstrating the extrinsic and intrinsic tenodeses for the opening phase in the two-stage reconstruction. Source: Reprinted with permission from "Restoration of Strong Grasp and Lateral Pinch in Tetraplegia Due to Spinal Cord Injury" by House JH et al, *Journal of Hand Surgery* 1976;1:152, Copyright © 1976, CV Mosby Co. *B–D,* Progressive MP and IP joint extension with active wrist flexion following the extensor tenodesis phase.

hours every morning for personal hygiene and dressing, the importance of shortening this time significantly can be understood.

Often these patients are not seen until well after their injury, and indeed no surgery should be undertaken until a minimum of a year after the injury or 6 months of neurological-level stability. Patients seen in the hand clinic are for the most part highly motivated and eager for upgrading. They have already exhib-

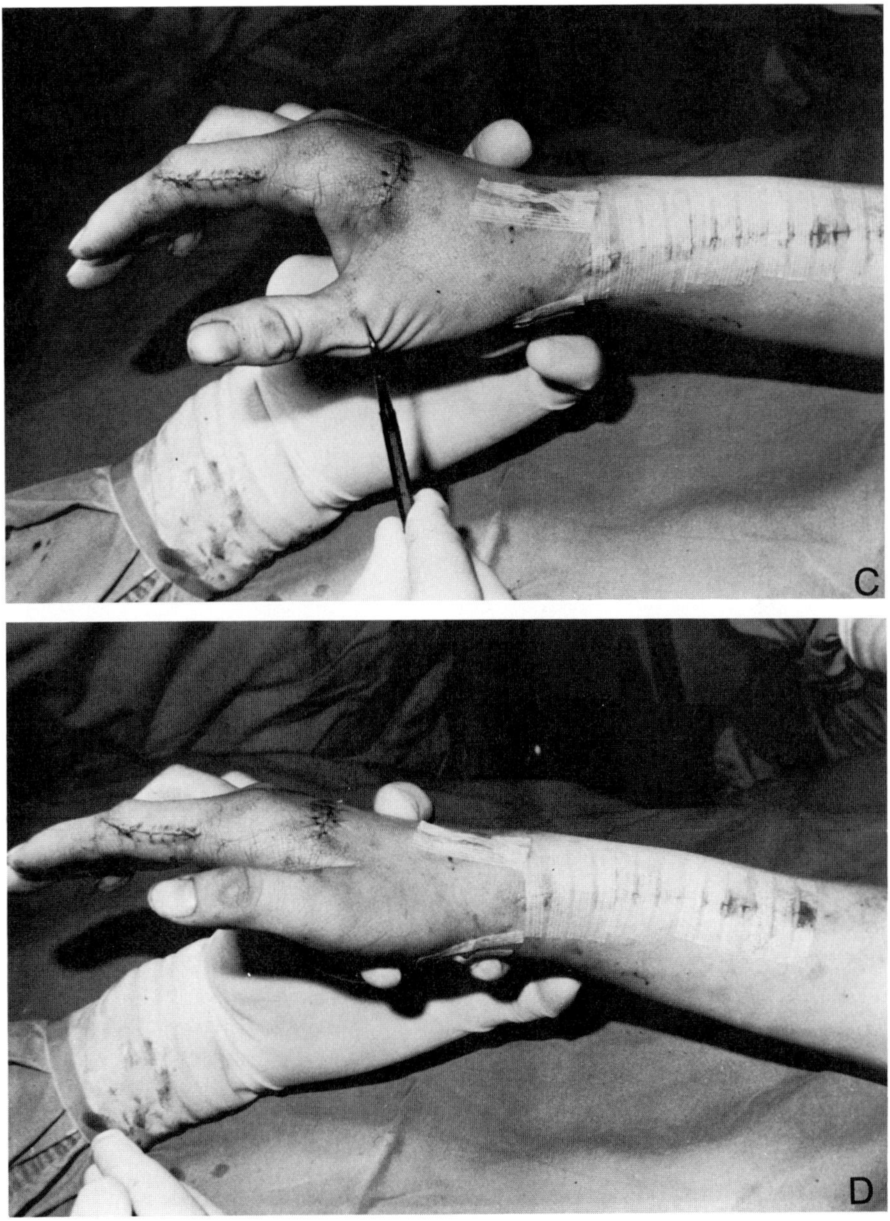

Fig. 18-9. Continued

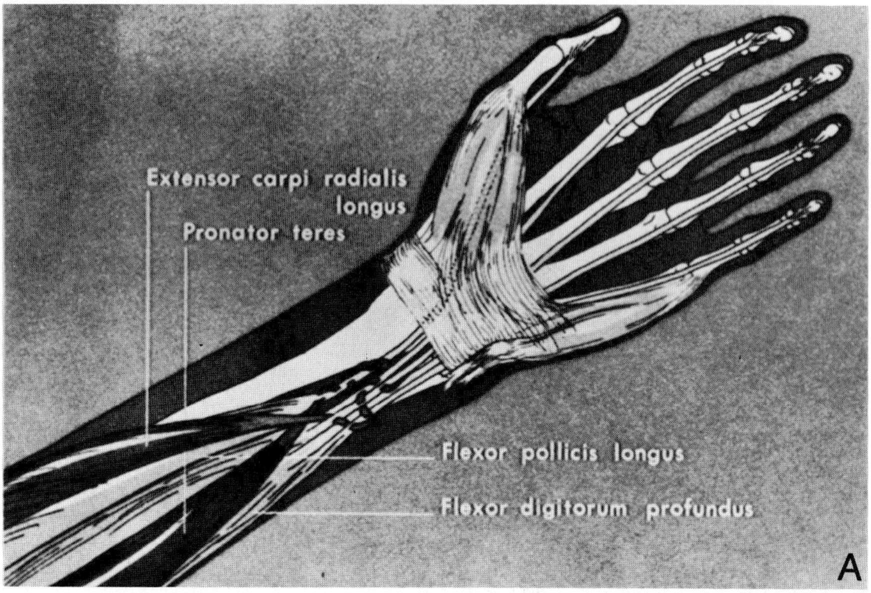

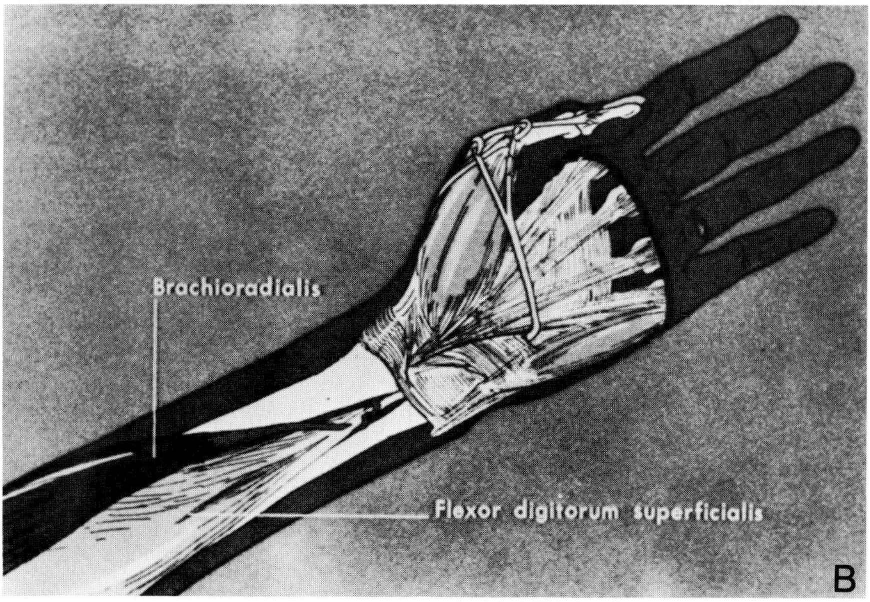

Fig 18-10. *A,* Schematic drawing of the tenorrhaphies of the extensor carpi radialis longus to the four digital flexor profundus tendons and the pronator teres to the flexor pollicis longus. *B,* Schematic drawing of the brachioradialis-to-ring flexor digitorum superficialis tenorrhaphy. The ring superficialis is harvested at the base of the ring finger and passed across the palm in an adductor route to an abductor insertion. Source: Reprinted with permission from "Restoration of Strong Grasp and Lateral Pinch in Tetraplegia Due to Spinal Cord Injury" by House JH et al, *Journal of Hand Surgery* (1976;1:152), Copyright © 1976, CV Mosby Co.

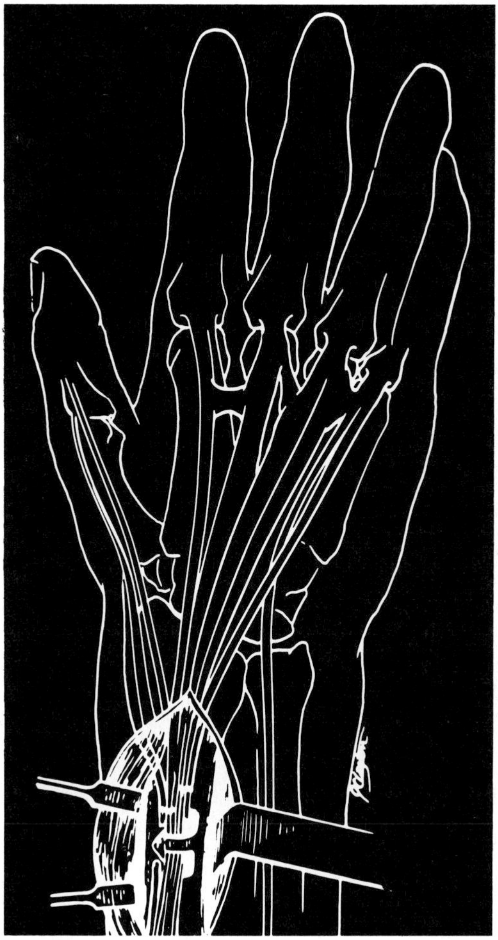

Fig 18-11. Balanced tenodesis of the extensor digitorum communis tendons of the index long and ring fingers into the radius, passing them under a bridge of bone so that tendon continuity is maintained. The extensor pollicis longus and the extensor digiti quinti are sectioned and sutured into the central tendon mass at the proper tension to preserve the transverse metacarpal arch. This leaves the abductor pollicis longus and extensor digitorum communis to the fifth finger intact, thereby preserving a musculotendinous unit in continuity to each digit.

ited what has been figuratively and accurately termed "creative adaptive behavior." If realistic and predictable functional gains can give them a higher level from which to exercise this creativity, then a major contribution has been made.

A team approach, including the spinal cord physician, the hand surgeon, the therapist, and the family counselor, is important so that realistic goals can be defined and achieved. It is not unfair to say that reconstructive surgery in this population should not be undertaken unless this team is intact. For example, we have found an area of great concern to be the period of dependency required during the surgery, cast immobilization, and therapy. These patients have worked very hard for their independence, and to take it away, even temporarily, can be a major psychological stress. The team interaction can make this dependency time much easier.

Finally, constant reevaluation of these patients is important so that the hand

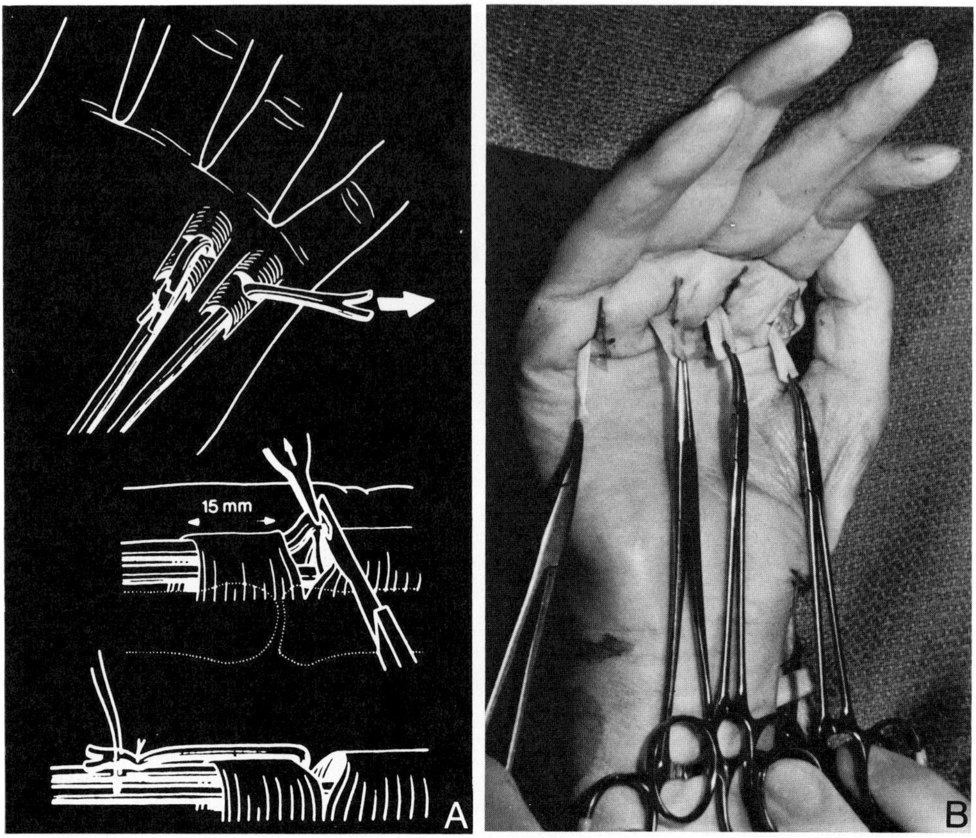

Fig 18-12. *A,* The "lasso" operation as described by Zancolli. The paralyzed flexor digitorum superficialis is brought back over the A1 pulley and sutured to itself, achieving a flexor tenodesis of the MP joints with active wrist extension. Source: Reprinted from *The Upper Limb in Tetraplegia* by Moberg E, with permission of Georg Thieme Publishers, Copyright © 1978. *B–D,* Progressive digital extension through wrist flexion after the extensor tenodesis phase. In this patient, the lasso procedure provides an MP flexion force with wrist extension that is relaxed during wrist flexion. The thumb CMC joint has been arthrodesed in this patient.

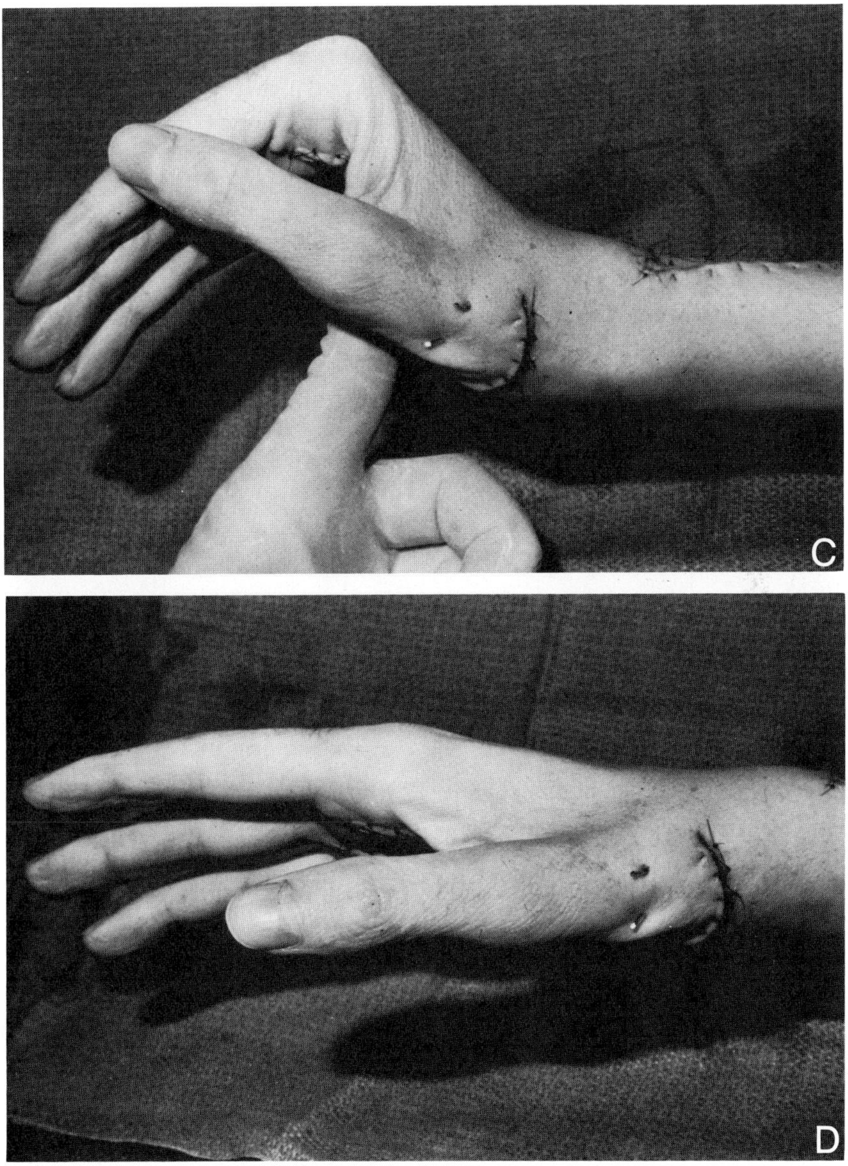

Fig. 18-12. Continued

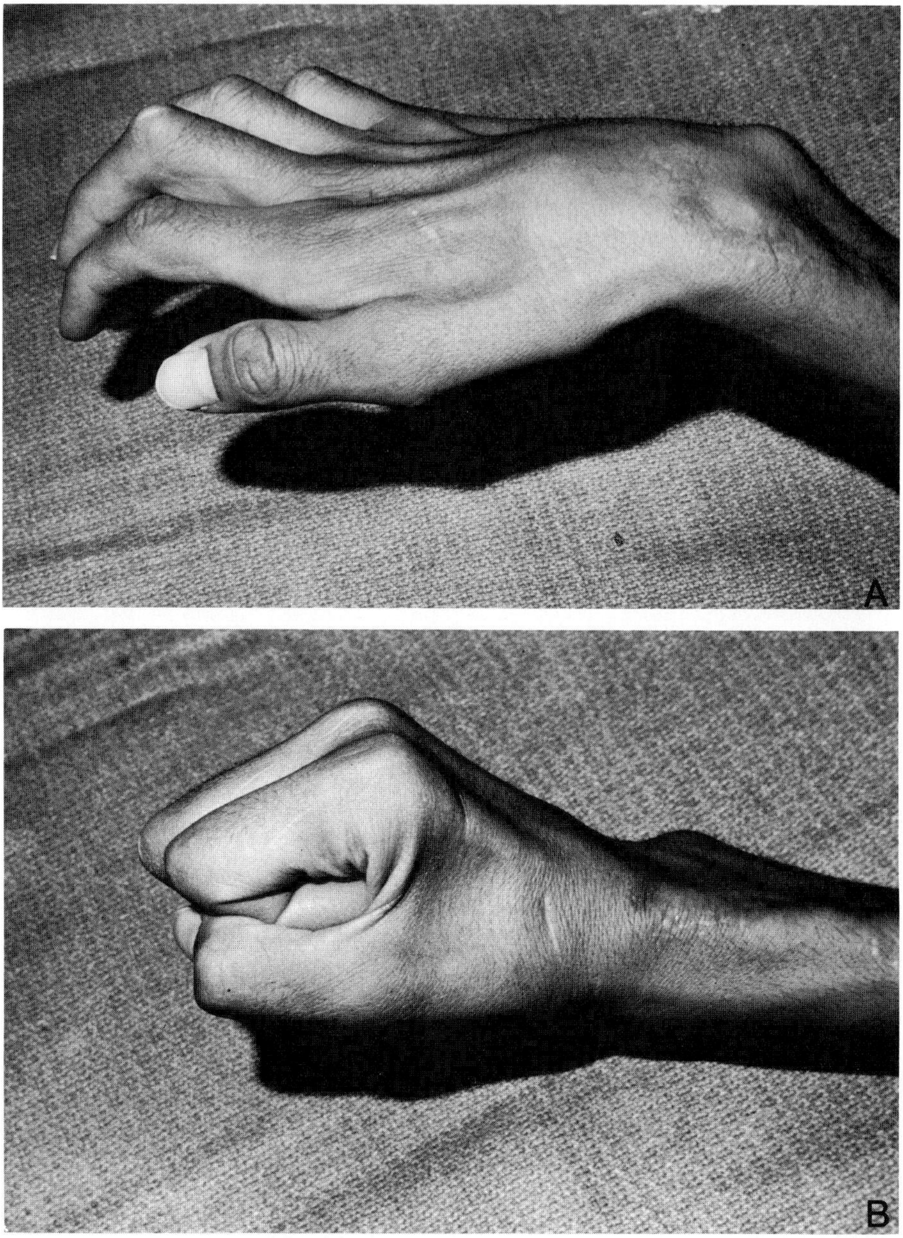

Fig 18-13. Opening (*A*) and closing (*B*) postures of the hand following the two-stage reconstruction. The extension is through tenodeses; the flexion pattern is active. Functional gains following two-stage reconstruction are many and include the ability for pinch and grasp of small objects (*C*) as well as power grip (*D*).

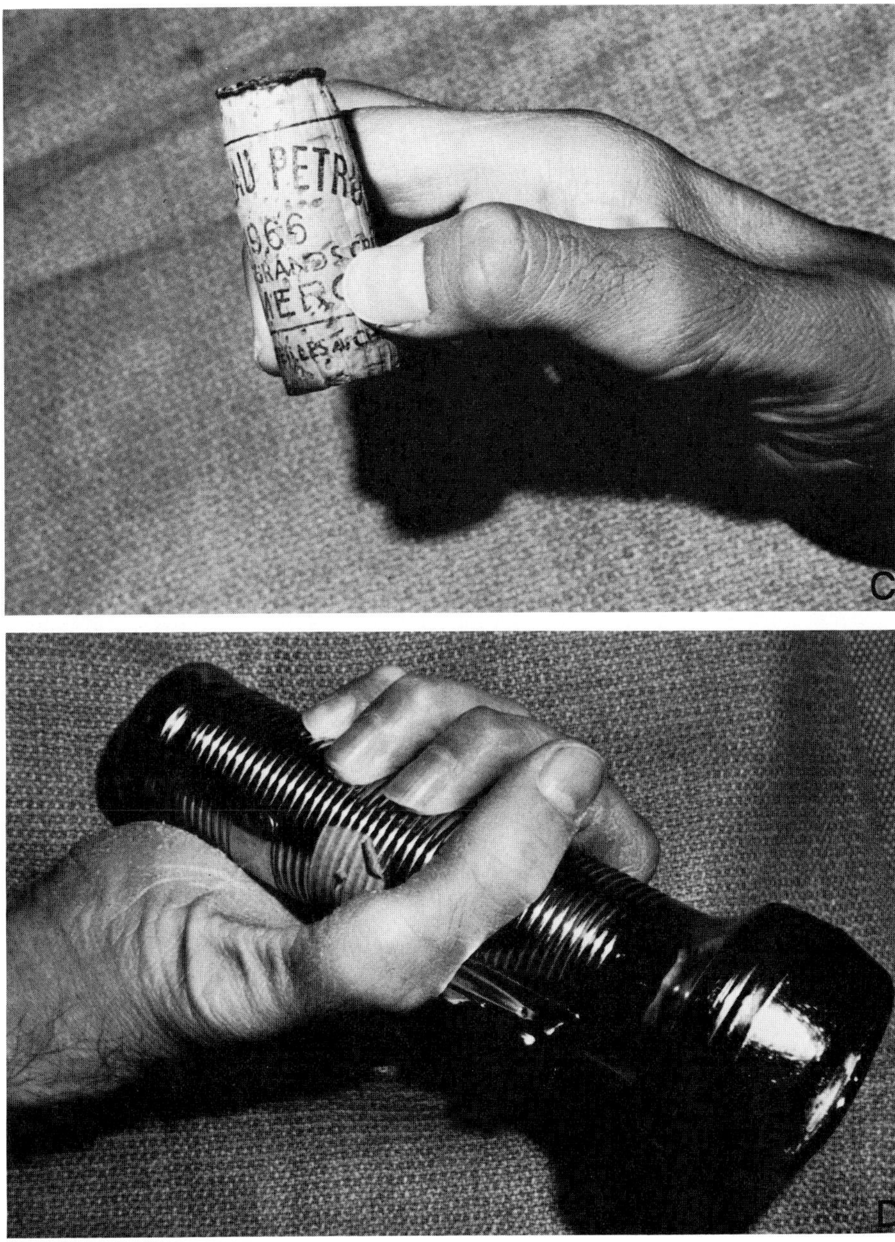
C
D

Fig 18-13. Continued

program can be upgraded continuously, not simply as regards the technical aspects of surgery, but in the total care of the patient. As a bottom line in our care, we look ultimately for patient satisfaction. This takes the form of three basic questions: Are you glad you had the surgery? Would you recommend it to others in your situation? and Would you do it again? If we can get an affirmative answer to these questions, we have succeeded.

References

1. Hanson RN, Franklin NR: Sexual loss in relation to other functional losses for spinal cord injuries. *Arch Phys Med Rehabil* 1976;57:291.
2. Nickel VL, Perry J, Garrett AL: Development of useful function in the severely paralyzed hand. *J Bone Joint Surg Am* 1963;45A:933.
3. Moberg E: *The Upper Limb in Tetraplegia—A New Approach to Surgical Rehabilitation.* Stuttgart, Georg Thieme Publishers, 1978.
4. Zancolli EA: Surgery for the quadriplegic hand with active, strong wrist extension preserved. A study of 97 cases. *Clin Orthop* 1975;112:101.
5. Lamb DW, Landry RM: The hand in quadriplegia. *Hand* 1971;3:31.
6. House JH, Gwatheney FW, Lundsgaard DK: Restoration of strong grasp and lateral pinch in tetraplegia due to spinal cord injury. *J Hand Surg* 1976;1:152.
7. Moberg E: Surgical treatment for absent single hand grip and elbow extension in quadriplegia. *J Bone Joint Surg Am* 1975;57A:196.
8. Freehafer AA, Mast WA: Transfer of the brachioradialis to improve wrist extension in high spinal cord injury. *J Bone Joint Surg Am* 1967;49A:648.

19

Supracondylar Fractures of the Phalanges of the Fingers and Thumb

Juan Manuel Fernandez-Vazquez

The hands of children are subject frequently to injuries, and Wood[1] has pointed out that "fractures of the phalanges, even though they occur in small bones and seem minor, can leave serious consequences if an adequate diagnosis and treatment are not established."

Leonard and Dubravcik[2] in 1970 published 236 cases of phalangeal fractures in children and found 38 phalangeal neck fractures, 9 of which needed open reduction because of subluxation or dislocation of the distal fragment; in 2 of these a rotation of 180° was noted. Bloem[3] in 1971 was the first to describe fracture of the neck of the phalanges in which the bone was rotated 90° and entrapped. In 1972 Dixon and Moon[4] published five cases; they explained the mechanism of injury and the importance of early adequate diagnosis and suggested open reduction and internal fixation.

Since then, few other articles dealing with this type of fracture have been written,[1,5-8] and astonishingly enough, the specialized textbooks in hand fracture offer only a few lines on the subject.[9-11]

Mechanism of Injury

The mechanism of injury described by Dixon and Moon[4] is certainly correct, as has been proved by the observation of several cases. The injured finger is trapped between two objects, producing shearing forces which, coupled with the hard withdrawal reaction of the hand, may open the fracture site enough for rotation to occur. This is followed by entrapment of the rotated condyle by the capsule and the collateral ligaments. The lack of tendon insertions in the distal aspect of the proximal and middle phalanges easily allows the rotation of the fragment (Fig 19-1).

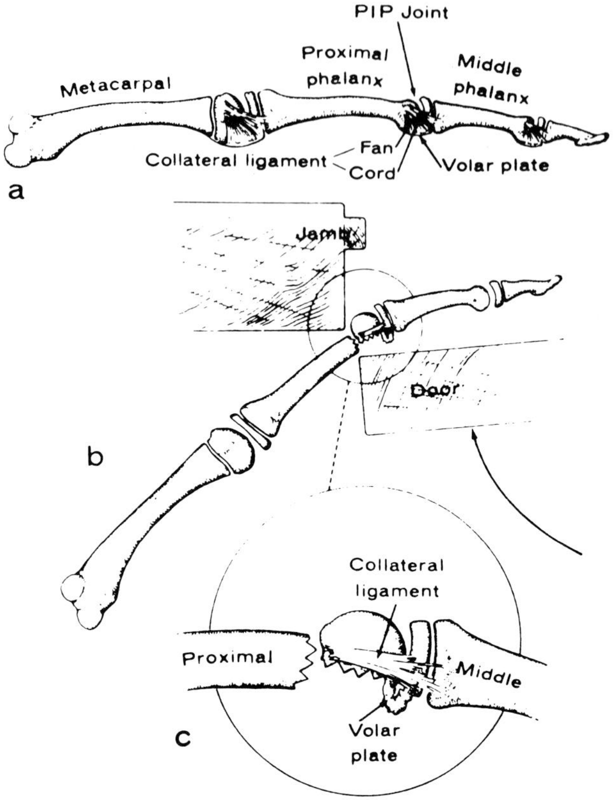

Fig 19-1. Mechanism of injury in supracondylar fracture of the finger phalanges. Source: Reprinted from *Clinical Orthopaedics and Related Research* 1972;83:155 by Dixon GL Jr and Moon NF with permission of JB Lippincott Co, © 1972.

Diagnosis

The involved digit appears swollen and may have some bruises over the dorsal aspect. The bones are more or less well aligned, but mobility is limited because of the swelling and pain. Color is normal and the finger is warm, but there can be some degree of cyanosis and even coldness of the fingerpad. Any attempt to move the finger actively or passively produces intense pain.

X-Rays

In any injury of the fingers it is imperative to obtain anteroposterior (AP) and lateral views, and then if necessary oblique views can be obtained. The AP view shows that the distal fragment has an ovoid shape and resembles the distal metacarpal epiphysis. The lateral view makes the diagnosis, showing the rotation and displacement of the distal fragment (Fig 19-2).

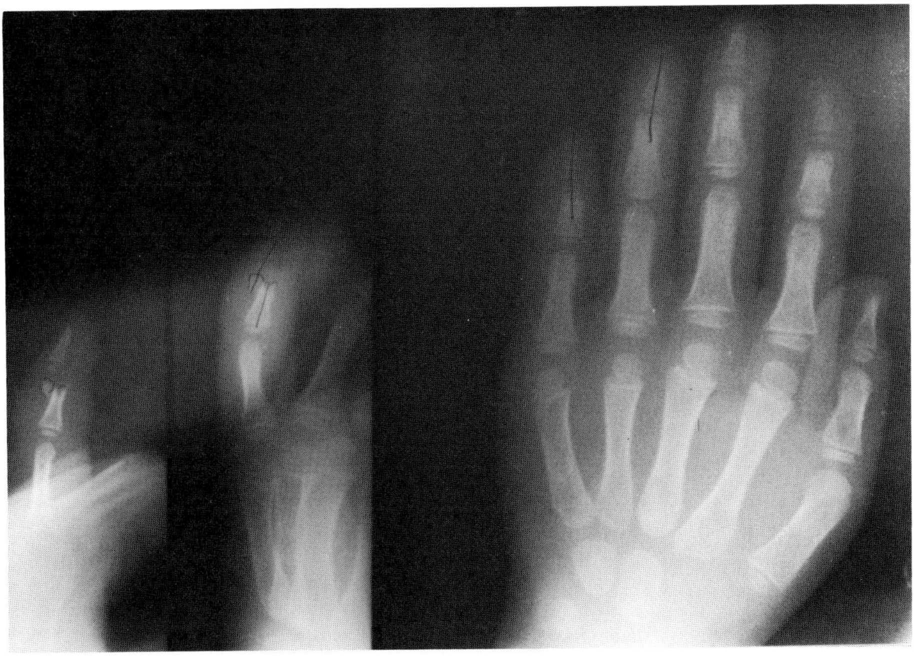

Fig 19-2. Lateral (left) and anteroposterior (right) views of a supracondylar fracture of the finger.

Treatment

As soon as the diagnosis has been established, prompt open reduction and Kirschner wire fixation are recommended. I have been using the dorsal approach, similar to that described by Pratt,[12] which gives a very good exposure and obviates the need to sever any of the collateral ligaments. Care should be taken to avoid injury to the extensor insertion.

Operative Technique

Through a dorsal zigzag or lazy curve incision the dorsal extensor tendon is split longitudinally or displaced laterally, the capsule is opened, and the rotated distal fragment is visualized. With a periosteal elevator and gentle traction on the finger the fragment is easily derotated and reduced. At this point a smooth Kirschner wire (0.035mm) is inserted. The stability of the fixation is tested by gentle motion of the joint, and if it is not secure another wire is driven in. The wound is closed and the wires are left protruding through the skin. A compression dressing is applied for 3 weeks followed by an aluminum splint for another

2 to 4 weeks until bone healing occurs. The Kirschner wires are then removed and gentle exercises are begun, keeping the aluminum splint in place until good motion is attained (Figs 19-3, 19-4).

Clinical Material

A 13-year retrospective chart review was undertaken of all patients diagnosed and treated with supracondylar fractures of the phalanges of the fingers and thumb. During this period I have treated 25 cases at the American British Cowdray Hospital and the National Institute of Orthopedics in Mexico City from January 1971 through December 1983. There were 18 males and 7 females ranging in age from 2 to 16 years (mean age 7.6 years). The mechanism of injury was entrapment of the finger or thumb in a door or similar mechanism (drawer, heavy falling objects) in 24, and the chain of a tortilla-making machine in 1 case. There were 10 cases of fractures of the thumb (the right thumb in 8 cases and the left in 2), 3 of the ring finger (2 right and 1 left), and 12 of the little finger (8 right and 4 left). The proximal phalanx was fractured in 23 cases and the middle phalanx in 2. All but one of the fractures were dorsally angulated or

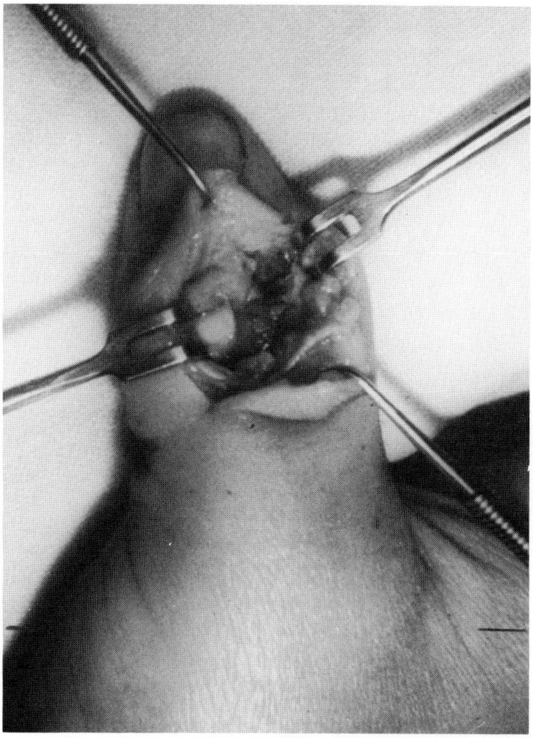

Fig 19-3. Intraoperative photograph showing rotated distal fragment of the phalanx.

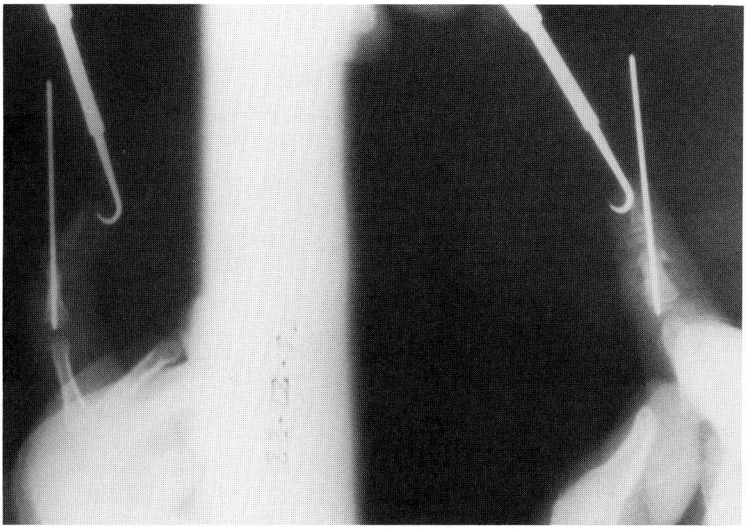

Fig 19-4. Intraoperative radiographs showing positioning of the Kirschner wire.

rotated; the exception was palmarly rotated and ended in amputation through the middle phalanx. There were no fractures of the index or middle fingers (Fig 19-5). Timė elapsed between injury and final treatment ranged from 3 hours to 4 weeks; the great majority (20 cases) were seen in the first 4 days.

All but three patients were treated with primary open reduction and Kirschner wire fixation. Two had late osteotomies and fixation, and one had an amputation through the middle phalanx.

Classification of Results

The results were classified according to the criteria published by Barton in 1979[8]:

- *Normal:* Digit completely normal with no symptoms and no signs.
- *Good:* A result satisfactory to patient and surgeon.
- *Fair:* A digit that was still useful but that either the patient or the surgeon regarded as less than good.
- *Poor:* Much pain or deformity or little function.

The results were classified as normal in 14 cases, good in 6, fair in 2, and poor in 3. The normal results were those cases treated during the first 4 days of injury, and the poor results occurred in two cases treated by osteotomy 3 and 4 weeks after injury and the one amputated case.

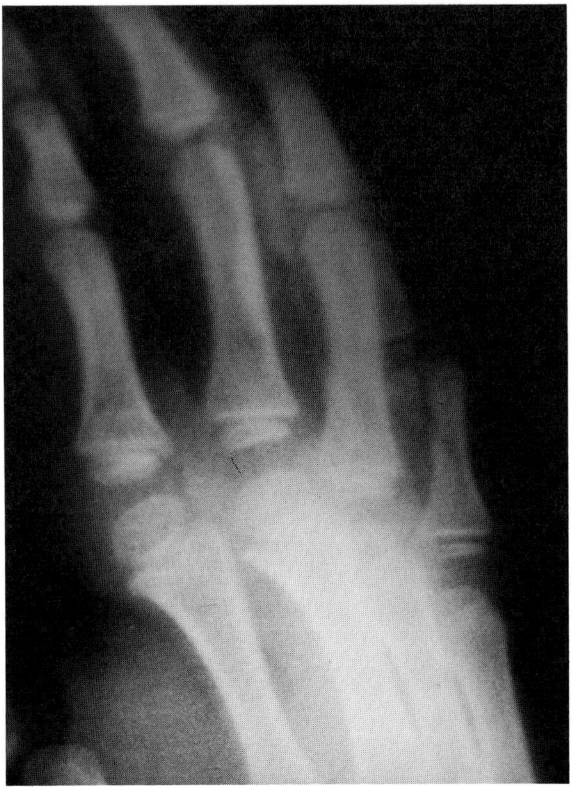

Fig 19-5. Fracture of the little finger with palmar rotation of the proximal phalanx and amputation through the middle phalanx.

Discussion

Supracondylar fracture of the phalanges of the fingers and thumb is a very severe injury that must be recognized and treated early if good results are to be achieved. It is probably more common than has been thought. The presence of circulatory deficit in two cases indicates the severity of the lesion and should make the surgeon aware of this complication.

One case of palmar displacement of the distal fragment not described previously and which ended in amputation was found, and it possibly indicates a different type of mechanism of injury. The patient was a 4-year-old boy whose little finger had been caught against a heavy rock.

The importance of prompt open reduction and Kirschner wire fixation has been emphasized by Dixon and Moon,[4] Leonard and Dubravcik,[2] and Wood.[1] It is also supported by this review and the method should be emphasized. Those patients who underwent surgery after 2 weeks obtained only fair or poor results.

References

1. Wood VE: Fractures of the hand in children. *Orthop Clin North Am* 1976;7:527–542.
2. Leonard MH, Dubravcik P: Management of fractured fingers in the child. *Clin Orthop* 1970;73:160–166.
3. Bloem JJAM: The treatment and prognosis of uncomplicated dislocated fractures of the metacarpals and phalanges. *Arch Chir Neerl* 1971;23:55–65.
4. Dixon GL Jr, Moon NF: Rotational supracondylar fractures of the proximal phalanx in children. *Clin Orthop* 1972;83:151–156.
5. Kilbourne BC: Management of complicated hand fractures. *Surg Clin North Am* 1968;48:201–213.
6. Leonard MH: Open reduction of fractures of the neck of the proximal phalanx in children. *Clin Orthop* 1976;116:176–179.
7. Barton NJ: Fractures of the phalanges of the hand. *Hand* 1977;9:1–10.
8. Barton NJ: Fractures of the shafts of the phalanges of the hand. *Hand* 1979;11:119–133.
9. Rang M: *Children's Fractures.* Philadelphia JB Lippincott Co, 1974, pp 145–149.
10. Sandzen SC Jr: *Atlas of Wrist and Hand Fractures.* Littleton, Mass, PSG Publishing Co, 1979, pp 254–261.
11. Weeks PM: *Acute Bone and Joint Injuries of the Hand and Wrist. A Clinical Guide to Management.* CV Mosby Co, 1981, pp 263–264.
12. Pratt DR: Exposing fractures of the proximal phalanx of the finger longitudinally through the dorsal extensor apparatus. *Clin Orthop* 1969;15:22–26.
13. Green DP, Rowland SA: Fractures and dislocations in the hand, in Rockwood, Green (eds): *Fractures.* Philadelphia, JB Lippincott Co, 1975, p 278.
14. O'Brien ET: Fractures of the metacarpals and phalanges, in Green DP (ed): *Operative Hand Surgery.* New York, Churchill Livingston, 1982, pp 604–612.

20

Extensor Carpi Radialis Longus Transfer for Rupture of the Extensor Pollicis Longus Tendon

Thomas G. Wadsworth

The extensor pollicis longus tendon appears on the dorsal surface of the muscle and enters a fibro-osseous tunnel on the ulnar side of Lister's tubercle, the third compartment of the extensor retinaculum. The tendon deviates obliquely and radially and then proceeds distally along the ulnar side of the thumb metacarpal and metacarpophalangeal joint; it then widens over the proximal phalanx and inserts into the base of the distal phalanx of the thumb.

Fibers of the short abductor and flexor pollicis brevis insert into the extensor apparatus, extending the interphalangeal joint on opposition of the thumb; occasionally, there is an accessory insertion of the extensor pollicis brevis into the distal phalanx and, in such circumstances, this musculotendinous unit can actively extend the thumb during abduction but not adduction. This can confuse the clinical picture with rupture of the extensor pollicis longus tendon.

The function of the extensor pollicis longus tendon is to extend the metacarpophalangeal, interphalangeal, and carpometacarpal joints of the thumb; contraction of this musculotendinous unit also aids adduction of the carpometacarpal and metacarpophalangeal joints[1].

The extensor pollicis longus tendon may be divided by a lacerating wound, but closed rupture of the tendon is more common. The injury was first described by Duplay[2] in 1876 and was further commented on as "drummer's palsy" by Dums[3] in 1896. Apart from drummers, tenosynovitis due to repetitive movement of the thumb can also be seen in other occupations such as woodcarvers, and on occasion the tendon ruptures. A further unusual cause of rupture of the tendon is a sudden, violent twisting injury of the forearm. In the past, tuberculosis, gonorrhea, and syphilis have been inculpated as causes of disease and rupture of the extensor pollicis longus tendon.

An important cause of rupture of the tendon is after Colles' fracture[4]; this more often occurs after an undisplaced or minimally displaced injury than one necessitating reduction. Rupture typically occurs 6 weeks to 3 months after the injury and is sometimes preceded by prodromal symptoms of pain and crepitus with active movement of the thumb. In the undisplaced or minimally displaced Colles' fracture, the extensor retinaculum is likely to be intact, if bruised, and in these circumstances increased pressure within the third dorsal compartment at the inner side of Lister's tubercule may jeopardize blood flow in the tendon and also interfere with the production of synovial fluid to the extent that the tendon may be deprived of nutrition via diffusional pathways. It may be that damage to the tendon at the time of fracture occurs by laceration against a spicule of bone, and there may be rupture of the mesotendon, producing ischemic necrosis of the tendon. Effusion or callus within the tunnel at the lower end of the radius may cause "strangulation" of the extensor pollicis longus tendon. Other causes that have been cited are distortion of the tunnel through which the tendon runs and angulation of the cortex with compression of the tendon against the extensor retinaculum. Also, the tendon may become adhered to callus and subsequently yield suddenly as a result of strain due to a forceful grasping movement. Direct blunt trauma to the tendon may cause rupture, as may indirect trauma by a fall onto the hand.

The extensor pollicis longus tendon is the tendon most commonly ruptured in rheumatoid disease; rupture is probably associated with the frequently seen proliferation of synovium in its long tendinous course and in the angular bend of the tendon around Lister's tubercule, the point where attrition rupture usually occurs. Rarely, the extensor pollicis brevis and abductor pollicis longus tendons may also rupture and, of course, rupture of the extrinsic extensor tendons of the fingers is fairly commonly seen in the rheumatoid patient with disease at the distal radioulnar joint. There may be significant deformity of the thumb, particularly the metacarpophalangeal and interphalangeal joints, as a consequence of rheumatoid arthropathy, thus compounding the deformity and loss of function due to rupture of the extensor pollicis longus tendon.

Rupture of the extensor pollicis longus tendon results in severe impairment of function of the hand. The thumb typically lies across the palm and cannot be adequately withdrawn in order that a proper grasping or pinch action can be accomplished. This is a much more serious deficit in the thumb than rupture of the long flexor tendon.

Included in the various methods of repair of the ruptured tendon are extensor indicis transfer; intercalated graft using the palmaris longus, plantaris, or fourth toe extensor tendon; extensor pollicis brevis transfer and splitting and transfer of a segment of the abductor pollicis longus tendon[5,6,7,8]. Another method is to translocate the proximal segment of the ruptured tendon out of the groove on the back of the radius and place it laterally and perform a direct anastomosis with the distal segment, this being a shorter route than the normal anatomical arrangement[9]. This is more suitable for very early cases before significant retraction of muscle has occurred, and suturing in this circumstance is best performed with the wrist dorsiflexed.

I have for 20 years used the extensor carpi radialis longus tendon as a transfer for closed rupture of the extensor pollicis longus tendon, the lesion almost invariably being at the level of Lister's tubercule at the radius. This method of repair was first described by Duplay[2] in 1876. The method is easy, the two tendons being similar in diameter and one overlying the other at the wrist (Fig 20-1).

A dorsiradial incision is used with preservation of the veins and terminal cutaneous branches of the radial nerve. The procedure is usually performed under general anesthesia and a pneumatic tourniquet. The proximal segment of the injured tendon is always retracted, often as much as 5 cm, and is usually not seen in the wound. The distal segment of tendon is identified and minimally resected. Next, a tendon suture is placed as far distally as possible in the extensor carpi radialis longus tendon in order to have a maximal length of tendon for subsequent transfer; the tendon is then divided close to its insertion at the base of the index metacarpal. The extensor carpi radialis longus tendon is sutured end-to-end into the distal segment of the ruptured extensor pollicis longus tendon (Fig 20-2). It is important not to overresect the injured tendon, and it is equally important to use the maximum length of the transferred extensor carpi radialis longus tendon; otherwise an extension deformity of the

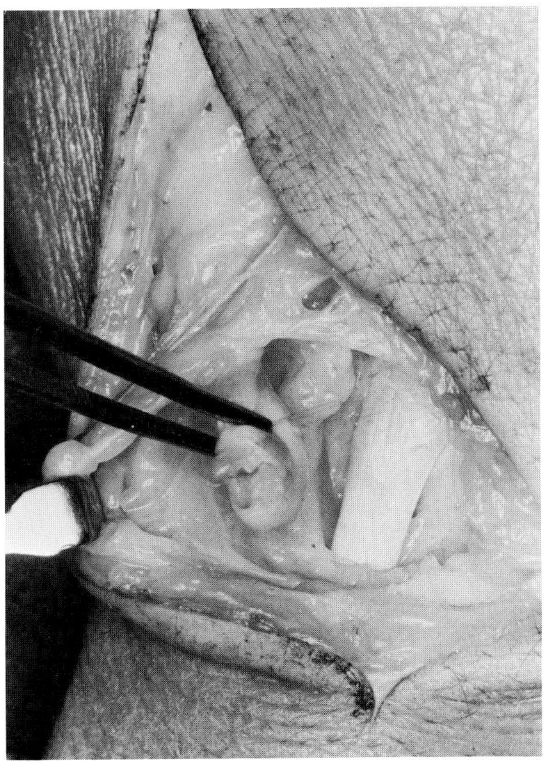

Fig 20-1. The extensor pollicis longus and extensor carpi radialis longus tendons are of similar girth and lie adjacent at the wrist.

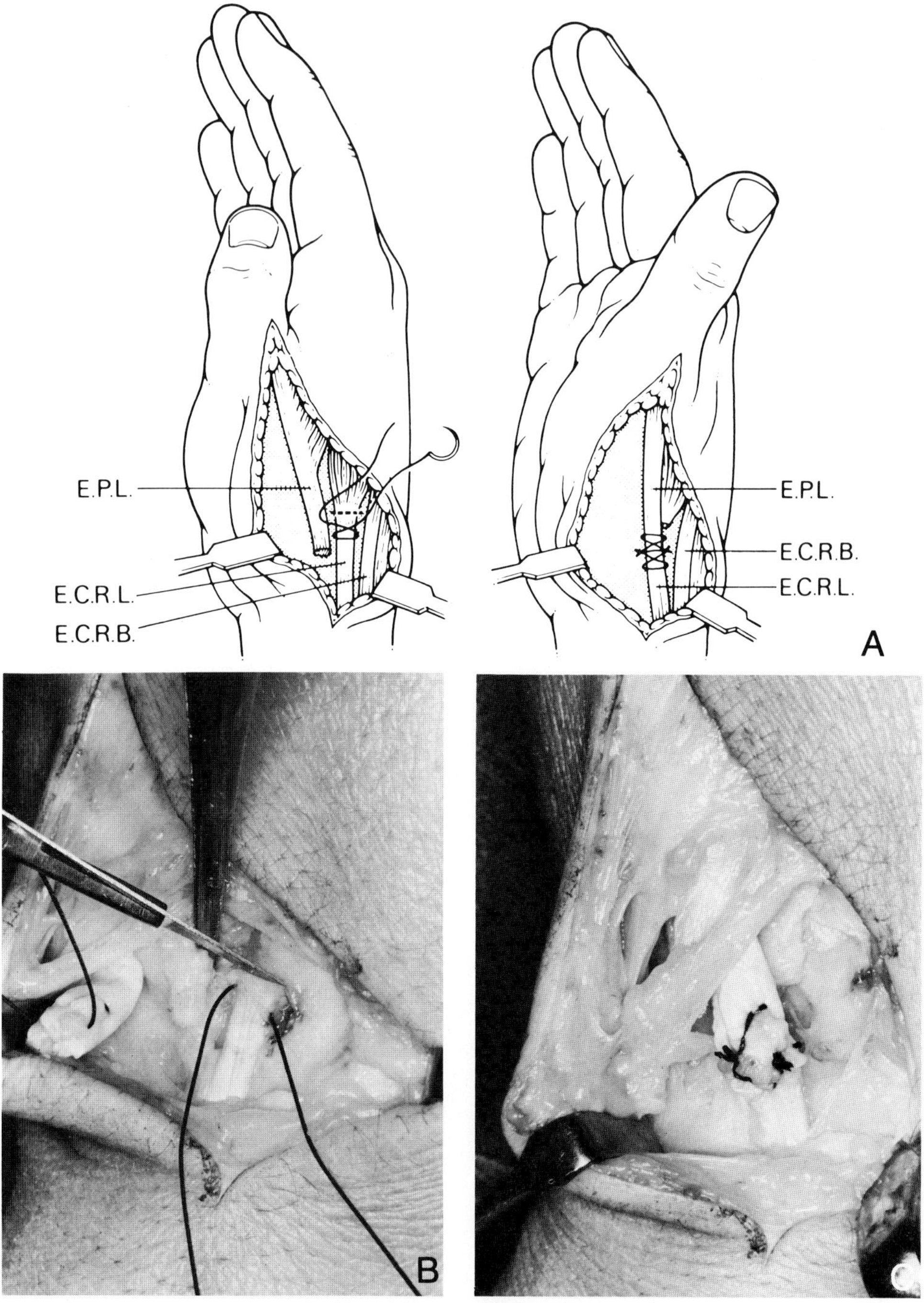

Fig 20-2. *A*, Schematic diagram of the simple technique of anastomosing the extensor carpi radialis longus (*E.C.R.L.*) to the distal segment of the ruptured extensor pollicis longus (*E.P.L.*) tendon. It is important to maintain adequate tendon length to avoid loss of flexion of the thumb. *E.C.R.B.*, extensor carpi radialis brevis. *B, C,* Intraoperative photographs.

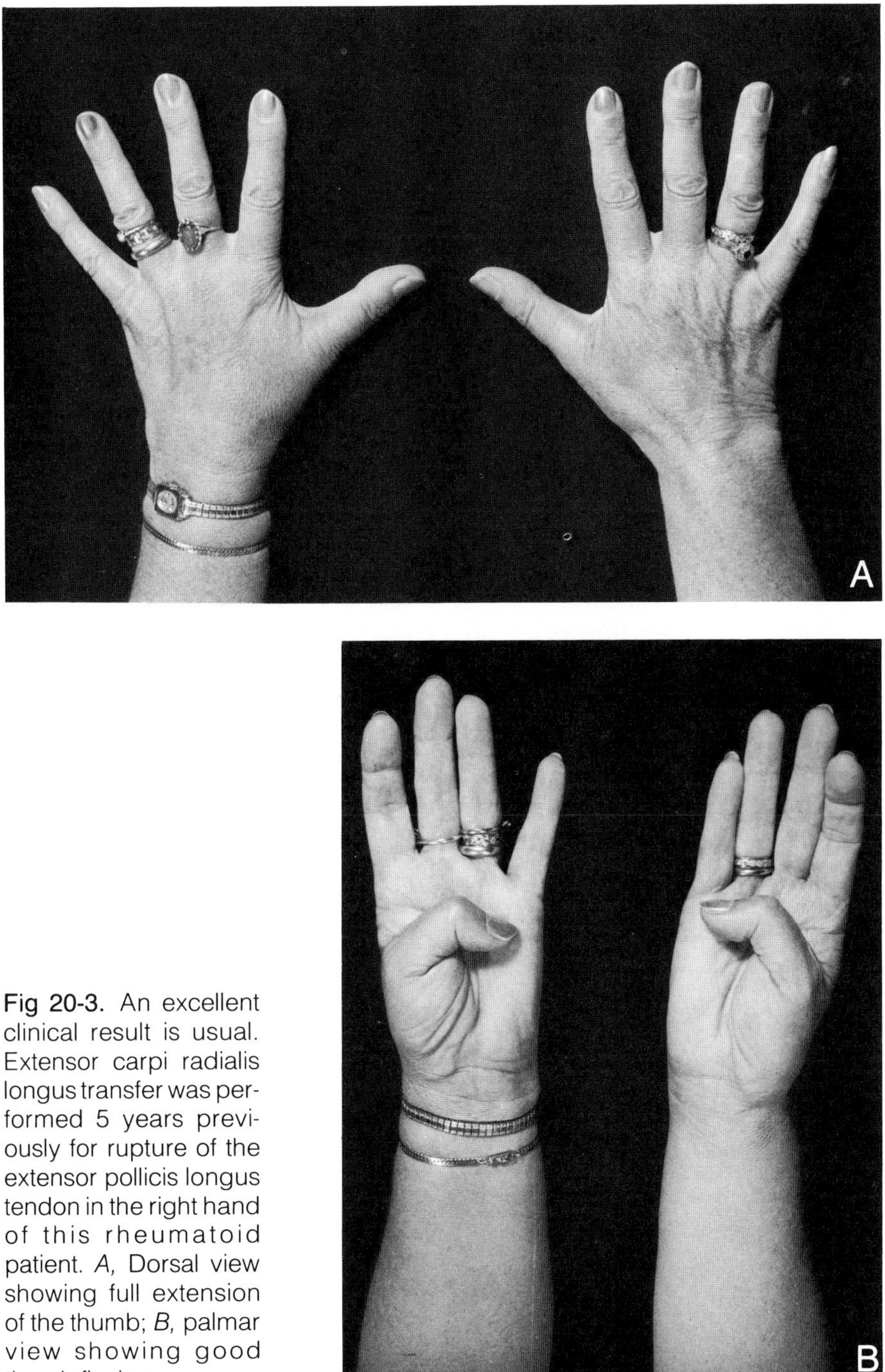

Fig 20-3. An excellent clinical result is usual. Extensor carpi radialis longus transfer was performed 5 years previously for rupture of the extensor pollicis longus tendon in the right hand of this rheumatoid patient. *A,* Dorsal view showing full extension of the thumb; *B,* palmar view showing good thumb flexion.

thumb may well result. The wound is closed in layers and a well-padded POP splint applied with the wrist in 20° dorsiflexion and the thumb in extension and abduction; this is maintained for 1 month. Thereafter, the patient goes on to a course of therapy, including wax baths and gripping and extension exercises.

Excellent results have been a feature of this technique in closed rupture of the extensor pollicis longus tendon (Fig 20-3). Good thumb flexion and minimal extensor lag are the usual result. Of course, with lesions distal to the radius, most often lacerating injuries, this method of repair is not applicable.

In the rare instance where the abductor pollicis longus and extensor pollicis brevis tendons are also ruptured, the extensor indicis should be transferred into the distal extensor pollicis longus tendon and the extensor carpi radialis longus transposed into the distal abductor pollicis longus while the extensor pollicis brevis stump is left free.

A commonly used method of repair for closed rupture of the extensor pollicis longus tendon is transposition of the extensor indicis. However, there are several advantages to using the extensor carpi radialis longus transfer:

- One incision is used.
- The extensor pollicis longus and extensor carpi radialis longus tendons are of similar girth and normally adjacent anatomically.
- The risk of index finger extensor lag and weakness is avoided.
- The extensor indicis can, in certain circumstances, be used for other purposes, eg, as a radial-deviating extensor transfer to the index finger.

Historically, the first recorded musculotendinous unit used to restore thumb extension after rupture of the extensor pollicis longus tendon was the extensor carpi radialis longus. It remains an excellent method of repair for lost thumb extension after closed rupture of the extensor pollicis longus tendon in the neighborhood of Lister's tubercle of the radius.

References

1. Chiron HS: A study of the functions of the extensor pollicis longus. *Bull Hosp Jt Dis Orthop Inst* 1973;34:84–91.
2. Duplay M: Rupture sous-cutanée du tendon du long extenseur du pouce de la main droite, au niveau de la tabatière anatomique. Flexion permanente du pouce. Rètablissement de la faculté d'extension par une opération (suture de l'extrémité du tendon rompu avec le premier radial externe). *Bull Mem Soc Chir Paris* 1876;2:788–791.
3. Dums F: Über Trommlerlähmungen. *Dtsch Militärarzt Z* 1896;25:145–155.
4. Trevor D: Rupture of the extensor pollicis longus after Colles' fracture. *J Bone Joint Surg Br* 1950;32B:370–375.
5. Heybroek G: Restoration of the extensor function of the thumb by tendon transposition. *Arch Chir Neerl* 1968;20:55–64.

6. Hamlin C, Littler JW: Restoration of the extensor pollicis longus tendon by an intercalated graft. *J Bone Joint Surg Am* 1977;59A:412–414.
7. Harrison S, Swannell AJ, Ansell BM: Repair of extensor pollicis longus using extensor pollicis brevis in rheumatoid arthritis. *Ann Rheum Dis* 1972;31:490–492.
8. Backhouse KM: Abductor pollicis longus musculo-tendinous split as a replacement motor for ruptured extensor pollicis longus. *Hand.* 1981;13:271–275.
9. Van Demark RE: Cottam GIW: Translocation tenorraphy of the extensor pollicis longus after spontaneous rupture in Colles' fracture. *Clin Orthop Rel Res* 1963;31:106–109.

21

Classification and Surgical Management of the Spastic Thumb

Juan Manuel Fernandez-Vazquez

The deformities present in the spastic thumb are the more handicapping elements affecting the cerebral palsy patient.[1-5] Much has been learned since Steindler's recommendation of arthrodesis of the metacarpophalangeal joint and Phelps's favoring of three-joint stabilizations as the only successful treatment for the thumb-in-palm deformity; studies published by Goldner,[2,6] Swanson,[5,7] Inglis,[4] Matev,[8] Samilson,[9] House,[3] Zancolli,[10,11] and others have opened new dimensions to the treatment of the spastic thumb.

Classification

The classification selected for this study was published by House et al[3] in 1981; this classification divides spastic thumb deformities into four different types.

- *Type 1:* "Simple" metacarpal adduction contracture. Mobility and varying degrees of voluntary control of the metacarpophalangeal and interphalangeal joints are present. The first metacarpal is held in adduction by a combination of spasticity and fixed contracture in the adductor pollicis and first dorsal interosseous muscles and the skin of the thumb cleft (Fig 21-1).
- *Type 2:* Metacarpal adduction contracture and metacarpophalangeal joint flexion deformity: The first metacarpal is fixed in adduction as described in type I deformity, and in addition the metacarpophalangeal joint is fixed in flexion by spasm and contracture of the flexor pollicis brevis. The interphalangeal joint is functionally mobile (Fig 21-2).
- *Type 3:* Metacarpal adduction contracture combined with metacarpophalangeal hyperextension deformity or instability: This defor-

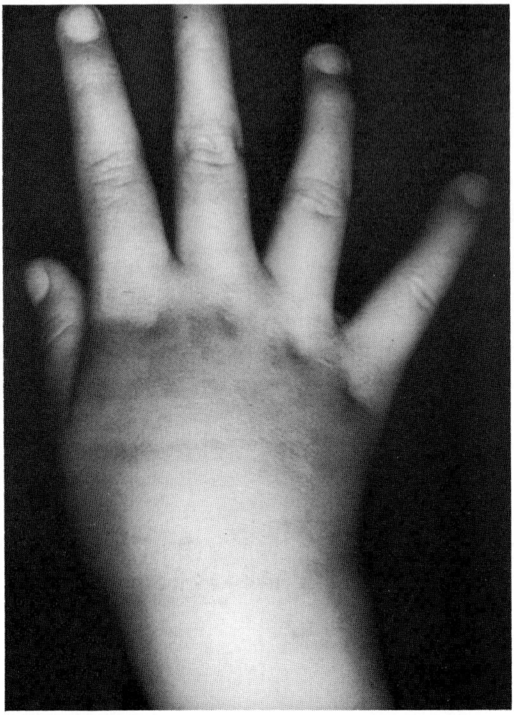

Fig 21-1. Type 1 spasticity of the thumb. Simple metacarpal adduction contracture.

mity results from the compensatory efforts of the extensor pollicis longus and extensor pollicis brevis acting across a hyperextensible metacarpophalangeal joint in the absence of spasticity of the flexor pollicis longus (Fig 21-3).

- *Type 4:* Metacarpal adduction contracture combined with metacarpophalangeal and interphalangeal flexion deformities: This deformity may be produced by isolated spasticity of the flexor pollicis longus, but more often it is the result of flexor pollicis longus spasticity combined with spasticity and contracture in the intrinsic muscles of the thumb as well (Fig 21-4).

Surgical Treatment

Inglis et al[4] have established that there are four main obstacles to useful function in the spastic thumb:

1. reduced sensation
2. fixed contractures

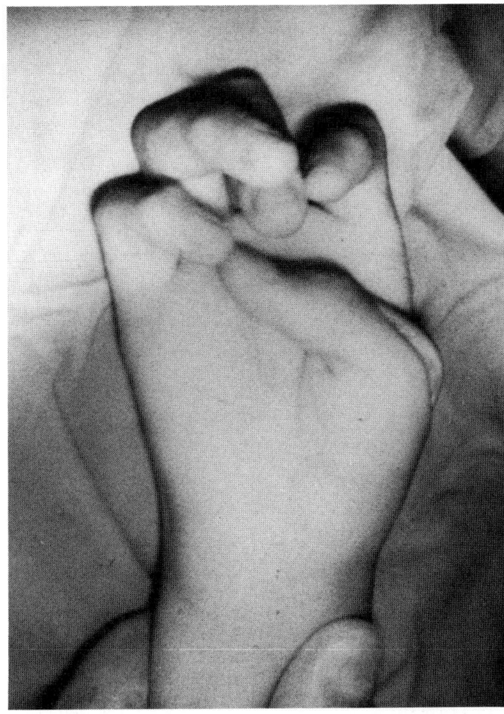

Fig 21-2. Type 2 spasticity. Metacarpal adduction contracture and metacarpophalangeal joint flexion deformity.

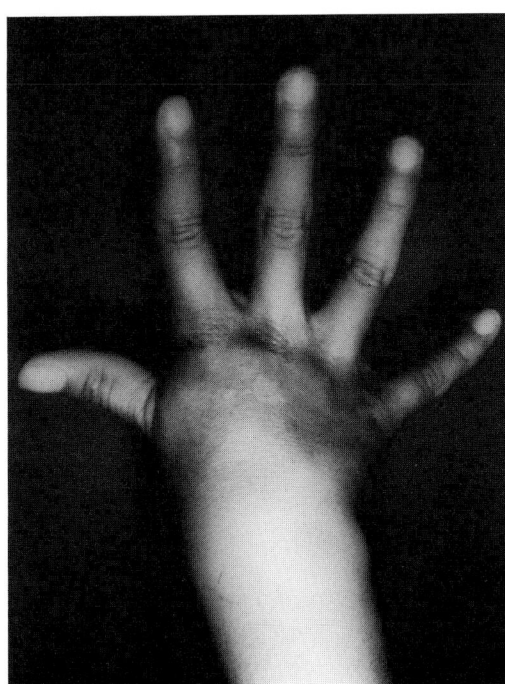

Fig 21-3. Type 3 spasticity. Metacarpal adduction contracture combined with metacarpophalangeal hyperextension deformity or instability.

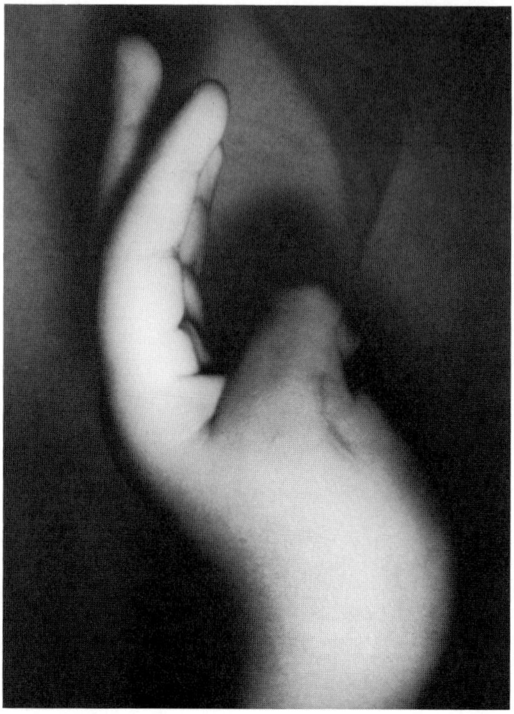

Fig 21-4. Type 4 spasticity. Metacarpal adduction contracture combined with metacarpophalangeal and interphalangeal flexion deformity.

3. muscle spasticity and paralysis or weakness
4. muscle imbalance.

Because of these, no single currently favored surgical procedure and no set combination of procedures is suitable to all cases. Three different types of surgical procedures are utilized in the management of the deformities present in the spastic thumb.

1. Release of contractures: Z-plasty for the first web space, release of the first dorsal interosseous muscle from the first metacarpal, release or division of the adductor pollicis muscle or tendon, release of the flexor pollicis brevis, lengthening of the flexor pollicis longus.
2. Augmentation of weak muscles: Tendon transfers or tenodesis of the brachioradialis, flexor carpi radialis, palmaris longus, or flexor superficialis tendon to the extensor pollicis longus or brevis or abductor pollicis longus, depending on which of the three joints of the thumb needs the augmentation; tendon transfer of the flexor pollicis longus to the radial side of the proximal phalanx to augment thumb abduction.

3. Skeletal stabilization: Skeletal stabilization of one of the three joints of the thumb can be done when there is no tendon transfer capable of stabilizing that particular joint.[12-20]

Clinical Materials

A retrospective study was carried out on patients surgically treated for deformities in the thumb afflicted with spastic paralysis. From 1971 through 1982, 50 patients with a diagnosis of spastic hemiplegia underwent surgery at the Hospital German Diaz Lombardo for Congenital Defects, Shriner's Hospital for Crippled children, the National Institute of Orthopaedics, and the American British Cowdray Hospital in Mexico City. There were 35 males and 15 females; their age at the time of surgery was from 6 to 16 years (mean age 10 years). The right thumb was surgically treated in 20 cases and the left in 30 cases.

The cases were classified as follows: type 1, 32 cases; type 2, 8 cases; type 3, 6 cases; and type 4, 4 cases.

All the patients were treated prior to surgery with different modalities of physical therapy and used opponens splints for a variable period of time ranging from 6 months to 12 months. In this study the preoperative goals were to correct the deformity and to improve function in 46 cases and to correct the deformity for hygienic purposes in 4 cases. From the chart review it was impossible to detect accurately the amount of sensorial deficit present before the surgical procedures were performed.

There were 96 surgical procedures performed in type I deformity: Z-plasty of the first web space in 32, stripping of the first dorsal interosseus muscle from the first metacarpal in 32, section of the adductor pollicis tendon in 31, and stripping of the adductor pollicis muscle from the third metacarpal in 1 case.

Surgical procedures were carried out on 24 type 2 cases: translocation of the extensor pollicis longus in 8, transfer of the palmaris longus to the extensor pollicis longus in 6, tendon shortening of the abductor pollicis longus in 8, and arthrodesis of the metacarpophalangeal joint in 2 cases.

Surgical procedures were utilized in 17 type 3 cases: radial translocation of the extensor pollicis longus in 6, transfer of the palmaris longus to the abductor pollicis longus in 4, tendon shortening of the extensor pollicis brevis in 4, arthrodesis of the metacarpophalangeal joint in 2, and Araico's internal wire splint[21] in 1 case.

Surgical procedures were performed on 23 type 4 cases: Z-plasty of the first web space in 4, stripping of the first dorsal interosseus muscle from the first metacarpal in 4, section of the adductor pollicis tendon in 4, section of the flexor pollicis brevis in 4, arthrodesis of the interphalangeal joint in 2, transfer of the palmaris longus to the extensor pollicis longus in 4, and Araico's internal wire splint[21] in 1 case (Fig 21-5). All the patients were immobilized in a dressing with a plaster splint above the elbow for 3 weeks, followed by a plaster cast thumb

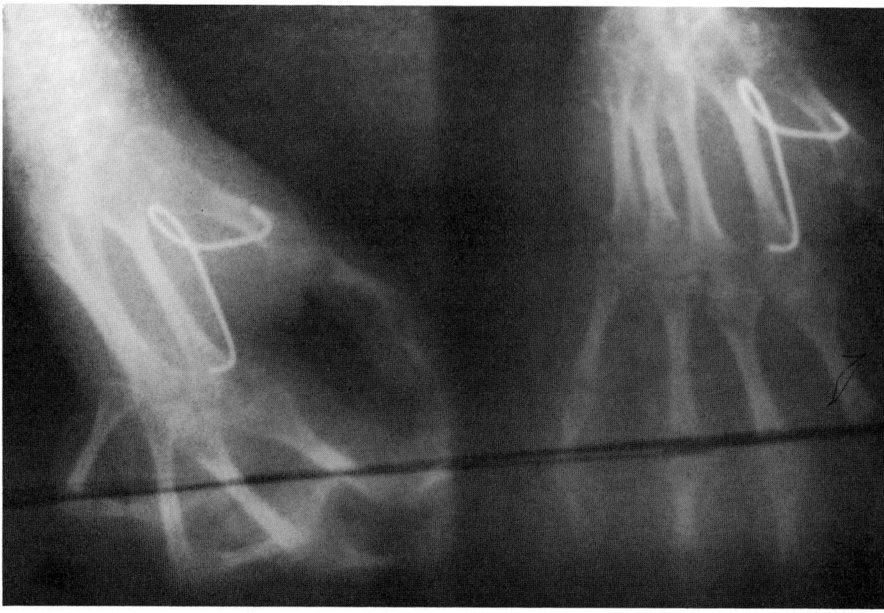

Fig 21-5. Araico internal wire splinting in type 4 thumb spasticity.

gauntlet for another 3 weeks. At that time physical therapy was instituted, and the patients were advised to wear an Orthoplast splint at least at night until growth maturity was reached.

Results

It is very difficult to assess the results of a single deformity in patients with multiple deformities afflicting the upper limb and contributing to the hand imbalance. Because the main objective of the surgical procedures was to correct the deformity and it was hoped, to improve function, a grading system consisting of three categories was utilized:

- *Good:* complete correction of the thumb deformity; the thumb was able to stand out from the palm and could perform pinch and grasp.
- *Fair:* a residual deformity of the thumb remained that did not interfere with the capacity to perform pinch and grasp.
- *Poor:* a residual or a recurrence of the deformity of the thumb remained that interfered with the capacity to perform pinch and grasp.

According to this classification, the postoperative results were: type I, 29 good and 13 fair; type II, 5 good, 2 fair, and 1 poor; type III, 2 good, 2 fair, and 2 poor; and type IV, 1 good, 2 fair, and 1 poor.

Discussion

It is obvious that function cannot be fully restored in these patients because of the neurological damage; however, any improvement in the overall appearance, mobility, and function of the hand is greatly appreciated by the patients and their parents. In many cases the simple fact of being able to clean one's hands more thoroughly is an important benefit that makes the surgical procedure justified.

The active nature of this disease makes the deformities prone to recurrence. It is therefore essential to followup closely and to instruct the patients to wear postoperative splints at least at night until the end of their growth period. Parents must be made aware of the important role they have in the treatment and aftercare of these patients.

The poor results were mainly related to the difficulty in assessing accurately the function of hands affected by cerebral palsy, and hence, to choice of an inadequate surgical procedure or to deficient postoperative management. All these problems have been diminished as more experience is gained by the treatment team.

Many other surgical procedures have been used for the correction of spastic thumbs: for instance, metacarpophalangeal capsulorrhaphy, brachioradialis tendon transfer, transposition of the flexor pollicis longus, and intermetacarpal bone block, but the author does not have any experience with these.

References

1. Cahuzac M, Nichil J, Claverie P, et al: La main hémiplégique de l'enfant I. M. C. *Rev Chir Orthop* 1973;59:321–334.
2. Goldner JL: Upper extremity tendon transfers in cerebral palsy. *Orthop Clin North Am* 1974; 5:389–414.
3. House JH, Gwathmey FW, Fidler MO: A dynamic approach to the thumb-in palm deformity in cerebral palsy. *J Bone Joint Surg Am* 1981; 63A:216–225.
4. Inglis AE, Cooper W, Bruton W: Surgical correction of thumb deformities in spastic paralysis. *J Bone Joint Surg Am* 1970; 52A:253–268.
5. Swanson AB: Surgery of the hand in cerebral palsy and muscle origin release procedures. *Surg Clin North Am* 1968; 48:1129–1136.
6. Goldner JL: The upper extremity in cerebral palsy, in Samilson RL (ed): *Orthopaedic Aspects of Cerebral Palsy.* New York, Harper and Row, 1975, pp 221–257.
7. Swanson AB: Surgery of the hand in cerebral palsy, in Flynn JE (ed): *Hand Surgery,* ed 3. Baltimore, The Williams & Wilkins Co, 1982, pp 476–488.

8. Matev IB: Surgical treatment of flexion-adduction contracture of the thumb in cerebral palsy. Acta Orthop Scand 1970; 41:439–455.
9. Samilson RL: Surgical improvement of the cerebral palsied upper limb. *J Bone Joint Surg Br* 1963; 45B:615–616.
10. Zancolli EA: *Structural and Dynamic Bases of Hand Surgery.* Philadelphia, JB Lippincott Co, 1968. pp 263–283.
11. Zancolli EA, Goldner LJ, Swanson AB: Surgery of the spastic hand in cerebral palsy: Report of the Committee on Spastic Hand Evaluation. *J Hand Surg* 8:766–772, 1983.
12. Chait LA, Kaplan I, Stewart-Lord B, et al: Early surgical correction in the cerebral palsied hand. *J Hand Surg* 1980; 5:122–126.
13. Filler BC, Stark HH, Boyes JH: Capsulodesis of the metacarpophalangeal joint of the thumb in children with cerebral palsy. *J Bone Joint Surg Am* 1976; 58A:667–670.
14. Greene MH: Operative procedures in the cerebral palsied hand. *J Bone Joint Surg Am* 1965; 47A:849–850.
15. Inglis AE: Upper extremity reconstruction in spastic paralysis and related neuromuscular disorders. *American Academy of Orthopaedic Surgeons Instructional Course Lectures* 1977; 26:127–133.
16. Keats S: Surgical treatment of the hand in cerebral palsy: Correction of thumb-in palm and other deformities. *J Bone Joint Surg Am* 1965; 47A:274–284.
17. McCue FC, Honner R, Chapman WC: Transfer of the brachioradialis for hands deformed by cerebral palsy. *J Bone Joint Surg Am* 1970; 52A:1171–1180.
18. Rennie WRJ, Carroll R: The value of extensor pollicis longus enforcement in the spastic adducted thumb. *J Bone Joint Surg Br* 1976; 58B:139.
19. Smith RA: Flexor pollicis longus abductor-plasty for spastic thumb-in deformity. *J Hand Surg* 1982; 7:327–334.
20. Van Rensburg W: Thumb-in-palm in cerebral palsy. *J Bone Joint Surg Am* 1971; 53B:562.
21. Araico JL, Valdes JL, Ortiz JM: An internal wire splint for adduction contracture of the thumb. *Plast Reconstr Surg* 1971; 48:339–342.
22. Lam SJS: A modified technique for stabilizing the spastic thumb. *J Bone Joint Surg Br* 1972; 54B:522–525.

22

Surgical Management of the Arthrogrypotic Thumb

Juan Manuel Fernandez-Vazquez

Arthrogryposis multiplex congenita is a disorder of unknown etiology recognized at birth. It was first described by Otto in 1841. Rosencranz in 1905 was the first to utilize the term *arthrogryposis,* and Stern and Lewin later popularized its use.[1-8] Since then other names have been proposed, such as amyoplasia congenita by Sheldon and myodystrophia foetalis deformans by Middleton.[5]

Arthrogryposis multiplex congenita is characterized by contracture of fibrotic muscles, producing stiffness of the joints with marked wasting of muscle and lack of subcutaneous tissue. Although motor function is very abnormal, sensation is normal and the patients have average or above-average intelligence. The disease seems to be more severe peripherally than centrally.[3,5,8-11]

The clinical appearance of the upper limb has been well documented,[7,11,12] and the deformities present in the thumb have been classically described as hypoplasia, clasping of the thumb into the palm with contracture of the first web space, absence of the extensor and abductor tendons, and laxity of the ulnar collateral ligament at the metacarpophalangeal joint.[1,2,4,5,8,13-16]

Treatment of the arthrogrypotic thumb remains unclear, as different recommendations are given in the literature: opening of the first web space with simple Z-plasty or four-flap Z-plasty with free full-thickness graft or pedicle grafts, either locally or distant;[4,8,12,17,18] osteotomy at the base of the first metacarpal or intermetacarpal bone graft;[8,15] tendon transpositions to augment abduction and opponens plasty utilizing the tendons of the flexor superficialis or the extensor indicis propius;[1,8] and arthrodesis of the carpometacarpal joint or the metacarpophalangeal joint to provide stability.[5,8,15]

Clinical Material

A retrospective study was undertaken of all patients with arthrogrypotic thumb deformities surgically treated from 1976 through 1982 at the Hospital German

Diaz Lombardo for Congenital disorders and the Shriner's Hospital for Crippled Children in Mexico City. As soon as the review was finished, it was evident that four different patterns of thumb deformities were present:

- *Group 1:* Simple adduction of the thumb with partial webbing of the first space (Figs 22-1, 22-2)
- *Group 2:* Flexion of the metacarpophalangeal joint with hyperextension of the interphalangeal joint, with absent or minimal adduction of the first metacarpal (Figs 22-3, 22-4)
- *Group 3:* Flexion of the metacarpophalangeal joint with absent or minimal adduction of the first metacarpal and partial webbing of the first space (Figs 22-4, 22-5)
- *Group 4:* Flexion of the metacarpophalangeal joint with adduction of the first metacarpal and webbing of the first space in the classic "clasped thumb" deformity (Figs 22-6, 22-7).

There were 13 patients with bilateral involvement of the thumbs; of these, 18 thumbs were surgically treated and are the basis of this report. Six of the patients were males and seven females; age at the time of surgery was between 3 and 14 years (average 7.5 years). The right thumb was surgically treated in 8

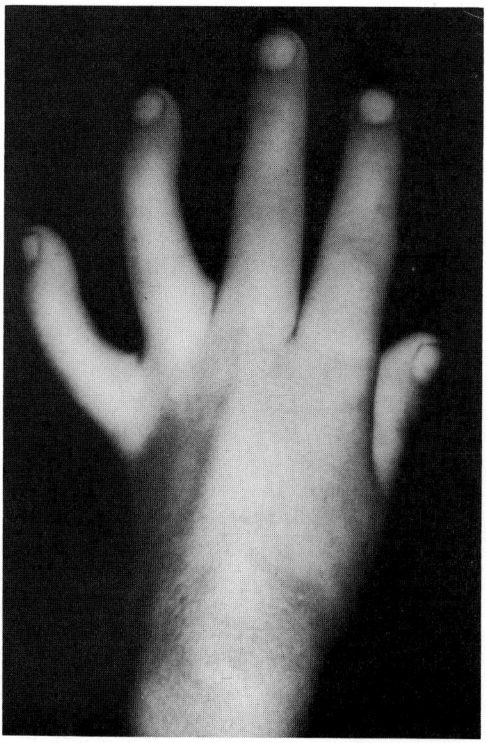

Fig 22-1. Simple arthrogrypotic adduction of the thumb with partial webbing of the first space.

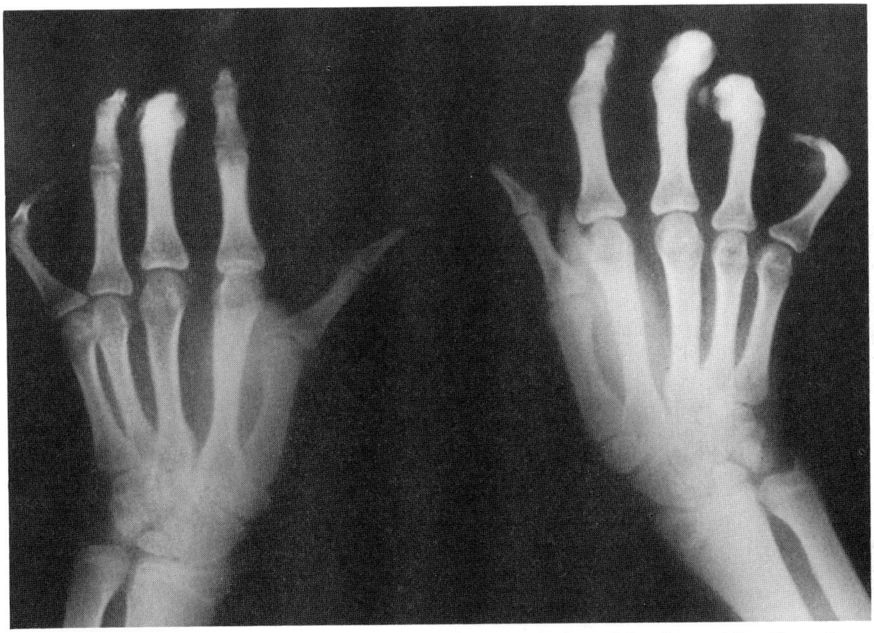

Fig 22-2. Radiographic view of simple arthrogrypotic adduction of the thumbs.

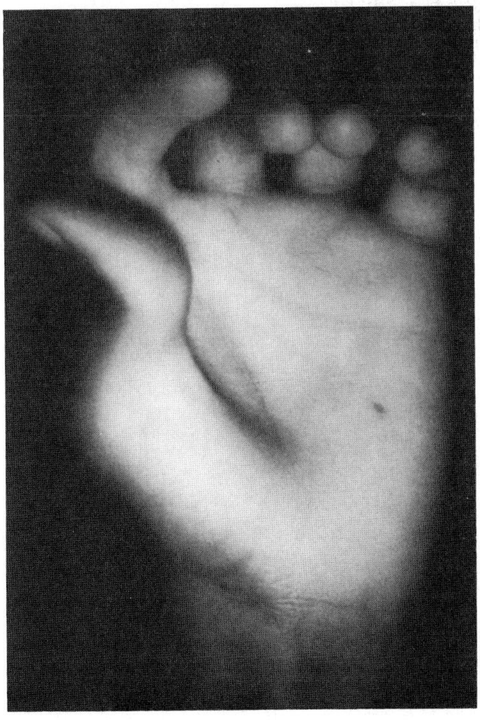

Fig 22-3. Flexion of the metacarpophalangeal joint with hyperextension of the interphalangeal joint.

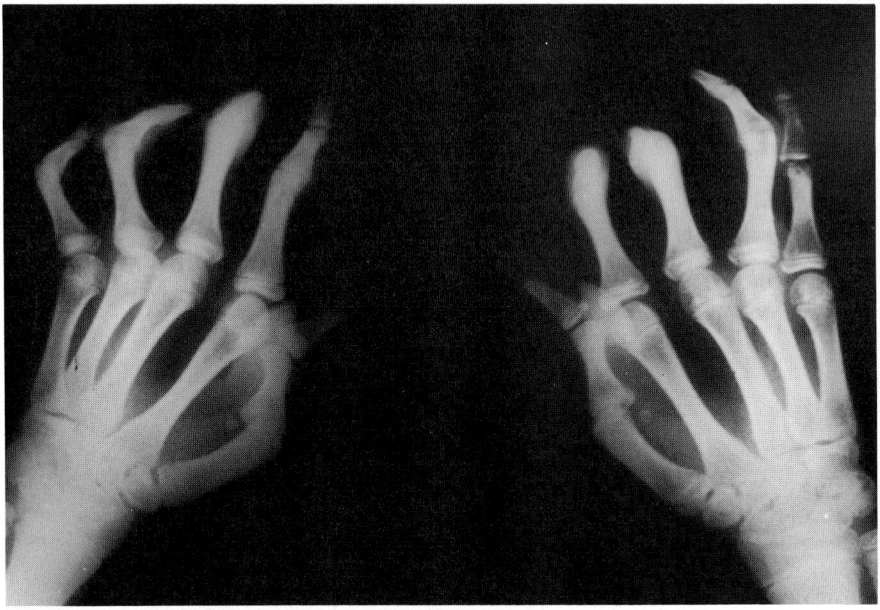

Fig 22-4. Radiographic view of the condition shown in Figure 22-3.

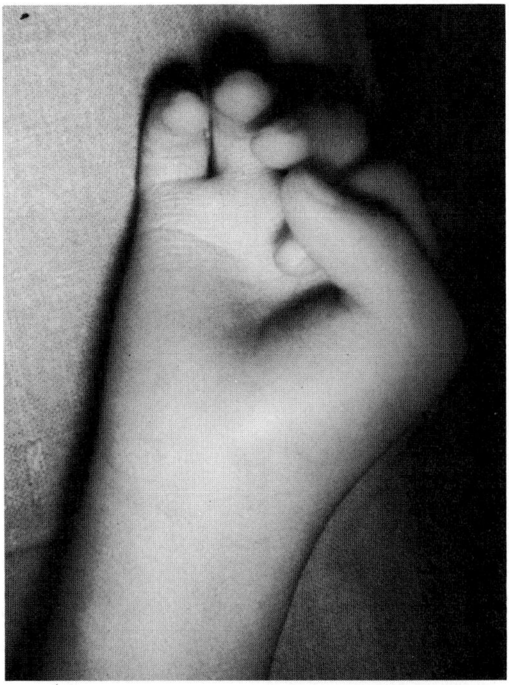

Fig 22-5. Flexion of the metacarpophalangeal joint with minimal adduction of the first metacarpal and partial webbing of the first space.

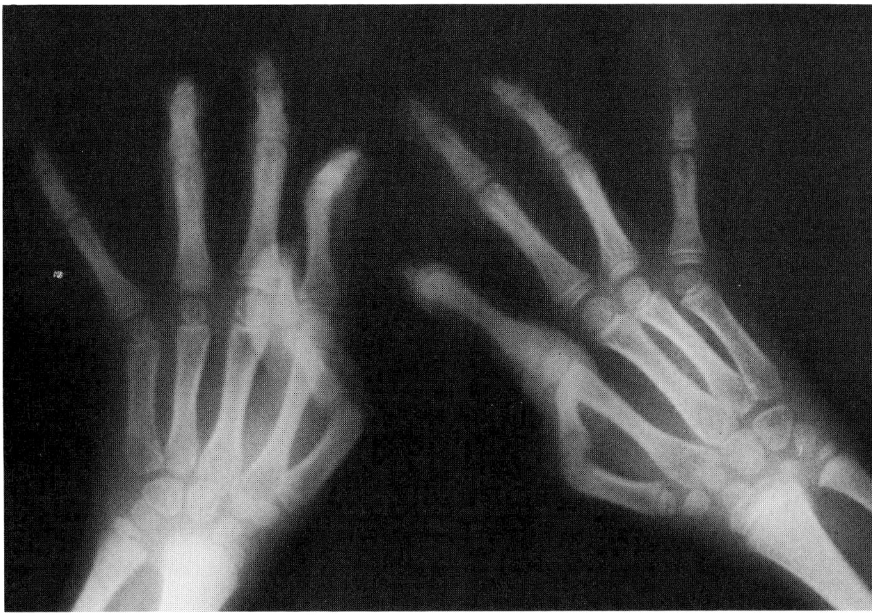

Fig 22-6. Classic "clasped thumb" deformity.

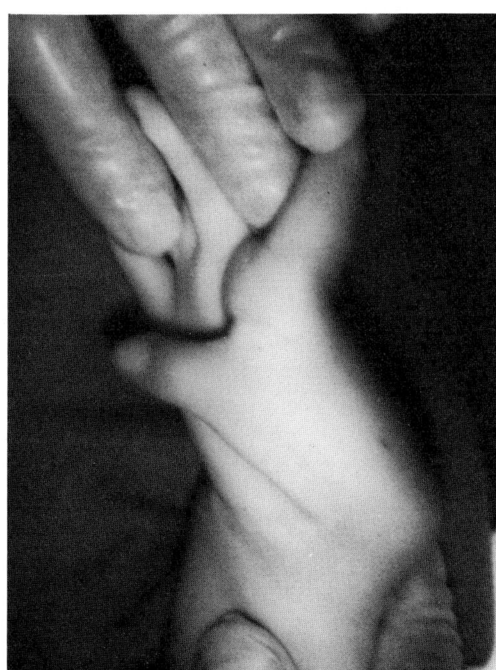

Fig 22-7. Radiographic view of clasped thumb deformity.

patients and the left in 10. According to the above classification, there were two thumbs in group 1, three in group 2, five in group 3, and eight in group 4.

Surgical Procedures

Before the patients were subjected to surgery, splinting was carried out for different periods of time averaging 6 months.

- *Group 1:* Surgery consisted of simple Z-plasty of the first web space with detachment of the first dorsal interosseous from the first metacarpal and section of the adductor pollicis brevis tendon in two cases.
- *Group 2:* Z-Plasty of the first web space with tendon section of the adductor and flexor pollicis brevis, plus arthrodesis of the metacarpophalangeal joint in 3 cases and full-thickness skin graft taken from the groin in 2 cases.
- *Groups 3 and 4:* The first web space was opened by a simple Z-plasty in 12 cases and local pedicle skin graft from the dorsoradial aspect of the index finger in 1 case. Full-thickness skin grafts were taken from the groin in 6 cases, detachment of the first dorsal interosseus and section of the adductor and flexor pollicis brevis tendons in 13, arthrodesis of the metacarpophalangeal joint in 13 cases, and in 1 case Araico's[19] internal wire splint was inserted because of a tendency to maintain the first web space contracture besides the sectioning of the previous described muscles.

All the Kirschner wires were left protruding from the skin. The hands were immobilized with a voluminous compression dressing and a plaster splint above the elbow for 3 weeks. At that time, the sutures were removed and a thumb plaster gauntlet was applied for another 3 weeks or until healing of the arthrodesis was achieved. Then the Kirschner wires were removed. The patients were advised to continue the immobilization at night with a splint for another 6 months.

Complications

There were no major complications. Two cases had partial necrosis of the full-thickness skin graft, which healed with local measures. Two patients developed contracture scars in the radiopalmar aspect of the metacarpophalangeal joint of the index finger; the scars did not interfere with the overall function of the hand.

No patient was made worse after surgery, and the patients and their parents were very pleased with the amount of correction of the deformity and the improved function obtained. The minimum follow-up after surgery has been 2 years and the maximum 6 years; three patients have reached osseous maturity, and no recurrence of the deformities has been documented.

Discussion

The deformities of the upper extremity in arthrogryposis multiplex congenita are difficult to correct, and many are due to a delay in the initiation of treatment. Tachdjian[10] recommends beginning at birth with small plaster casts followed by bivalved night casts. Williams[8] is convinced that aggressive surgical treatment in infancy and childhood is more successful than previously accepted methods of care.

The objectives of the treatment are to correct the deformity present and, if possible, to increase motion both actively and passively. Usually the former can be obtained, but the latter is very difficult in the hand because of the deficiency in the motor muscles, the wrong line of muscle pull, and the joint surfaces being oriented at a wrong angle,[8] which explains why the tendon transfers used to improve the abduction and extension of the thumb have consistently failed.

Dangles et al[1] reported good results in four cases treated with tendon transpositions to improve opposition of the thumb; they used the ring finger flexor superficialis tendon in three cases and the extensor indicis propius in one. Mead et al[5] were the first to recommend metacarpophalangeal joint fusion plus widening of the first web space with pedicle grafts. From this review it is evident that at least four different types of thumb deformities are present in arthrogryposis multiplex congenita, and these explain fully the great variety of surgical procedures recommended in the literature. Usually patients are very cooperative, and a good deal of benefit can be obtained when the deformities are corrected. A good understanding of the different pathological changes found in the arthrogrypotic thumb is mandatory in order to select the appropriate surgical treatment.

References

1. Dangles CJ, Bilos ZJ: Surgical correction of thumb deformity in arthrogryposis multiplex congenita. *Hand* 1981;13:55–58.
2. Drummond DS, Siller TM, Cruess RL: Management of arthrogryposis multiplex congenita. *American Academy of Orthopaedic Surgeons Instructional Course Lecture* 1974;23:79–95.
3. Friedlander HL, Westin GW, Wood WL Jr: Arthrogryposis multiplex congenita. *J Bone Joint Surg Am* 1968;50A:89–112.
4. Gibson DA, Urs DK: Arthrogryposis multiplex congenita. *J Bone Joint Surg Br* 1970;52B:483–493.
5. Mead NG, Lithgow WC, Sweeney HJ: Arthrogryposis multiplex congenita. *J Bone Joint Surg Am* 1958;40A:1285–1309.

6. Shariff FK, Horoupian D, Greenlaw RK: Arthrogryposis multiplex congenita. *Clin Orthop* 1973;94:263–267.
7. Weeks PM: Surgical correction of upper extremity deformities in arthrogrypotics. *Plast Reconstr Surg* 1965;36:459–465.
8. Williams P: The management of arthrogryposis. *Orthop Clin North Am* 1978;9:67–88.
9. Hansen OM: Surgical anatomy and treatment of patients with arthrogryposis. *J Bone Joint Surg Br* 1961;43B:855.
10. Tachdjian MP: *Pediatric Orthopedics.* Philadelphia, WB Saunders Co, 1972, pp 232–243.
11. Weeks PM: Surgical correction of arthrogrypotic deformities of the upper extremity. *J Bone Surg Am* 1967;49A:579–580.
12. Greene MH: Cryptic problems of arthrogryposis multiplex congenita. *J Bone Joint Surg Am* 1963;45A:885–886.
13. Bayne LG: Arthrogryposis, in Green DP (ed): *Operative Hand Surgery.* New York, Churchill Livingstone, 1982, pp 306–308.
14. Gibson D, Urs K: Arthrogryposis. *J Bone Joint Surg Br* 1969;51B:191.
15. Kelikian K: *Congenital Deformities of the Hand and Forearm.* Philadelphia, WB Saunders Co, 1974, pp 585–592.
16. Lloyd-Roberts GC, Lettin AWF: Arthrogryposis multiplex congenita. *J Bone Joint Surg Br* 1970; 52B:494–508.
17. Flatt A: *The Care of Congenital Hand Anomalies.* St Louis, CV Mosby Co, 1977, pp 61-62.
18. Meyn M, Ruby L: Arthrogryposis of the upper extremity. *Orthop Clin North Am* 1976;7:501-509.
19. Araico JL, Valdes JL, Ortiz JM: An internal wire splint for adduction contracture of the thumb. *Plast Reconstr Surg* 1971;48:339-342.
20. Smith RJ: Hand deformities with arthrogryposis multiplex congenita. *J Bone Joint Surg Am* 1973;55A:883.

23

Extensor Tendon Injuries

Robert L. Horner

Extensor tendon injuries are much more common than flexor tendon injuries. Surgeons in general have respect for flexor tendon injuries and frequently feel that extensor tendon injuries are easier to handle and better results can be obtained. However, there are major pitfalls where severe imbalance of the hand can occur following a seemingly trivial injury.

Areas of major concern include (Fig 23-1):

- *The hand:* Associated problems of the underlying bone, such as fractures of the metacarpals, can cause adherence, resulting in hand stiffness, with not only lack of good extension but lack of flexion.
- *The metacarpophalangeal joints:* There is the concern of infection from teeth wounds received during a fistfight.
- *The proximal interphalangeal joints:* A boutonnière deformity can occur.
- *The distal interphalangeal joints:* A mallet finger deformity can occur.

This chapter will discuss the general principles that apply to all types of extensor tendon injuries and then emphasize specific injuries that can cause complex problems.

Anatomical Considerations

Forearm

The wrist extensors arise from origins both distal and proximal to the elbow. Innervation is from the radial nerve with motor branches arising not only above but also below the elbow. The musculotendinous junctions are at various levels

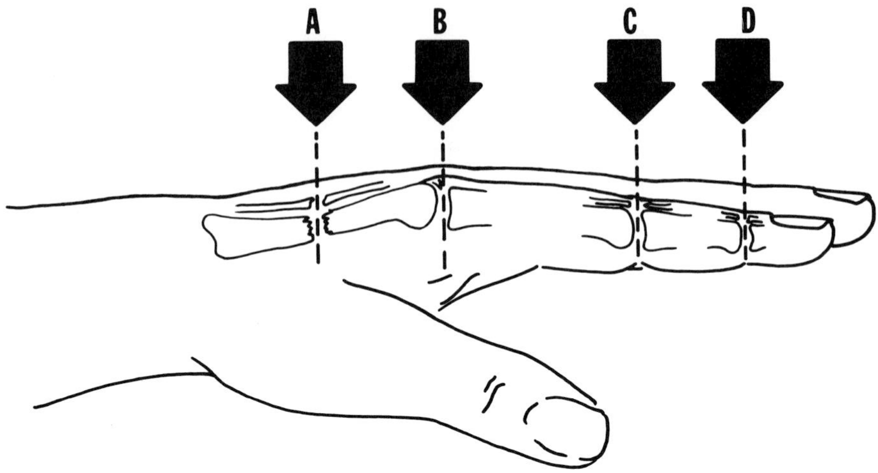

Fig 23-1. Areas of special problems with extensor tendon injuries.

in the forearm, and the extensor tendons are covered with a layer of paratenon. The paratenon provides the cut ends with active tissues that will proliferate and attempt to restore continuity, but if the wrist is not splinted during the healing process, the extensor mechanism will be too long and efficiency of the wrist extension will be lost. There are fascial bands and tendinous structures high in the forearm that are important for proper musculotendinous tension and function and that can be repaired.

Wrist

The extensor retinaculum over the dorsum of the wrist is a complex ligamentous system with compartments that guide the movement of the tendons as they pass over the dorsum of the wrist. This pulley system is unyielding, and cut tendons in this area present problems similar to those of flexor tendons in the digital sheaths. Any enlargement at the tendon junction will cause impingement. Ingrowth of adhesions will cause adherence.

Metacarpals

Tendon injuries at the metacarpal level are usually associated with damage to underlying bone as well as to the overlying skin. Because all of the adjacent tissues will heal with one continuous scar, adherence is a particular problem in this area, since there is minimal paratendinous tissue. The skin is only a millimeter away superficially and the bone only a little further away.

A helpful, but sometimes confusing feature is the presence of the intertendinous bands (Fig 23-2) which allow finger extension even when an isolated

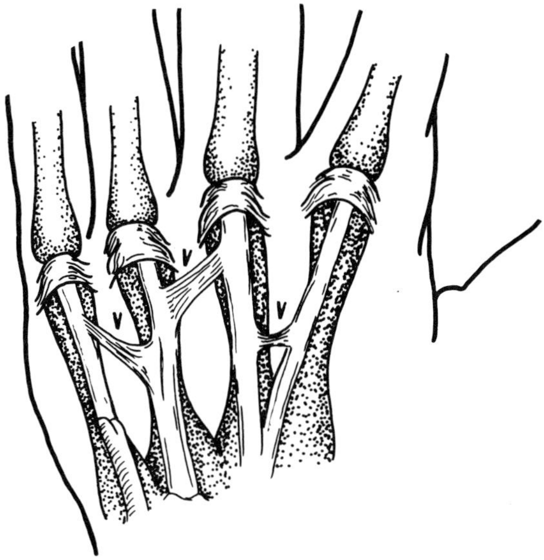

Fig 23-2. The intertendinous bands, or juncturae tendinum, (*arrows*) can transmit force from an intact tendon to a cut tendon, resulting in confusion in diagnosis. They can also cause an abnormal ulnar pull with fifth metacarpal depression when closing the hand, resulting in dislocation of an extensor tendon.

extensor tendon is completely cut. Another factor is the presence of two extensor tendons to each of three of the digits (thumb, index, and little fingers). This allows independent extension of these digits, but it should be remembered that the extensor digitorum tendons to the index and long fingers have quite independent motion. Thus, even with loss of the extensor indicis, complete index finger extension may still be possible when the other digits are flexed.

Metacarpophalangeal Joint

At the metacarpophalangeal joint level, the extensor tendons take on a more complex structure, with the blending of the extrinsic and intrinsic extensors into the dorsal mechanism. The intrinsic muscles exert flexion force through their bony attachments and by their insertions into the dorsal apparatus, whereas the extrinsic extensors extend the same joint by force around the base of the proximal phalanx through the sagittal fibers of the extensor mechanism, attaching to the volar plate.

The centralization of the extensor tendon over the dorsum of the metacarpophalangeal joint depends on the integrity of the fibers of the sagittal bands. The angle of pull of the extensor tendons, especially in the long finger, is such that there is an ulnar deviation force on the extensor tendon, and this is aggravated by the pull of the intertendinous bands from the little and ring finger extensors as the ulnar metacarpal heads descend during flexion. Some people have marked flexibility of their fourth and fifth metacarpals, and this can accentuate the deforming force and become a factor in recurrence of ulnar displacement of the extensor tendons.

Proximal Phalanx

Because of the convexity of the underlying phalanx and the overlying extensor mechanism (Fig 23-3), it is virtually impossible to cut the entire width of the extensor mechanism at this level without significant bony damage. If there are fractures of the proximal phalanx they should be stabilized enough to permit early motion and avoid adherence of the damaged tendon to the underlying bone.

Proximal Interphalangeal Joint

The central portion of the extensor mechanism can be completely detached from the base of the middle phalanx, and for a few days the lateral bands will still provide full extension of the proximal interphalangeal joint. As the weak triangular portion of the extensor mechanism stretches with overuse, the lateral bands will separate and migrate palmarly until their route is on the flexor side of the axis of motion of the proximal interphalangeal joint. Then the extensor mechanism will no longer act as a proximal interphalangeal joint extensor, but will only pull the middle phalanx into more flexion. The end result is that the head of the proximal phalanx will "buttonhole" through the attenuated extensor mechanism, resulting in a boutonnière deformity (Fig 23-4). The structure of the proximal interphalangeal joint is such that the palmar portion of the collateral ligaments will become contracted and the volar plate adheres. A fixed deformity will result. The oblique fibers of the retinacular system will thicken, and flexion of the distal interphalangeal joint will soon be limited.

Distal Interphalangeal Joint

A cut or rupture of the tendon in the area of the distal interphalangeal joint will be overpulled by the strong opposing flexors, resulting in a mallet deformity

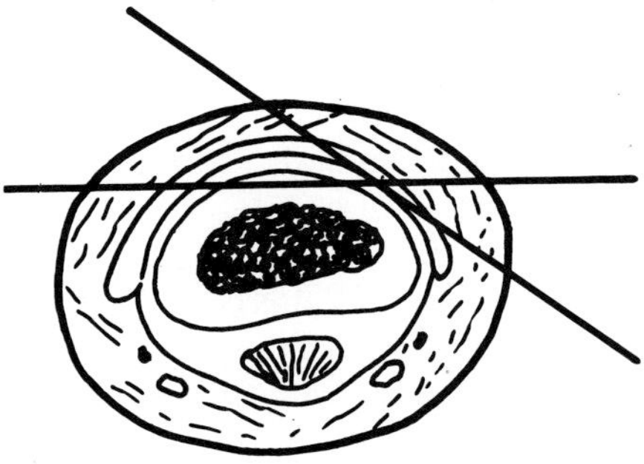

Fig 23-3. Cross section of the proximal phalanx. The lines represent saw cuts or knife cuts showing how the convexity of the extensor mechanism against the underlying bone protects against lacerations of the entire width of the extensor mechanism.

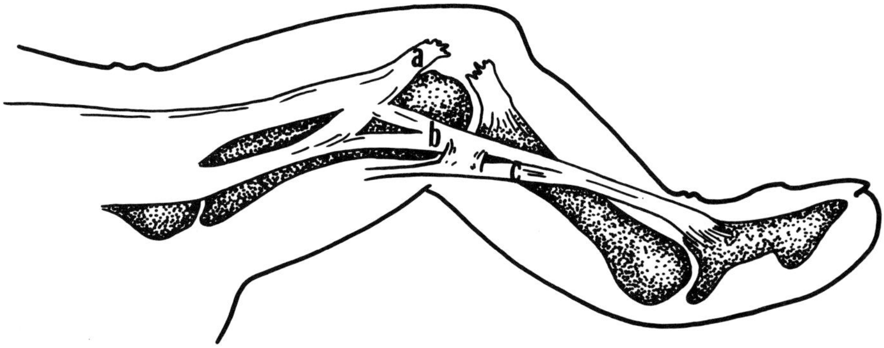

Fig 23-4. Boutonnière deformity. *a,* Ruptured or lacerated central slip; *b,* palmarly displaced lateral band, preventing active proximal interphalangeal joint extension; *c,* contracted oblique retinacular ligament, resulting in hyperextension deformity of the distal joint.

(Fig 23-5). The overlying skin is thin, presenting problems for proper splinting because pressure is not tolerated well.

Wound Healing Considerations

Outside their fibrous sheaths, cut tendons have a marked tendency to proliferate. A cut extensor tendon will try to "satisfy its ends" and reestablish its continuity. The tendon will heal, but the tension will not be proper if splinting has not been adequate.

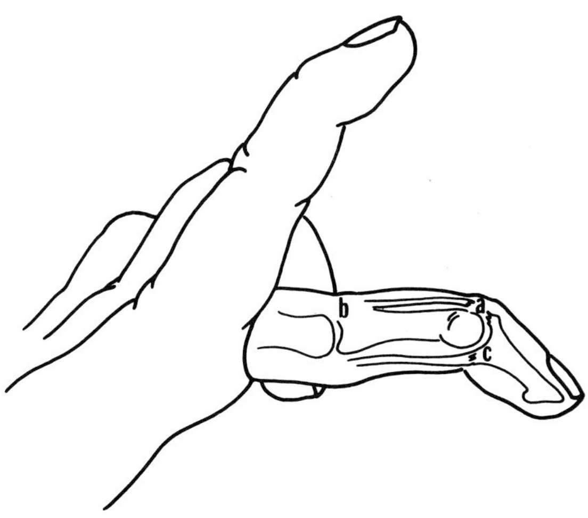

Fig 23-5. Mallet finger deformity. *a,* Ruptured or lacerated extensor mechanism at the base of the distal phalanx; *b,* associated mild hyperextension of the proximal interphalangeal joint; *c,* overpull of the intact flexor digitorum profundus tendon, resulting in the "drop" finger deformity.

Biomechanical Considerations

Even with a healed tendon, function will not be good if there is an increase in length (resulting in an extensor lag), or if there has been too much shortening (resulting in lack of flexion). The normal excursion of extensor tendons is very short, so that even a length discrepancy of as little as 2 to 3 mm will result in a functional loss. The digital extensors attach close to the joints, and because of the short lever arms, tension is much more critical when dealing with extensor tendon injuries. In contrast, flexor tendons have excursions of several centimeters, and the moment of motion at the joint is usually 1 or 2 cm.

The difference is in the nature of the extensor tendons, which are thin when compared to their opposing flexors, and the strengths of the muscles are markedly different. The extensor tendons of the digits are not designed for strength but for positioning. The tendon attachments are designed for speed in positioning so that the digits can be placed so the stronger flexors can then grasp and pinch. If flexion is not controlled by proper splinting, the weak, tenuous extensors will be overstretched or ruptured, and deformity will result.

Splinting of the joint must be carefully controlled during a 6-week period for extensor tendons, whereas 3 ½ to 4 weeks will usually suffice for flexor tendons.

Mechanisms of Injury

Blunt trauma can result in extensor tendon rupture. Swelling, pain, and stiffness due to associated injury can obscure the nature of the problem early. A partial tendon rupture can progress to a complex lesion as the joint capsule and intact tendinous structures stretch.

Open injuries can be due to knives, saws, burns, or any object that can cause crushing. Each type of wound presents its own complicating factors, and it is important to know as much as possible about the injury, because decisions concerning proper care must be based on a good knowledge of the patient, the wound, and the condition of the surrounding tissues.

Diagnosis

Many extensor tendon injuries are obvious, but a high level of suspicion is necessary for complete evaluation. All of the modalities of physical diagnosis have a role, but specific techniques are often required. An adequate account of the injury will help in all cases. Careful inspection of swelling and finger position overlying an area of tendon damage is necessary for a proper choice of treatment. A skin laceration over an extensor tendon will require direct inspection, and surgical extension of the wound is almost always necessary for complete evaluation.

Palpation over the base of the middle phalanx may reveal tenderness, which often is the first sign of partial central slip rupture. Even when there is a full range of motion there can be a complete extensor digitorum laceration. It is important to determine any lack of strength in order to elicit any subtle laceration masked by the force exerted through the intertendinous bands from the adjacent tendons.

Longitudinal compression on the bones of the hand and forearm may elicit pain from unsuspected fractures of the underlying bones. Careful palpation over the dorsum of the digit, hand, and forearm may reveal tenderness over retracted tendon ends. Palpable and even audible crepitation over the dorsum of the forearm can indicate tendon attrition that can result in eventual tendon rupture. Tenderness over the wrist may indicate a tenosynovitis developing in the compartments of the dorsal retinaculum.

Treatment

Closed mallet finger deformities can be treated by external splinting, and even old injuries at the distal joint level respond to closed methods of treatment.

Three basic types of splints can be used. Usually a molded plastic Stack splint is the most convenient (Fig 23-6A). Moleskin adhesive lining of a portion of the splint may be helpful for giving a proper fit when one size is too tight and the next larger size without the padding would be too loose. Providing an instruction sheet to the patient and his or her family will help ensure compliance. If the physician and the staff have confidence in the splinting, the patient will understand the importance of the conservative program and will cooperate for the 6 weeks or more that may be necessary.

Padded metal splints can be used palmarly (Fig 23-6B) or dorsally. Motion of the proximal interphalangeal joint is encouraged, and any splint should immobilize only the distal joint.

Uninterrupted distal joint extension is required. Just one flexion motion in the early weeks could overstretch the immature healing tissue and mean that the 6-week period of immobilization has to be started again. Protection against excessive hyperextension and pressure is needed to prevent an ulcer from developing over the dorsum of the base of the distal phalanx.

After the 6-week initial period of full-time splinting, careful monitoring is needed for another 2 months. During this time, the splint may be needed at night, when driving, and when the patient is engaging in strenuous activity. The patient can be given a short cardboard pattern outlining the finger position when at full, active extension of the distal joint. Each evening the patient can hold the pattern along the dorsum of the finger and detect any loss of extension. If a lag is developing, the patient can start using the splint again full-time for another 4 weeks and then can monitor progress and receive further treatment as needed.

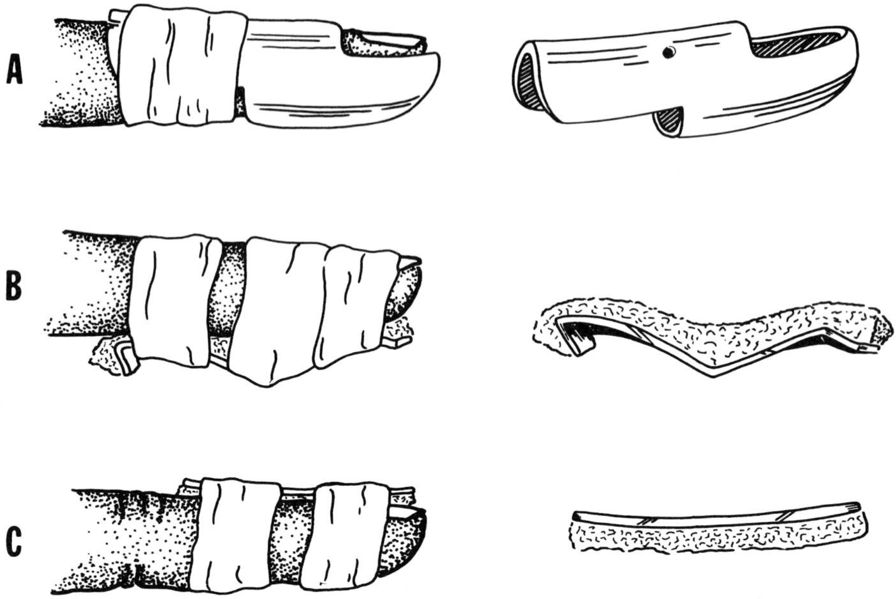

Fig 23-6. Splints for closed mallet finger deformities. *a,* Stack splint; *b,* palmar splint to support the distal joint in full extension; *c,* dorsal splint in full extension. All of these splints allow proximal interphalangeal joint motion. The dorsal splint allows tactile function of the distal finger pad.

Open mallet finger deformities require intramedullary 0.035-inch Kirschner wire fixation in full extension (Fig 23-7). The pin can be inserted by a power drill after making a 5-mm distal incision just palmar to the nail. The pin is passed 1 cm proximal to the distal joint. The position is confirmed by x-ray examination. The pin should be left protruding about 3 mm, and an external splint should be used so that the danger of pin breakage is minimized.

Boutonnière Deformity

Closed injuries are treated by splinting of the proximal interphalangeal joint in full extension (Fig 23-8). Metacarpophalangeal and distal joint flexion should be encouraged. If there is no active proximal interphalangeal joint extension, but there is full passive extension, open central slip repair should be considered, even in a closed injury.

Closed splinting is difficult if there is a dorsal wound, so an internal splint in the form of an oblique 0.045-inch Kirschner wire (Fig 23-9) should be inserted if there is a dorsal incision or wound.

Surgery will not help a boutonnière deformity if there is a fixed flexion deformity. A passive range of extension must be obtained preoperatively by progressive splinting.

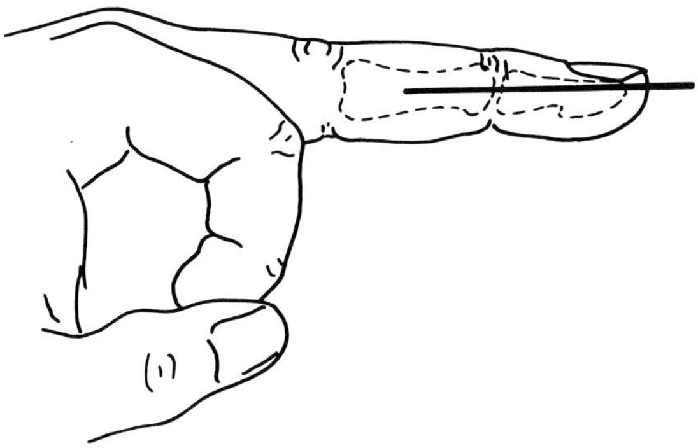

Fig 23-7. Closed mallet deformity treated with percutaneous intramedullary Kirschner wire fixation across the distal interphalangeal joint.

Serial casting (Fig 23-10), using 1.5-cm-wide strips of rolled, extra-fast-setting plaster of Paris may be the most effective way of correcting a fixed deformity. The patient or an assistant pulls the finger lengthwise into extension as the plaster is applied directly on the skin. No pressure is exerted over the dorsum of the joint, so ulceration is unlikely to develop. The patient must understand the need to avoid undue pressure, and hand elevation may be necessary to prevent swelling in the cast. Ideally the plaster will be changed twice a week until full passive extension is possible. A removable splint can then be used for an additional 4 weeks, and surgery may not be necessary, for full correction is often obtained by the splinting program. The extensor mechanism can often readjust its length if a passive range of motion is maintained. Surgery is performed if a persistent lag of the proximal interphalangeal joint is noted, meaning that there is better passive extension than active extension. Surgery should only be done if necessary, and then the minimal amount of surgery that achieves a good correction is the best.

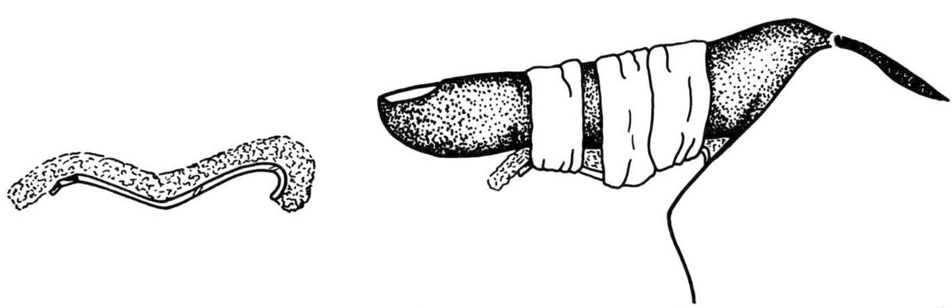

Fig 23-8. Closed boutonnière deformity treated by a palmar-padded metal splint holding the proximal interphalangeal joint in extension but allowing distal interphalangeal joint flexion.

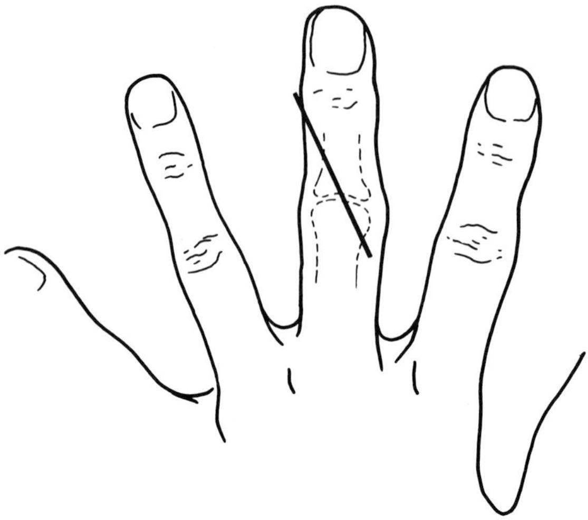

Fig 23-9. An open boutonnière deformity or central slip laceration with potential boutonnière deformity is best treated by an oblique Kirschner wire holding the proximal interphalangeal joint in full extension.

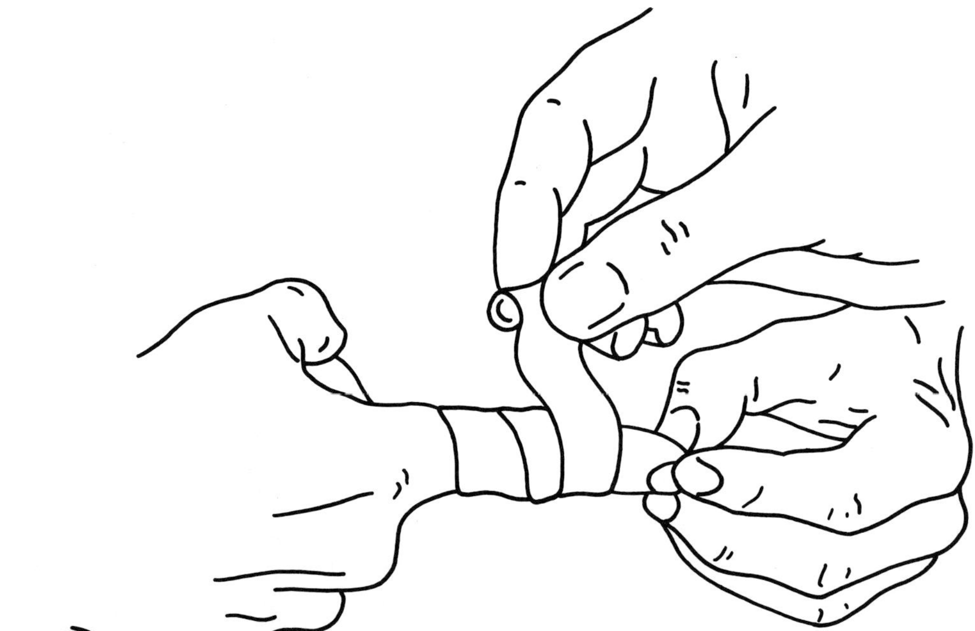

Fig 23-10. Serial casting using plaster of Paris bandages to immobilize the proximal interphalangeal joint in as much extension as can be obtained while the patient places traction of his or her own finger while the plaster is reapplied.

A fixed boutonnière deformity is a difficult problem, and often full correction is not possible. Prolonged splinting programs are usually preferable to the unacceptable alternatives of surgery in the face of fixed deformity, fusion, or amputation.

Metacarpophalangeal Joint

Extensor tendon injuries at the metacarpophalangeal joint level are frequently associated with contaminated wounds. Early tendon repair should not be done if there is any suspicion that the wound may have been caused by a human tooth. Joint destruction and chronic bone infection are real possibilities with this type of wound, and tendon repair should be delayed until any wound healing problems are solved. Proper splinting without direct tendon suture may be preferable.

Splinting of the wrist in extension is essential so that tension is removed from the damaged tendon without having to hold the metacarpophalangeal joint in full extension. Splinting the metacarpophalangeal joint completely straight for 2 weeks will result in contracture of the collateral ligament and the dorsal capsule, limiting future flexion. The tendon junction will be protected if the wrist is splinted in 45° extension and the metacarpophalangeal joints are held in 25° of flexion for 4 weeks. Any subsequent lag of extension can be treated by the use of a night splint in full metacarpal extension part-time during the next 4 to 6 weeks.

Metacarpals

Wounds in the metacarpal area should be excised, extended, and repaired as needed. The extensor tendons should be repaired by buried knot or removable suture techniques. Any associated fracture should be stabilized completely so that early protective motion can be begun. Complete immobilization of a damaged tendon over a fracture will result in scarring that will not only preclude good digital extension, but also prevent adequate flexion. Good bone and tendon fixation combined with a careful program of hand therapy has the best chance of resulting in function.

Wrist

Tendon junctions will not glide through the compartments of a damaged retinacular system. Single-tendon injuries are best treated by excision of the overlying ligaments and careful suturing.

Multiple-tendon injuries should be treated by transfer of the retinaculum deep to the damaged tendons. The proximal forearm fascia will prevent "bowstringing" of the tendons as the wrist is extended, and the overlying subcutaneous fat will allow gliding that would have been prevented if the retinacular system were still there.

Forearm

Repair of all structures is important. Often complete restoration of muscle and tendinous function can be obtained by meticulous repair of all structures using fine sutures and loupe magnification.

Postoperative Treatment

The key to proper care is adequate splinting in a proper position. Lacerations of the extensor tendons over the forearm or hand do not require that the interphalangeal joints be immobilized. Elbow motion combined with elevation and interphalangeal joint flexion should be encouraged. Well-sutured tendons over the dorsum of the wrist can be allowed to glide during controlled therapy sessions, as the metacarpophalangeal joints are held temporarily in full extension, and the wrist is allowed to be brought into 20° of extension instead of the usual 45°.

As healing progresses, careful monitoring of an extension lag is necessary. Later measurements need to be taken of fingertip-to-palm distances to ensure that there is a gradual resumption of full flexion.

Conclusion

Extensor tendon injuries at all levels require careful evaluation and treatment. The patient and the family need to understand the necessity of proper immobilization, elevation, and gradual exercises. The final result is usually not known until 3 to 4 months after the injury. Good results can be obtained by careful attention to details.

Acknowledgment

Special thanks are expressed to Stephen J. Nazario, Porter Memorial Hospital, Denver, Colorado, for the illustrations.

24

Pathomechanics of the Finger Metacarpophalangeal Joint in Rheumatoid Arthritis

Thomas G. Wadsworth

In the normal individual an intricate musculotendinous system, with fine interplay among its elements, is combined with the architecture of the bones and joints which together make up the arches of the hand and allow for a fine but vulnerable balance. By contrast, in the rheumatoid hand the restraining ligamentous tissue is lengthened, balance is compromised and there is deranged mechanical equilibrium; daily use of the hand in these circumstances compounds the progress of the deformity[1].

Common deformities of the metacarpophalangeal joint of the finger in the rheumatoid patient include ulnar drift, subluxation and dislocation, rotation of the digit (particularly pronation of the index finger), distortion of the hood mechanism, and dislocation of the extrinsic extensor tendon, usually ulnarward.

The natural history of rheumatoid synovitis of the joint begins with synovial proliferation, which may herniate laterally[2]. Expansion of the joint occurs and the disease leads to laxity of the collateral ligaments, the capsule, and the volar plate. The stage is then set for subluxation and dislocation of the joint (Fig 24-1 and 24-2). Stretching of the radial sagittal fibers of the extensor hood results in loss of central extensor balance, and there is medial migration of the tendon. Ulnar drift is thereby perpetuated and increased, the joint sometimes becoming locked in flexion (Fig 24-3). Radial deviation of the wrist significantly increases the risk of ulnar drift of the fingers, and a combination of the two deformities is classic in the rheumatoid hand and wrist.

Subluxation of the metacarpophalangeal joint is increased by intrinsic and flexor muscle contraction. Tightening of the intrinsic mechanism results in a tendency toward proximal interphalangeal (PIP) joint hyperextension. The extent of this deformity depends upon the degree of normal elasticity of the capsule and ligaments and the degree of rheumatoid involvement in the particular joint.

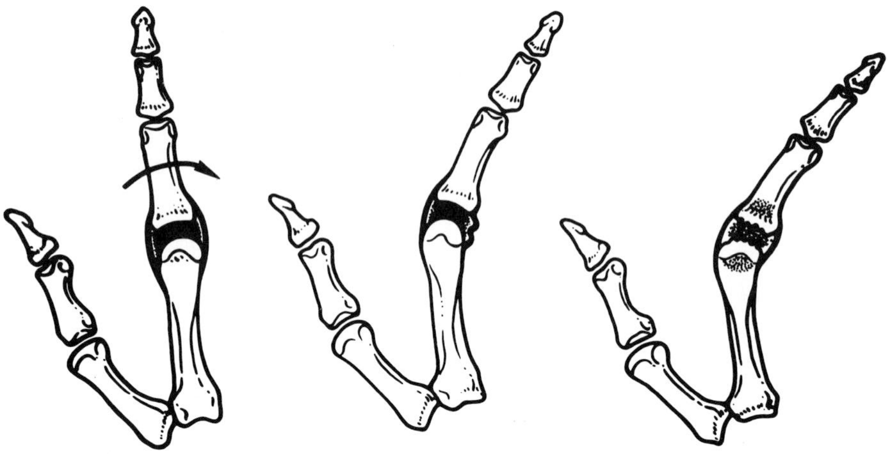

Fig 24-1. Synovitis expands the metacarpophalangeal joint, leading to stretching of the collateral ligaments and capsule. Instability results with the potential for subluxation and ulnar drift. Rotation of the index finger can occur with pronation deformity, shown in this palmar view. Pannus formation is also shown.

There is normal inclination toward slight ulnar drift of the fingers at rest in the average individual, greatest in the index finger. Normally this is correctable, but if not, hand function is threatened. There is lateral mobility of the joint in extension because the collateral ligaments are lax; this mobility is lost at 70° of flexion and beyond as the ligaments become taut. Importantly, the index radial collateral ligament tends to resist abnormal rotation and ulnar deviation of the digit.

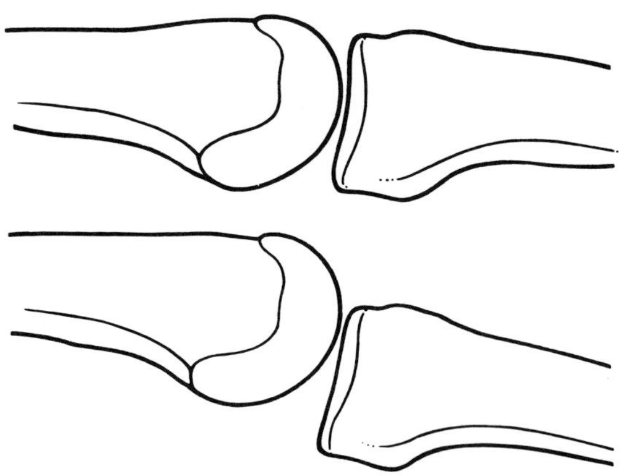

Fig 24-2. Forward subluxation of the proximal phalanx on the metacarpal head, a result of rheumatoid expansion of the joint.

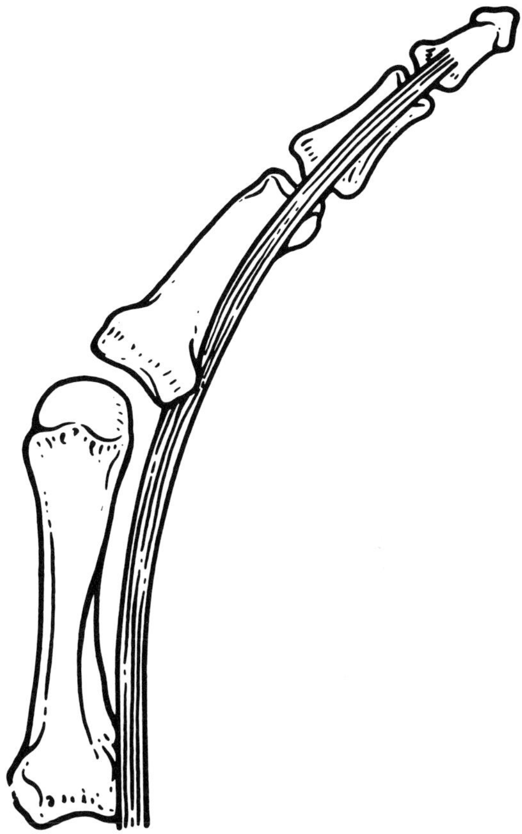

Fig 24-3. Medial deviation of the extensor tendon perpetuates and increases the ulnar drift of the finger. Centralization of the tendon is an important part of the reconstruction of such a joint. In an extreme case, the joint may be locked in flexion.

There is a clear relationship between radial deviation of the carpus and metacarpus and ulnar drift of the fingers[3]; arthrodesis of the wrist with only 5° of radial deviation can result in significant risk of ulnar drift of the fingers in the rheumatoid patient. With pathological ulnar drift, the ulnar intrinsic mechanism tightens and drift is thereby accelerated. In these circumstances active extension of the fingers by the patient results in tightening of the PIP joints in extension by the intrinsic mechanism; the extrinsic extensor tendon pulls primarily on the middle phalanx through the central slip insertion, and the stage is set for swan-neck deformity.

Ulnar drift in the rheumatoid patient is produced by a dynamic imbalance of forces within the hand acting on the intercalated joint system of the hand and wrist. There is a zigzag collapse deformity of the wrist and the metacarpophalangeal joint, with gradual progressive sliding ulnarward of the extrinsic extensor tendon at the metacarpophalangeal joint. Integrity of the radial collateral ligament of the index metacarpophalangeal joint is important in controlling ulnar drift deformity of the fingers. With regard to the flexor tendons, ulnar torque on the inner side of the palm produces a dislocating force on the metacarpophalangeal joints. Laxity of the metacarpophalangeal joint ligaments, capsule, and volar plate can lead to palmar and ulnar deviation of the pulley entrance which is accentuated by flexor synovitis, an often common feature in the rheumatoid patient (Fig 24-4). Additionally, the ulnar interossei are generally stronger than the radial interossei. Therefore, in addition to extensor tendon forces on the back of the hand, the flexor tendons play their part in producing pathological ulnar drift of the fingers in the rheumatoid patient. Trigger finger release can compound this problem by increasing the deviating forces on the flexor tendons. A proximal pulley should be left in order to minimize the risk of initiating or perpetuating ulnar drift of the fingers.

Within the joint, synovial pannus crosses the articular surfaces and infiltrates deep into the bone, so that the articular cartilage is attacked from above and below (Fig 24-1). These changes in the articular cartilage can lead to fibrous and even bony ankylosis in deformity.

Involved in ulnar drift of the fingers in the rheumatoid patient are synovitis of the metacarpophalangeal joint, the extrinsic extensor tendons, the flexor tendons, and the intrinsic tendons and descent of the fourth and fifth metacarpals with volar displacement of the extensor carpi ulnaris tendon.

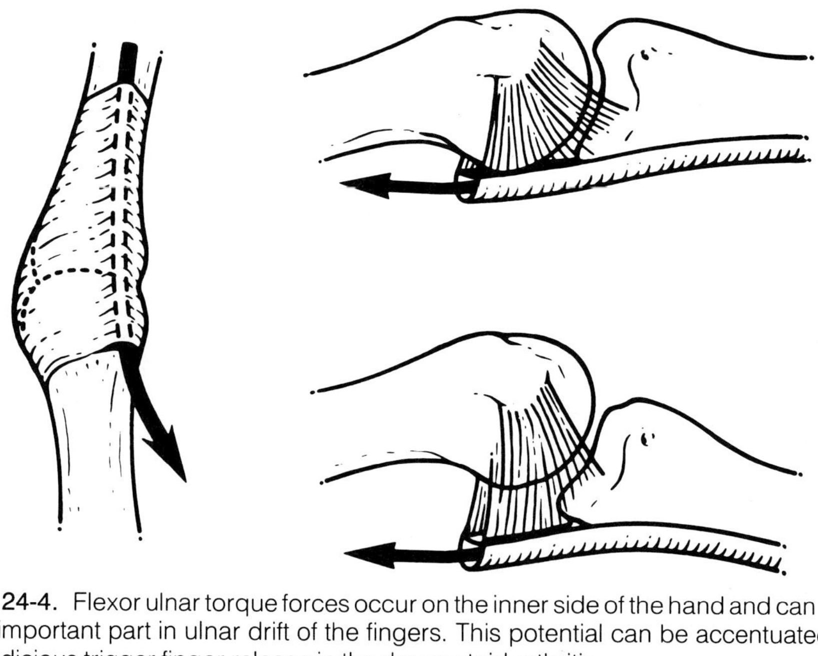

Fig 24-4. Flexor ulnar torque forces occur on the inner side of the hand and can play an important part in ulnar drift of the fingers. This potential can be accentuated by injudicious trigger finger release in the rheumatoid arthritic.

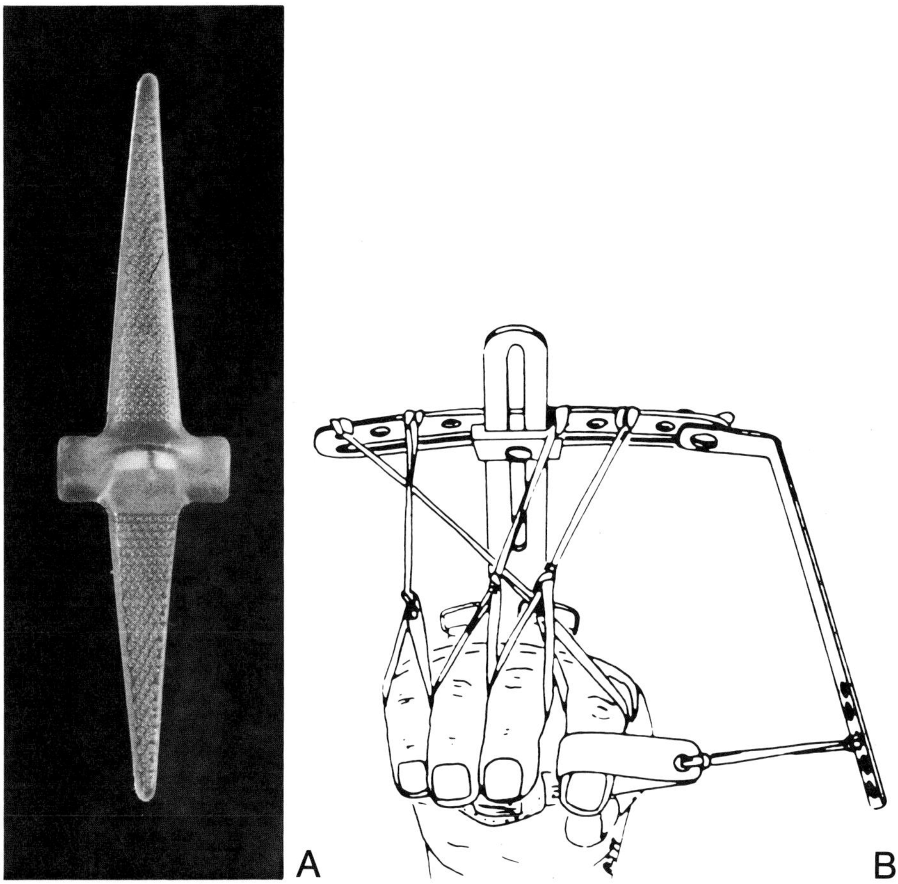

Fig 24-5. Of the available implants for the severe arthritic metacarpophalangeal joint, the Swanson flexible prosthesis (*A*) is the most successful; stem fracture and silicone synovitis have been unusual in the author's experience thus far. Such prostheses have largely replaced the several forms of resection arthroplasty.[1,5,6,7] An active exercise program with appropriate bracing (*B*) is essential in the postoperative phase of treatment.

Accompanying arthritic change in the wrist is important. Also, dorsal displacement of the ulnar head, with erosion, as a consequence of disease at the inferior radioulnar joint leads to risk of rupture of the extrinsic extensor tendons of the fingers, and this can increase the difficulty of correcting ulnar drift. Of course, limitation of forearm rotation and wrist movement compounds the patient's problems, and disease proximally in the elbow and shoulder is a further complicating factor in many patients.

The aim of treatment in ulnar drift of the fingers is to counterbalance radial pressure pinch and similar forms of grip by providing sufficient lateral stability

Arthroplasty of the MP Joint

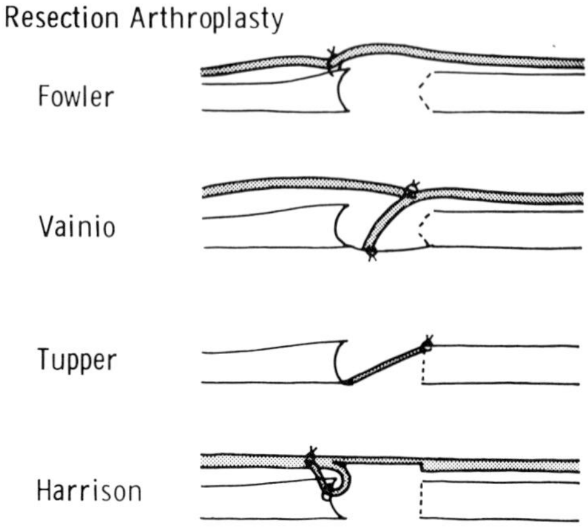

Fig 24-6. Types of resection arthroplasty of the metacarpophalangeal joint.

for the fingers. Where there is mild to moderate ulnar drift, synovectomy, using a radial incision in the extensor hood, is performed and relocation of the extrinsic extensor mechanism achieved by release of the medial longitudinal band and radial overlap of the extensor hood, while creation of retinacular ligaments can be considered. The ulnar intrinsic tendon should be released if tight and can be used as an intrinsic radial transfer to the adjacent finger with radial transfer of the extensor indicis to the proximal phalanx of the index finger. In some patients the radial collateral ligament may be effectively shortened and reattached to the phalanx and metacarpal. Where ulnar drift is severe and function significantly impaired, prosthetic replacement of the joint is usual in addition to soft-tissue reconstruction; destruction of the articular surfaces is an indication for implant surgery. The Swanson flexible implant is the most popular prosthesis at this time[4]; stem fracture and silicone synovitis are unusual complications in the author's experience thus far (Fig 24-5).

Frequently, when the metacarpophalangeal joints of the hand are severely involved in rheumatoid disease, the PIP joints are relatively spared, and in such circumstances resection arthroplasty in the past has improved the overall function of the hand (Fig 24-6); the author favors the Fowler resection arthroplasty[1,5,6,7]

References

1. Flatt AE: *Care of the Arthritic Hand,* ed 4. St Louis, CV Mosby Co, 1983.
2. McMaster M: The natural history of the rheumatoid metacarpo-phalangeal joint. *J Bone Joint Surg Br* 1972;54B:687–697.

3. Clayton ML, Ferlic DC: Tendon transfer for radial rotation of the wrist in rheumatoid arthritis. *Clin Orthop Related Res* 1974;100:176–185.
4. Swanson AB: *Flexible Implant Arthroplasty in the Hand and Extremities.* St Louis, CV Mosby Co, 1973.
5. Fowler SB: Arthroplasty of metacarpo-phalangeal joints in rheumatoid arthritis. *J Bone Joint Surg Am* 1962;44A:1037–1038.
6. Tupper JW: The volar plate arthroplasty for rheumatoid arthritis. Proceedings of the Fifteenth Annual Meeting of The Japanese Society for Surgery of the Hand. 24:1972
7. Vainio K, Reiman I, Pulkki T: Results of arthroplasty of the metacarpo-phalangeal joints in rheumatoid arthritis. *Reconstr Surg Traumatol* 1967;9:1–7.

25

Volar Approach to the Stiff Proximal Interphalangeal Joint in Swan-Neck Deformity

Nashaat Naam and John A. Boswick, Jr.

Swan-neck deformity of the fingers often causes significant disability of the hand function. The deformity is characterized by hyperextension of the proximal interphalangeal joint and extension lag at the distal interphalangeal joint. It is commonly associated with flexion deformity of the metacarpophalangeal joint (Fig 25-1). Swan-neck deformities have been classified by Nalebuff and Millender[1] into four types: In type I, the proximal interphalangeal joint is flexible in all positions; in type II, flexion of the proximal interphalangeal joint is limited in certain positions; in type III, proximal interphalangeal joint flexion is limited in all positions of the finger; in type IV, stiffness of the proximal interphalangeal joint is associated with advanced radiological changes. To understand the pathomechanics and surgical treatment of swan-neck deformities their functional anatomy and pathophysiology should be carefully examined.

Functional Anatomy

The proximal interphalangeal joint is a simple hinge joint. The capsule is reinforced volarly and laterally, but it is lax and supple dorsally. It takes a long time for shortening or contracture of the soft and pliable dorsal part of the capsule to occur.[2] The volar plate, a fibrocartilaginous structure, is attached distally to the volar border of the base of the middle phalanx. Proximally it extends to the neck of the proximal phalanx, creating a proximal pouch, the retrocondylar recess[2-4]. The collateral ligaments are triangular in shape. They extend from the lateral fossa of the proximal phalangeal head to the lateral surface of the base of the middle phalanx. They are at a constant tension whether the joint is flexed or extended. This explains the absence of lateral movements in the flexed or extended proximal interphalangeal joint. Actual

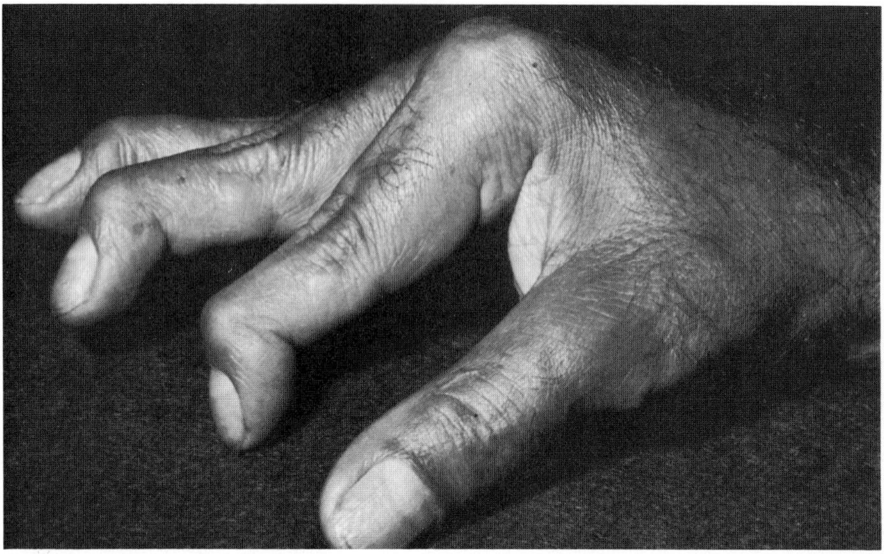

Fig 25-1. Swan-neck deformity with hyperextension of the proximal interphalangeal joint and flexion of the distal interphalangeal joint. Note flexion of the metacarpophalangeal joint.

shortening of the collateral ligaments is a less important cause of stiffness of the proximal interphalangeal joint than adhesions between the ligaments and the underlying proximal phalangeal head.[5] The transverse retinacular ligament originates from the volar aspect of the capsule of the proximal interphalangeal joint and the flexor tendon sheath and extends dorsally and laterally to attach to the lateral margin of the extensor mechanism on each side of the proximal interphalangeal joint. The oblique retinacular ligament arises from the flexor tendon sheath at the level of the distal one fourth of the proximal phalanx and crosses over the proximal interphalangeal joint to insert with the lateral extensor tendon into the dorsum of the distal phalanx.[6] The extensor mechanism at this level consists of the strong central slip, which is inserted into the base of the middle phalanx, and the lateral bands, which gain insertion into the base of the distal phalanx. The capsule is attached to the extensor mechanism by fibrous tracts, which are strongest near the middle phalanx. Because of its strength and wide insertion, the central slip acts as a dorsal ligament opposing the volar plate.[4]

Pathophysiology

Several factors may contribute to the production of swan-neck deformity in rheumatoid and nonrheumatoid hands. Flexion deformity of the distal interphalangeal joint secondary to rupture of the distal extensor tendon, producing a mallet deformity, may result in secondary hyperextension of the proximal interphalangeal joint. Synovitis of the proximal interphalangeal joint is probably one of the main factors causing swan-neck deformity. The proliferating synovial tissue fills the volar compartment and the retrocondylar recess, causing limitation of the mobility of the volar plate. Later on, adhesions in the retrocondylar recess between the volar plate and the proximal phalanx cause more limitation of the volar plate movement. Furthermore, the volar plate support is weakened allowing hyperextension of the proximal interphalangeal joint.[5,7,8] Dorsal extension of the proliferating synovial tissue may cause erosion of the retinacular ligaments, resulting in dorsal subluxation of the lateral bands and subsequent hyperextension of the proximal interphalangeal joint. Adhesions between the extensor mechanism and the ligaments and the bone produce varying degrees of stiffness of the joint.

Flexor tenosynovitis is well recognized as an important factor in producing swan-neck deformities in rheumatoid hands. Initially active flexion is limited without limitation of passive flexion. In some patients, limitation of passive flexion may develop later because of lack of motion, synovitis of the proximal interphalangeal joint, or periarticular adhesions.[9] Synovitis of the metacarpophalangeal joint causes attenuation of the extensor digitorum communis insertion into the base of the proximal phalanx, allowing a more effective pull on the base of the middle phalanx. Volar subluxation of the metacarpophalangeal joint may result from the action of the long flexors. The intrinsic muscles become shortened as a result of the metacarpophalangeal subluxation, causing a greater pull on the central slip over the proximal interphalangeal joint. The net effect is a dorsal subluxation of the lateral bands, producing hyperextension of the proximal interphalangeal joint and flexion of the distal interphalangeal joint.[10] Several other factors may contribute to the production of swan-neck deformities such as extensor tendon contracture, capsular or collateral ligament contracture, imbalance of the intrinsic muscles, and intra-articular fibrous or ankylosis.[11] True intra-articular causes are rarely responsible for stiffness of the proximal interphalangeal joints of rheumatoid patients.[12] Swan-neck deformity is often the result of pathological changes in more than one structure, and according to the degree of involvement of each element a different kind of swan-neck deformity results. All these factors must be taken into consideration in evaluating patients with such deformities.

Surgical Approaches

Surgical treatment of swan-neck deformity is dependent upon understanding the various pathological processes involved and should be aimed as much as possible at correcting the primary cause. Various surgical approaches have been described. Harrison described a dorsal approach in which the transverse retinacular ligament is incised between the lateral bands and the oblique retinacular ligament. The dorsal capsule is exposed and divided, avoiding injury of the central slip. The collateral ligaments are released on both sides.[5] Other dorsal approaches have been described by Gould, Kaplan, and Young.[13-15] Curtis and Rhode and Jennings use a lateral approach to expose and retract the retinacular ligaments, and then the collateral ligaments are divided on each side of the joint.[16,17] In the bilateral midlateral incision described by Sprague, the retinacular ligament is divided and repaired following correction of the deformity.[18]

Volar Approach

Through studying the functional anatomy and pathomechanics of swan-neck deformity it becomes evident that a volar approach to the proximal interphalangeal joint has several advantages. First, it allows a more direct approach and an adequate release of volar plate adhesions and adhesions between the collateral ligaments and the proximal phalangeal head. Second, it preserves the retinacular ligament complex, which is essential for proximal interphalangeal joint stability. Third, through the volar approach a superficialis tenodesis can be performed at the same time as an additional step to limit the last degrees of proximal interphalangeal joint extension and help prevent recurrence of the deformity.[7]

The proximal interphalangeal joint is approached through a Bruner zigzag incision. The flexor sheath is exposed and entered between the A2 and A4 pulleys. The flexor tendons are retracted to one side, exposing the volar plate. Incisions are made on both sides of the volar plate at its junction with the collateral ligaments (Fig 25-2). Volar plate adhesions especially in the retrocondylar recess are released with a Frrer elevator, making sure to keep the proximal and distal attachments of the volar plate intact. The adhesions between the collateral ligaments and the proximal phalangeal head are freed, and then the contracted collateral ligaments are released until full passive movement of the joint is obtained. Usually between 25% and 50% of the volar aspect of the collateral ligaments needs to be released. The rest of the correction can be achieved by manipulation. Tenodesis of one slip of the superficialis tendon might then be done. Occasionally, a dorsal incision is needed for extensor tenolysis.

Motion is started early postoperatively, usually within 24 to 48 hours of surgery. Dynamic traction is used to allow active movements of the proximal interphalangeal joint through all but the last 30° of extension. Traction is usually continued for 3 to 4 weeks, but it may take longer to achieve the maximum range of motion.

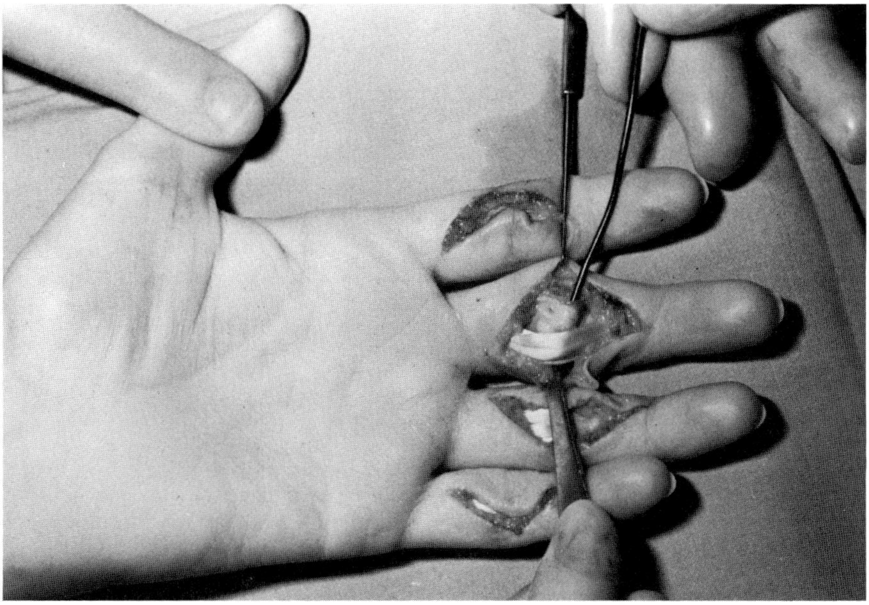

Fig 25-2. Through a Bruner zigzag incision the flexor tendons are exposed and retracted. Incisions are made on the lateral aspect of the volar plate at its junction with the collateral ligament. The volar plate is bluntly dissected off the proximal phalanx, releasing adhesions in the retrocondylar recess.

Results

The volar approach was used in treating 58 stiff proximal interphalangeal joints in 18 hands of 13 patients. There were six males and seven females. Their ages ranged from 31 to 78 years, with an average of 61 years. The patients were followed for an average of 21 months (6 to 47 months). Simultaneous superficial tenodesis was done in 14 fingers. The average preoperative range of motion was $+5°$ extension and 22° flexion. Postoperatively, the average range of motion was $-9°$ extension and 71° flexion. The total arc of motion not only increased from 27° to 62° postoperatively but also became more functional with greater flexion. (Fig 25-3). Patients who have gross destruction of the articular surfaces are not candidates for soft-tissue arthroplasty; however, moderate intra-articular changes are not contraindications to such operations. The original pathological process may progress in the joints after soft-tissue operations leading to progressive joint destruction and recurrence of the stiffness. Joint replacement or arthrodesis may be indicated in those joints with gross intra-articular destruction.

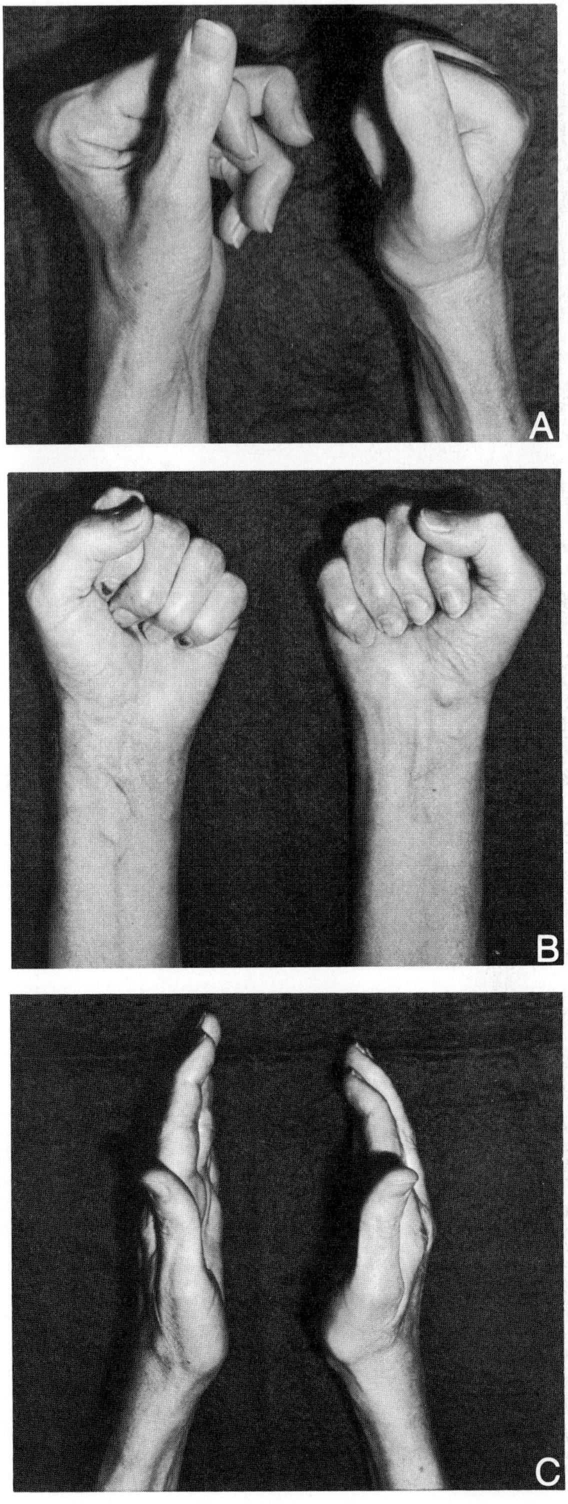

Fig 25-3. *A*, Preoperative view showing swan-neck deformities of the left index, long, ring, and little fingers; *B* and *C*, postoperative views showing excellent range of motion in flexion and extension.

References

1. Nalebuff EA, Millender LH: Surgical treatment of the swan neck deformity in rheumatoid arthritis. *Orthop Clin North Am* 1975;6:733–752.
2. Kuczynski K: The proximal interphalangeal joint. *J Bone Joint Surg* 1968;50B:656–663.
3. Harrison SH: The proximal interphalangeal joint in rheumatoid arthritis. *Hand* 1971;3:125–130.
4. Dubousset JF: The digital joints, in Tubiana R (ed): *The Hand.* Philadelphia, WB Saunders Co, 1981, pp 191–201.
5. Harrison DH: The stiff proximal interphalangeal joint. *Hand* 1977;9:102–108.
6. Milford LW: The retaining ligaments of the digits of the hand, in Tubiana R (ed): *The Hand.* Philadelphia, WB Saunders Co, 1981 pp 232–235.
7. Scott FA, Boswick JA: Palmar arthroplasty for the treatment of the stiff swan neck deformity. *J Hand Surg* 1983;8:267–272.
8. Scott FA: Management of swan neck deformity in rheumatoid disease, in Boswick JA (ed): *Current Concepts in Hand Surgery.* Philadelphia, Lea & Febiger, 1983, pp 247–253.
9. Millis HB, Millender LH, Nalebuff EA: Stiffness of the proximal interphalangeal joints in rheumatoid arthritis. *J Bone Joint Surg* 1976;58:801–805.
10. Welsh RP, Hastings DE: Swan neck deformity in rheumatoid arthritis of the hand. *Hand* 1977;9:109–116.
11. Curtis RM: Capsulectomy of the interphalangeal joints of the fingers. *J Bone Joint Surg Am* 1954;36:1219–1232.
12. Helal BH: Extra-anticular causes of proximal interphalangeal joint stiffness in rheumatoid arthritis. *Hand* 1975;7:37–40.
13. Gould JS, Nicholson BC: Capsulectomy of the metacarpophalangeal and proximal interphalangeal joints. *J Hand Surg* 1979;4:482–486.
14. Kaplan EB: *Functional and Surgical Anatomy of the hand,* ed 2. Philadelphia, JB Lippincott Co, 1965.
15. Young VL, Wray RC, Weeks PM: The surgical management of stiff joints in the hand. *Plast Reconst Surg* 1978;62:835–841.
16. Curtis RM: Management of the stiff proximal interphalangeal joint. *Hand* 1969;1:32–37.
17. Rhode CM, Jennings WD: Operative treatment of the stiff proximal interphalangeal joint. *Am Surg* 1971;37:44–59.
18. Sprague BL: Proximal interphalangeal joint contractures and their treatment. *J Trauma* 1976;16:259–265.

26

Mallet Finger: A Review of Treatment and Some Observations on the Microvascular Anatomy of the Distal Digital Extensor Tendon

Richard A. Warren, Neville R.M. Kay, and David G. Ferguson

Mallet finger is a common condition that is frequently dismissed as unimportant. It usually occurs in the middle-aged or elderly female or the young active male, and the principal associated disability is often described as cosmetic. This is not invariably the case. A mallet finger in the little finger of the right hand of a professional violinist would effectively limit his or her career or demand an adaptation in the bowing technique such that the ring finger is used in lieu of the little finger. Moreover, in an age increasingly dominated by the computer keyboard, mallet fingers can be more than a cosmetic disability to many working patients. Many treatments have been described for mallet finger, but few surgeons would attempt formal operative repair. More recently, this view has been challenged and the technique of dermatotenodesis has been popularized.

In 1974, one of us (N.R.M.K.) began treating a series of patients in whom closed tendon rupture had produced a mallet finger and in whom treatment by conservative techniques had failed. These patients were treated by Kirschner wire fixation of the distal interphalangeal joint in hyperextension for 6 weeks, and the results of a small series of patients were subsequently presented to the British Society of Surgery of the Hand. The concept of an avascular area of tendon at the common site of rupture was postulated, and it was noted that other tendons, principally the supraspinatus tendon, had been shown to have a similar area of relative avascularity. Injection studies of a hand amputated for tumor of the forearm produced four specimens in which the microvascular anatomy of the extensor tendon was studied, and although the techniques were unsatisfactory these initial inquiries were sufficient to prompt one of us (R.A.W.) into an extensive investigation of the microvascular anatomy of the extensor tendon insertion based on cadaveric injection studies, microvascular dissection, and histological examination of the preparation.

This chapter reviews some of the common treatments of mallet finger. A small series of patients is presented in whom closed treatment had failed but who were successfully treated by percutaneous Kirschner wire fixation, and some of the complications of that technique are indicated and the microvascular anatomy of the extensor tendons is briefly described. Our findings would appear to support the concept that there is an area of relative avascularity of the extensor tendon at the site where it commonly ruptures. The clinical implications that result from this concept are briefly discussed.

Review of the Treatments of Mallet Finger

The variety of recommended treatments for mallet finger is witness to the lack of success of any one method. If the tendon ruptures (as distinct from pulling off a small fragment of bone), this rupture usually occurs a few millimeters proximal to the osseotendinous insertion on the terminal phalanx.[1-3] The divided tendon does not retract because of its more proximal attachments,[3] and therefore almost all forms of treatment depend upon immobilizing the distal interphalangeal joint in extension or slight hyperextension for a sufficient length of time for healing to take place. Treatment of mallet finger can be divided into two principal groups, namely, closed splintage and operation.

Closed Splintage

The classic method of treatment by immobilization in a plaster of Paris cast is still practiced. The work of Bunnell[4] was influential and showed that the distal extensor tendon was relaxed if the distal interphalangeal joint of the finger was in extension and the proximal interphalangeal joint was in flexion. Stark[5] described a plaster of Paris cast designed to hold the distal interphalangeal joint in extension and the proximal joint in 60° of flexion, and he described a series of 78 patients treated by this method. The patients in this series had relatively recent injuries, and this factor has subsequently been shown to improve the apparent success rate,[3,6] although the criteria described for improvement were not stringent. Nonetheless, some 33% were reported as showing a good result, and a further 55% were improved by this plaster of Paris technique.

Despite these results and the simplicity of treatment, the use of a plaster of Paris cast is not universal. Experience has shown that holding the distal interphalangeal joint in extension causes pressure on the skin over the distal interphalangeal joint, and necrosis of the skin is a recognized complication of this technique.[2,7]

Ingenious splints have been designed to hold the proximal interphalangeal joint in flexion in the Bunnell fashion,[8,9] but the work of Kaplan[3] disputed the Bunnell theory and showed that the extensor tendon is fully relaxed when both the proximal and the distal interphalangeal joints are in extension. There followed a profusion of splints for immobilizing the distal interphalangeal joint only. These included a metal tube[10], a simple pad and strapping,[11] and a splint constructed from the inner tube of an automobile tire.[12] Two of these splints are worthy of special mention, namely, the Stack splint[2] and the Abouna splint.[6]

The Stack splint is a simple, molded polyethylene device available in a variety of sizes (Pryor & Howard Co., United Kingdom). It is comfortable, durable, easily washable, and reusable. This splint is probably the most popular in current use in the United Kingdom because of its comfort, durability, and simplicity. Crawford[13] reported a long-term follow-up of 151 patients treated with the Stack splint and showed that in some 65% of patients the results were good and in an additional 27% the mallet finger deformity was improved (Fig 26-1).

The Abouna splint (Peacock Co., United Kingdom) is constructed from steel wire and coated with rubber. In a study of 110 unselected patients of all ages and including both new and late injuries (up to 11 weeks), Abouna and Brown[6] reported a high success rate of some 72%, with a further 13% of patients who showed some improvement. Unfortunately, this success rate has not been repeated by other workers, and the Abouna splint is not popular in the United Kingdom.

Operative Methods

The problems and variable success with closed splintage have led to many attempts at developing an acceptable surgical procedure. It is acknowledged that in such a minor condition the potential is great for surgery to do more harm than good.[14]

Direct tendon suture for open injuries to the extensor tendon have been described in standard textbooks.[1,15] One of the first operative techniques to gain wide acceptance in the surgical treatment of closed tendon ruptures was that of Pratt.[16] This method adhered firmly to the Bunnell theory and fixed the distal interphalangeal joint in extension and the proximal joint in flexion by means of a single Kirschner wire. The wire was driven through the terminal phalanx and the distal interphalangeal joint through the soft tissues of the volar aspect of the middle and proximal phalanges, penetrating the bone of the proximal phalanx (Fig 26-2). Pratt reported that 6 (50%) out of 12 patients treated by this method were cured, the remaining 6 (50%) being improved.

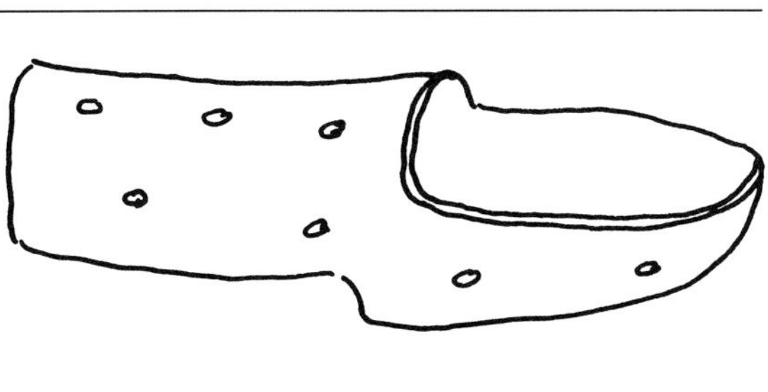

Fig 26-1. A Stack mallet finger splint.

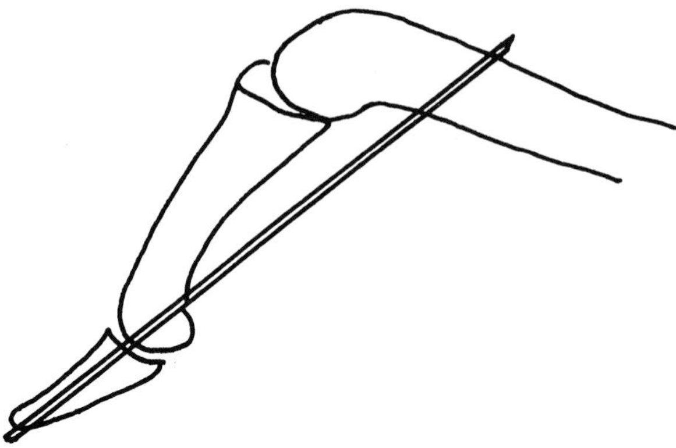

Fig 26-2. The Pratt technique of stabilization of the distal interphalangeal joint in extension and the proximal interphalangeal joint in flexion.

However, Cascells and Strange[17] reported a high complication rate with the original Pratt technique, especially subsequent pain and restriction of flexion at both the proximal and distal interphalangeal joints. They advised a simple technique using a short Kirschner wire to fix the distal joint only. Using this technique Cascells reported cures in 9 (45%) of 20 patients studied, with a further 7 (35%) cases showing useful improvement.

A variation on the theme of fixing the distal interphalangeal joint with Kirschner wires was described by Weinberg et al.[18] This method avoids penetration of the joint proper by fixing two wires through the skin into the dorsal aspect of the middle and distal phalanges at either side of the distal interphalangeal joint at 90° to the long axis of the finger (Fig 26-3). The protruding wires are then firmly tied together thereby holding the distal joint in slight hyperextension. Of 15 patients treated by this technique, 9 (60%) were cured and the remaining 6 (40%) were improved.

Tenodermodesis[19] is an extension of the simple subcutaneous silk suture method described by Hillman.[20] Iselin suggested that the operation be used only for those patients who have failed to benefit from closed splintage. A wedge of tissue including the skin and the extensor tendon is excised from the dorsal aspect of the distal interphalangeal joint and the defect closed by several nonabsorbable through-and-through sutures which penetrate the skin, tendon, and joint capsule. In a series of 26 cases, 13 patients (50%) were cured and 8 (31%) were improved.

Finally, arthrodesis of the persistently painful distal interphalangeal joint is occasionally necessary, but the method advocated by Rosenzweig,[21] namely, amputation, has never been necessary in the author's experience.

Kirschner Wire Stabilization of the Distal Interphalangeal Joint

Patients, especially women, find the results of conservative splintage for the treatment of mallet finger disappointing. Many of these patients are concerned

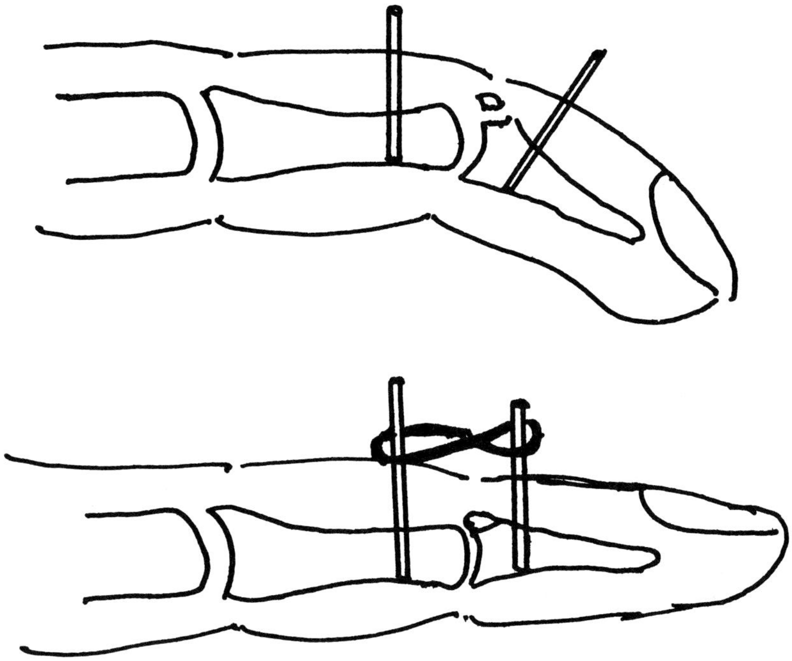

Fig 26-3. The Weinberg technique of stabilization of the distal interphalangeal joint.

about the functional loss consequent to an unstable distal interphalangeal joint, and the cosmetic aspect of the deformity does not pass unnoticed, particularly in female patients. In an attempt to improve the results, a small number of patients in whom conservative splintage had failed and in whom there was no radiographic evidence of a bony "pull-off" fragment from the distal phalanx Kirschner wire were offered stabilization of the distal interphalangeal joint in extension for a period of 6 weeks. It was believed, on theoretical grounds at least, that there might be a relative area of avascularity. If this were so, direct surgery to the extensor tendon might compound this relative avascularity and the sutures would effectively strangle the available blood supply. This would certainly appear to be a logical explanation for the relatively poor results associated with direct extensor tendon repair at this level. On the other hand, stabilization of the distal interphalangeal joint in extension should allow the scar to mature and permit adequte revascularization.

The distal interphalangeal joint was stabilized with a Kirschner wire under digital nerve block and radiographic control. It is worth noting that if the distal interphalangeal joint had to be fixed in hyperextension, then the Kirschner wire would have to pass through the condyles of the middle phalanx. If the Kirschner wire passes along the medullary canal of the distal and middle phalanx, then the distal interphalangeal joint is effectively fixed in slight flexion (Fig 26-4).

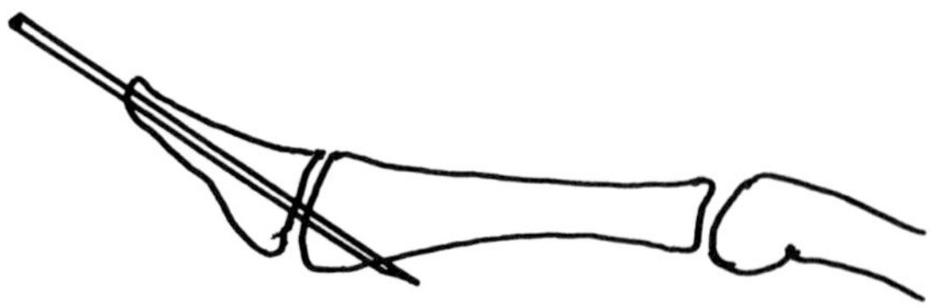

Fig 26-4. Correct placement of Kirschner wire for stabilization of the distal interphalangeal joint in extension.

The Kirschner wire was left in situ for 6 weeks, and it was deemed necessary to protect the wire with a splint, for otherwise patients undertaking such activities as boat building and plastering could fracture the wire. The initial small series of 16 patients consisted of 11 in whom conservative treatment had failed and 5 new patients (within 6 weeks of injury). The results showed that in the new patients a normal finger was achieved. In the 11 late cases, which presented between 9 weeks and 20 weeks after injury, over 50% achieved a normal finger. Two additional late cases were significantly improved, giving an 80% improvement rate. Three fingers were somewhat stiff but had an active range of flexion of 30° to 35°.

The complications associated with this technique were malposition of the Kirschner wire and fracture of the wire on one occasion. Sepsis was not recorded, although one patient had a somewhat red pulp for a week. It has to be emphasized, however, that this was a highly select group of patients, and elderly patients who had clinical and radiographic evidence of arthritis of their distal interphalangeal joint were excluded. Most surgical series of mallet fingers are small, indicating a high degree of selectivity.

Table 26-1 shows some of the published results of various treatments.

Table 26-1. Results of Various Methods of Treatment of Mallet Finger

Method	*Reference*	*No. Patients*	*Good Result (%)*	*Improved Result (%)*	*Failures (%)*
Abouna splint	6	110	72	13	15
Stack splint	13	151	65	27	8
Kirschner wire external fixation	18	15	60	40	
Kirschner wire (long) internal fixation	16	12	50	50	
Tenodermodesis	19	26	50	31	19
Kirschner wire (short) internal fixation	17	20	45	35	20
Oakley splint	10	30	40	53	7
Plaster cast	5	78	33	55	12

Significance of Results of Treatment of Mallet Finger

If one leaves aside the exceptionally good results claimed by Abouna for his splint, which to date do not seem to have been confirmed by independent studies, the published cure rates vary from approximately one third to two thirds, with an average of about 50%. This means that whereas some patients may be improved, approximately half are not cured. Although mallet finger is a relatively minor condition, these results leave room for improvement. Most work is concentrated on finding a better splint or a better operation, on the assumption that if a damaged tendon is immobilized in opposition to itself or to the bone from which it has been avulsed for a sufficient time, healing will occur. If it were shown that the distal digital extensor tendon had a deficient blood supply, this might explain the poor result of conservative and surgical treatment. This concept stimulated the authors to embark on a study of the microvascular circulation of the distal extensor tendon and its osseotendinous junction. Avascular areas have been shown in other tendons, notably the supraspinatus tendon and the long-headed biceps.[22]

The Blood Supply of the Distal Extensor Tendon of the Finger

Von Kolliker[23] declared that tendons had no blood supply, and it was Ludwig[24] who first showed that intratendinous blood vessels do exist. It was not until 70 years later that Edwards[25] and Brockis,[26] stimulated by a desire to improve techniques of tendon surgery in the hand, published their classic observations on the blood supply of tendons. These studies dealt with both flexor and extensor tendons in humans and animals, and interest was concentrated on the flexor tendons lying within their synovial sheath. This concentration on the flexor tendons continued with Peacock[27] and continues today.[28,29] Much less interest has been shown in extensor tendons, and when these have been studied, attention has been focused on the manus and the carpus.[30,31] Gigis and Kuczynski[32] gave a very good description of the blood supply of the distal interphalangeal joint of the human finger but did not report on the supply of the distal extensor tendon to any significant extent.

These studies used a variety of techniques including injection of colloidal silver, which was developed photographically,[26] injection of India ink,[30] alloy-coated resin examined under the electron microscope,[28] and injection of radioactive phosphorus-32.[33]

Materials and Methods

To date, 16 fingers from three cadavers have been studied. A tight tourniquet was applied just above the wrist and a cannula introduced into the radial artery at the wrist. The venous network on the dorsum of the hand was also cannulated. The circulation was washed out with 1,500 mL of heparinized 0.9% saline solution introduced into the radial artery, the effluent being carried away via the cannulated dorsal veins. Two of the washed-out hands from different cadavers were injected via the radial artery with a latex solution containing red dye (Latex Injection Mass, Philip Harris Ltd., United Kingdom), which was coagulated by immersion of the hand in a buffered formalin solution for several days. Another two hands from different cadavers were injected in a similar fashion with gelatin solution containing orange dye (Speedball Coloured Ink), which was also coagulated in buffered formalin solution. The hands injected with red latex were dissected under the dissecting microscope at a magnification of 20 × to display the fine vessels supplying the distal extensor tendon. The distal phalanx, extensor tendon, and surrounding tissue were dissected from the eight fingers injected with orange gelatin. The specimens were decalcified by immersion in ethylenediaminetetraacetic acid dehydrated with alcohol and were then embedded in resin from which 10μ sections were cut. The sections were stained with toluidine blue for examination under the light microscope.

Observations

The blood supply to the distal extensor tendon and osseotendinous junction was remarkably constant in the eight fingers that had been injected with red latex (Fig 26-5). The radial and ulnar sides were symmetrical other than for a tendency for the digital artery and its branches to be slightly larger on the radial side. The blood supply is entirely from the digital artery proper, the small dorsal digital artery's branches reaching no further than the proximal phalanx. A constant feature is a dorsal branch of the digital artery arising at the level of the neck of the middle phalanx, to divide into a deep (usually posterior) and a superficial branch (usually anterior). The deep branch forms with its fellow from the opposite side a network on the periosteum on the dorsal aspect of the middle phalanx, giving an occasional branch to the underside of the extensor tendon. The superficial branch has far more branches, which it sends to both the paratenon immediately above the extensor tendon and the tendon proper. These branches anastomose with their opposite neighbors and with branches from an arcade arching over the terminal phalanx between the insertion of the extensor tendon and the nail bed. This terminal dorsal arcade is formed from recurrent branches from either digital artery proper and branches from the superficial dorsal branch. The number of vessels observed on the surface and undersurface of the extensor tendon at the level of the distal interphalangeal joint is not so great as more proximally, and, significantly, the vessel-containing connective tissue—the paratenon, which envelops the tendon—was progressively less prominent as one approached the distal limit of the tendon.

The specimens for histological analysis (those injected with orange gelatin) were cut on the microtome to give serial 10μ sections at 1-mm intervals from the tip of the terminal phalanx (Fig 26-6). Under the light microscope, penetration

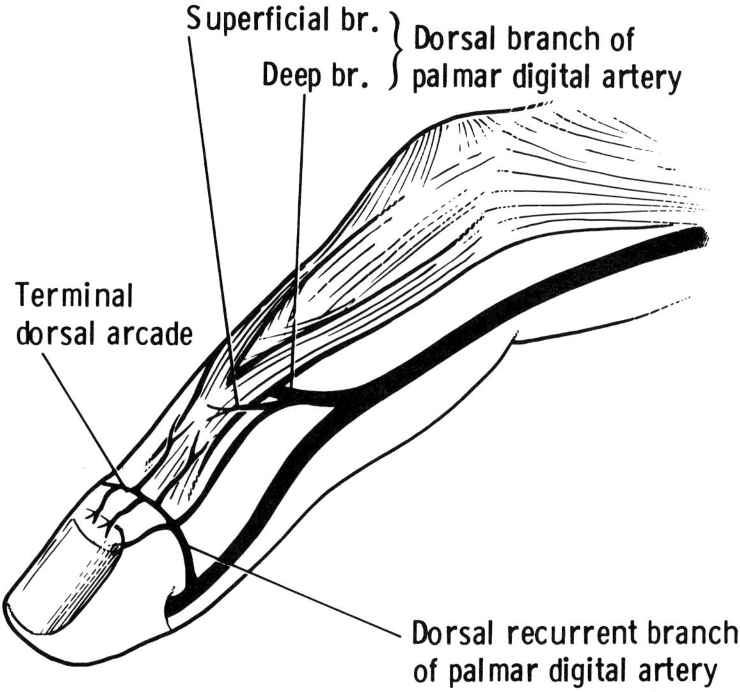

Fig 26-5. Anatomical arrangement of the blood vessels in the distal segment of the extensor tendon.

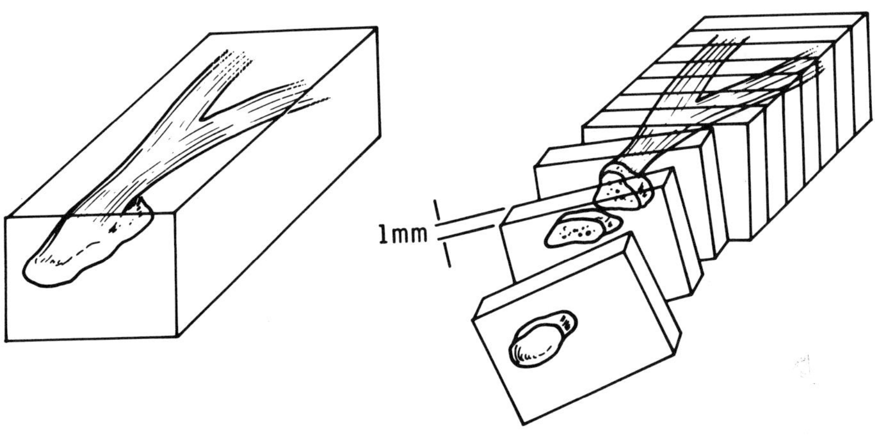

Fig 26-6. Method of preparation of the histological specimens.

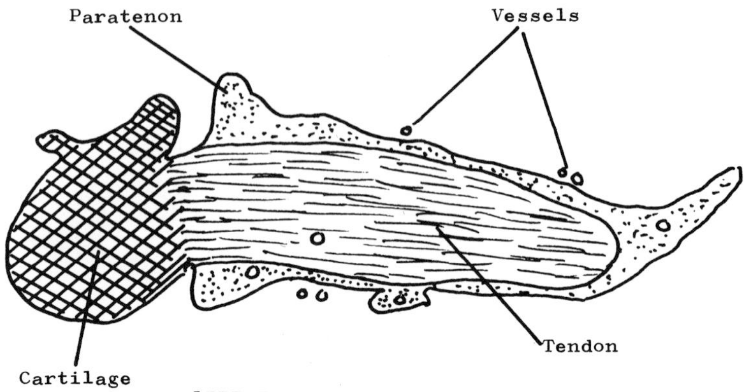

Fig 26-7. Schematic diagram of histological specimen showing extensor tendon insertion into the terminal phalanx with associated blood vessels.

of the vessels with gelatin was seen to be good and most revealing. The orange dye and blue counterstain defined and distinguished the vessels from other structures, allowing them to be studied closely. Two noteworthy observations were apparent, both suggesting that the last 5 mm of the distal extensor tendon does have a deficient blood supply compared with the same tendon only 20 mm more proximal: First, it was confirmed that there is less vessel-containing paratenon surrounding the distal extremity of the extensor tendon (Fig 26-7), and the tendon is partly inserted into the avascular cartilage of the articular

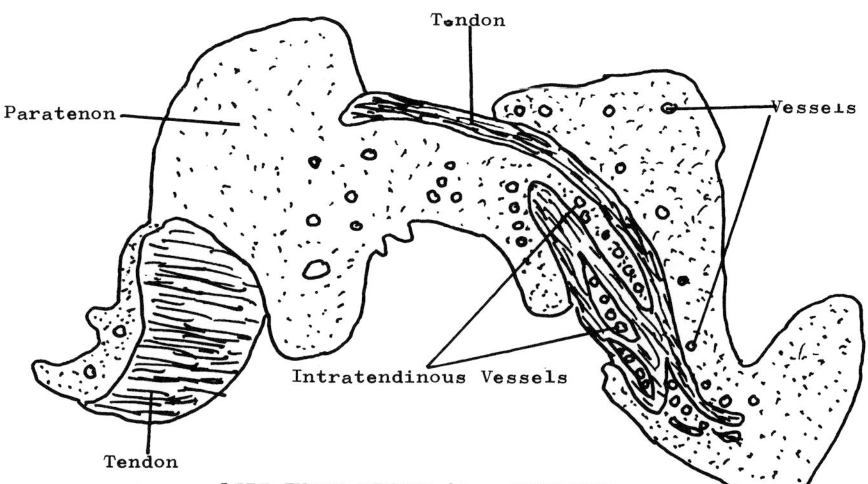

Fig 26-8. Schematic diagram of tendons and associated vessels around the proximal interphalangeal joint.

surface of the terminal phalanx. The paratenon surrounding the tendon at the level of the proximal interphalangeal joint (Fig 26-8) is more profuse and proportionately more vascular. The second and perhaps most significant observation of all was that there were very few vessels demonstrable within the distal portion of the tendon proper at the level of the distal interphalangeal joint (Fig 26-8), whereas there were a large number of vessels within the tendon proper at the level of the proximal interphalangeal joint, and these were often arranged in layers (Fig 26-8).

These observations were remarkably consistent in the fingers so far examined, suggesting that there is indeed an area of deficient blood supply in the distal digital extensor tendon at the level of the distal interphalangeal joint.

References

1. Barron JN, Saad MN: *The Hand—Operative, Plastic and Reconstructive Techniques,* vol 3. Edinburgh, Churchill Livingstone, 1980.
2. Stack HG: Mallet finger. *Hand* 1969;1:83–89.
3. Kaplan EB: Anatomy, injuries and treatment of the extensor apparatus of the hand and the digits. *Clin Orthop* 1959;13(no 27): 24–41.
4. Bunnell S: *Surgery of the Hand.* Philadelphia, JB Lippincott Co, 1945.
5. Stark HH, Boyes JH, Wilson JN: Mallet finger. *J Bone Joint Surg Am* 1962;44A:1061–1068.
6. Abouna JM, Brown H: The treatment of mallet finger. *Br J Surg* 1968; 55:653–667.
7. Hallberg D, Lindholm A: *Acta Chir Scand* 1960;119:260.
8. Fowler FD: New splint for the treatment of mallet finger. *JAMA* 1959;170:945.
9. Spigelman L: New splint for management of mallet finger. *JAMA* 1953;153:1362.
10. Mikic Z, Helal B: The treatment of the mallet finger by the Oakley splint. *Hand* 1974;6(no 1):76–81.
11. Ellis M: *The Casualty Officer's Handbook,* ed 3. London, Butterworths, 1969.
12. Joshi BB: Simple and economical splints for the hand (using readily available materials), in Pulvertaft RG (ed): *Operative Surgery: The Hand,* ed 3. London, Butterworths, 1977.
13. Crawford GP: The molded polythene splint for mallet finger deformities. *J Hand Surg* 1984;9A:231–237.
14. Littler JW: The voice of polite dissent. *Plast Reconstr Surg* 1976;58:439–450.
15. Pulvertaft RG (ed): *Operative surgery: The Hand,* ed 3. London, Butterworths, 1977.
16. Pratt DR: Internal splint for closed and open treatment of injuries of the extensor tendon at the distal joint of the finger. *J Bone Joint Surg Am* 1952;34A:785–789.
17. Cascells SW. Strange TB: Intramedullary wire fixation of mallet finger. *J Bone Joint Surg Am* 1957;39A:521–526.
18. Weinberg H, Stein HC, Wexler MR: A new method of treatment for mallet finger. *Plast Reconstr Surg* 1976;58:347–349.
19. Iselin F, Levame J, Godoy J: A simplified technique for treating mallet fingers: Tenodermodesis. *J Hand Surg* 1977;2:118–121.
20. Hillman FE: *JAMA* 1956;161:1135.
21. Rosenzweig N: *S Afr Med J* 1950;24:831.

22. Rathbun JB, MacNab I: The microvascular pattern of the rotator cuff. *J Bone Joint Surg Br* 1970;52B:540–553.
23. Von Kolliker A: *Mikroskopische Anatomie oder Gewebelehre des Menschen.* Leipzig, W Engelmann, 1850.
24. Ludwig C, Schweigger-Seided F: *Die Lymphgefässe der Fascien und Schnen*''; Leipzig, Hirzel, 1872.
25. Edwards DAW: The blood supply and lymphatic drainage of tendons. *J Anat* 1946;80:147–152.
26. Brockis JG: The blood supply of the flexor and extensor tendons of the fingers in man. *J Bone Joint Surg Br* 1953;35B:131–138.
27. Peacock EE: A study of the circulation in normal tendons and healing grafts. *Ann Surg* 1959;149:415–428.
28. Takasugi H, Akahori O, Nishihara K, et al: Three dimensional architecture of blood vessels of tendons demonstrated by corrosion casts. *Hand* 1978;10(no 1):9–15.
29. Zbrodowski A, Gajisin S, Grodecki J: The anatomy of the digitopalmar arches. *J Bone Joint Surg Br* 1981;63B:108–113.
30. Zbrodowski A, Gajisin S, Grodecki J: Vascularization and anatomical model of the mesotendons of the extensor digitorum and extensor indicis muscles. *J Anat* 1980;130:697–705.
31. Zbrodowski A, Gajisin S, Grodecki J: Vascularisation of the tendons of the extensor pollicis longus, extensor carpi radialis longus and extensor carpi radialis brevis muscles. *J Anat* 1982;135:235–244.
32. Gigis PI, Kuczynski K: The distal interphalangeal joints of human fingers. *J Hand Surg* 1982;7:176–182.

27

Comprehensive Rehabilitation of the Diseased and Injured Upper Extremity

Laurence A. Kirwan
and John A. Boswick, Jr.

It is well recognized that many minor injuries and disease processes of isolated joints and areas of the hand often result in severe impairment of function of the upper extremity. This chapter reviews the principles of rehabilitation of the upper extremity following disease and injury and presents techniques of management that will prevent or minimize loss of motion and decrease impairment of function.

Restoration of hand function and pain relief are the goals of rehabilitation of the diseased or injured upper extremity. The upper limb must be considered as a whole. Emotional instability and neuroticism are factors that predispose a patient to chronic pain. These must be evaluated and treated also.

Rehabilitation, as defined by the *Oxford English Dictionary,* is "the action of replacing a thing or restoring it to its previous condition or status." It may be argued that it is impossible to improve on a normal hand and that an injured hand is never normal again. If so, the term *rehabilitation* is incorrect. The aim of therapy is a level of recovery consistent with our previous experience of what is "possible." Often this will fall short of the preinjury or predisease level of function.

Two statements that encapsulate our philosophy and practice over the past decade are that "Early motion prevents stiffness," and that "The best form of occupational therapy is the person's own work."

"All uninjured parts should be kept unrestrained and free to move."[1] Patients are instructed on the operating table at the termination of surgery and again in the recovery room to exercise their shoulder and elbow as well as the unsplinted parts of their affected hand. The patient should actively abduct the shoulder to the side of the head and flex the elbow until the fingers touch the shoulder, in addition to exercising the wrist and fingers, 4 to 5 minutes every hour while awake. As postoperative pain and inflammation settle, exercises are performed for longer periods of time (25 to 30 minutes) two to three times daily.

The stiff hand is frequently stiff in several joints—the wrist, the metacarpophalangeal (MP) joints, the interphalangeal (IP) joints—rather than one or two individual ones. Stiffness may follow trauma or disease such as an infection or an arthropathy, for example, rheumatoid arthritis, dermatomyositis, or systemic lupus erythematosus.

The indications for rehabilitation are:

- a stiff hand with loss of motion in one or more joints in the hand, wrist, elbow, or shoulder
- loss of strength
- loss of dexterity
- sensory impairment—either diminished sensibility (protective or discriminative) or increased sensibility (hypersensitivity)
- swelling (edema)
- amputation, requiring reeducation, with or without a prosthesis
- pain
- emotional disturbance.

Acute Pain Versus Chronic Stiffness

Stiffness is sometimes described as acute or chronic. Acute stiffness is a result of the acute pain and the edema that follow injury or disease. It can usually be treated quickly with short-term measures, such as elevation and analgesics. In contrast, chronic stiffness is often painless unless attempts are made to move the tissues. Chronic stiffness does not result from pain or edema but is due to structural changes, for example, contractures of ligaments or adhesions of the joint capsule and tendons. Treatment is lengthy and the return of function is often incomplete. Peacock[2] described the fixation, which can occur in chronic stiffness, of joint ligaments to bone by new collagen synthesis in areas normally free of such attachments.

Preliminary measurements and tests are an integral part of therapy. They include grip and pinch strength, two-point discrimination, and active and passive range of motion. Serial measurements enable one to monitor progress and adjust therapy as indicated.

The causes of limitation of motion are tight skin, tight tendons or muscles, tight ligaments, tight joint capsules, and obstructions to motion such as adhesions (within a tendon sheath or a joint) or a bony block.

Tight Skin

Skin tightness can be distinguished by blanching of the overlying skin when the joint is stretched, for example, the dorsum of the MP joints following burn injury. Adherence of skin to underlying structures is diagnosed by observing skin puckering when the underlying tendons, ligaments, or muscles move.

Tight Tendons or Muscles

Tight extrinsic tendons and muscle-tendon units are diagnosed by examining for a tenodesis effect. For example, if the deep flexors are tight, as in Volkmann's ischemic contracture, wrist extension results in flexion of the MP and IP joints, which cannot be extended unless the wrist is flexed. Tightness of the intrinsic muscles is diagnosed by testing for laxity of flexion at the proximal interphalangeal (PIP) joint when the MP joint is extended. Differential tightness of the radial and ulnar intrinsics can be evaluated by deviation of the finger at the MP joint in an ulnar or radial direction, respectively. A tight oblique retinacular ligament (Landsmeer's ligament) is diagnosed by testing for laxity of the distal interphalangeal (DIP) joint when the PIP joint is extended.

Tight Ligaments

The collateral ligaments of the MP joints are tight in flexion and lax in extension. Contracture of these ligaments in extension prevents active or passive flexion of the joint. In contrast, the collateral ligaments of the IP joints are of the same length in all positions. Contractures of these ligaments may result in loss of flexion or extension dependent on a variety of factors (Table 27-1).

Tight Joint Capsules

Tight capsules, like tight ligaments, are detected when motion at the joint is unaltered by motion at adjacent joints. Adhesions between the volar plate and the overlying bone in the cul-de-sac proximal to the joint space may limit flexion or extension depending on the position in which the adhesions form.[3]

Obstructions to Motion

Adhesions within a joint or a tendon sheath, exostoses, or malunited fractures may be responsible for loss of joint motion. If the obstruction is springy, it is likely that movement can be improved, but if the block is abrupt, it is unlikely to improve with nonoperative therapy. Passive range that exceeds active range is due to tendon injury, tendon adhesions, or nerve injury.

A good range of motion is still possible in the IP joints, even with signs of significant radiological derangement. The reason for stiffness in such cases should be sought in tight collateral ligaments, tight intrinsics, or in other causes rather than bony incongruity (Table 27-1).

Specific Rehabilitation Techniques

A variety of techniques are used to restore function and rehabilitate the diseased or injured upper extremity. They include:

- active motion
- active assisted motion
- passive motion
- splinting (dynamic and static)
- sensory reeducation
- compression
- massage
- elevation
- biofeedback
- heat
- pain reduction
- drugs.

Active Motion

When the splint is removed at approximately 3 weeks after a tendon repair, active motion is allowed in the line of pull of the muscle tendon unit. Gentle

Table 27-1 Causes of PIP Joint Stiffness in Flexion and Extension

Flexion
Check-rein ligaments
PIP joint synovitis or effusion
Digital, wrist, or palmar flexor tenosynovitis (including trigger finger)
Flexor contracture or adhesions
Collateral ligament contracture or adhesions
Volar plate adhesions to bone
Capsular contracture (PIP joint)
Bony block
Joint fibrosis, ankylosis, or articular incongruity
Palmar skin contracture
Extension
Intrinsic muscle contracture or adhesions
Intrinsic tightness secondary to MP joint synovitis or contracture
Intrinsic muscle shortening secondary to mallet deformity (DIP joint)
PIP joint synovitis or effusion
Digital, wrist, or palmar flexor tenosynovitis
Distal profundus entrapment
Extensor contracture or adhesion
Collateral ligament contracture or adhesions
Volar plate adhesions to bone
Capsular contracture (PIP joint)
Retinacular ligament contracture or adhesions
Bony block
Joint fibrosis, ankylosis, or articular incongruity
Dorsal skin contracture

active motion is allowed in the opposite direction also. No further splintage is recommended unless the patient is untrustworthy because of infirmity or personality disorder or because his or her occupation may place unreasonable stress on the repair. Gentle resistive exercises are not permitted until approximately 6 weeks after repair.

Aggressive resistive exercises as well as passive stretching in a direction opposite to the pull of the repaired tendon are permitted 8 weeks after tendon surgery (repair or transfer). When restoring motion it is unnecessary to achieve 90° of flexion at the MP joints. Although normal MP joints will flex to 90°, the normal functional range is 75° at the index and middle fingers, 80° at the ring finger, and 80° to 85° at the little finger. Similarly, less flexion is required at the PIP joints of the index and long fingers and relatively more in the ring and little fingers. The index and long fingers are important for pinch, whereas the ring and little fingers are more important for power grip.

Improvement in active motion is the best sign of patient progress. Active motion is the safest and most effective exercise. If it achieves satisfactory results, there is no indication for other forms of treatment. However, in certain cases active motion may be harmful, for example, following tendon repair or transfer where active contraction may weaken or rupture the repair if applied too early. Active exercise such as making a fist has the added advantage of aiding venous return and decreasing edema.

Graded exercises against resistance are used to increase the strength and pull-through of tendons, provided they are well healed. The increased force will stretch adhesions more effectively than will unresisted active exercises alone. Resistive exercises are also of use in rehabilitating muscles after nerve injury.

Overly aggressive therapy by the patient or the therapist can cause an "overuse" syndrome resulting in an acute inflammatory reaction. Before initiating an exercise program, active or passive, any inflammatory response should have resolved, and edema in the limb must be reduced using one of the methods described later.

Active contraction may be hindered by co-contraction of antagonistic muscles. This may be a conscious or a subconscious attempt by the patient to prevent movement that he or she fears. Co-contraction can be avoided by showing the patient which muscles are contracting and by the use of biofeedback instruments. Electrodes that record muscle contractions are used to let patients know when they are contracting the muscle-tendon unit that has been injured or diseased (agonist) or its antagonist (co-contraction; see "Biofeedback" below).

Early motion prevents stiffness. It has been our policy to instruct the patient regarding exercises immediately after surgery, while still in the operating room, and again in the recovery room. The patient is instructed to move all the unsplinted parts of the hands, as well as the shoulder and the elbow. Initially, exercises should be performed for 4 to 5 minutes every hour while awake and later less frequently for 25 to 30 minutes two to three times daily. An early, aggressive exercise program will prevent most of the complications of immobilization. Between active exercises, the parts may be splinted to prevent deformity. This is especially important in the burned upper extremity where adduction contractures of the shoulders, flexion contractures of the elbows and wrists, hyperextension deformities of the MP joints, flexion contractures of the IP joints, and adduction deformities of the thumb (Fig 27-1) may develop.

In the unburned patient, complications such as frozen shoulder may be prevented by early active motion. When active motion is impossible, passive exercises will help to retain a full range of motion. If the patient understands and is able to follow instructions, he or she need not be seen again until the dressing needs changing, which may be 2 to 3 weeks after surgery. If the patient fails to follow the initial instructions, he or she is seen as often as necessary until the exercises are being performed correctly.

Active Assisted Motion

When indicated, the proper use of active assisted motion plays a major role in the rehabilitation of the injured or diseased upper extremity. It is commonly used after tendon or joint surgery. It enables patients to increase the gains they might achieve with active motion alone. The best example of this is the so-called "blocking" of joints. If the available excursion of a tendon is used in flexing, or extending a joint proximal to the site of tendon injury, the excursion at the site of repair will be minimal. To increase distal tendon excursion, the proximal

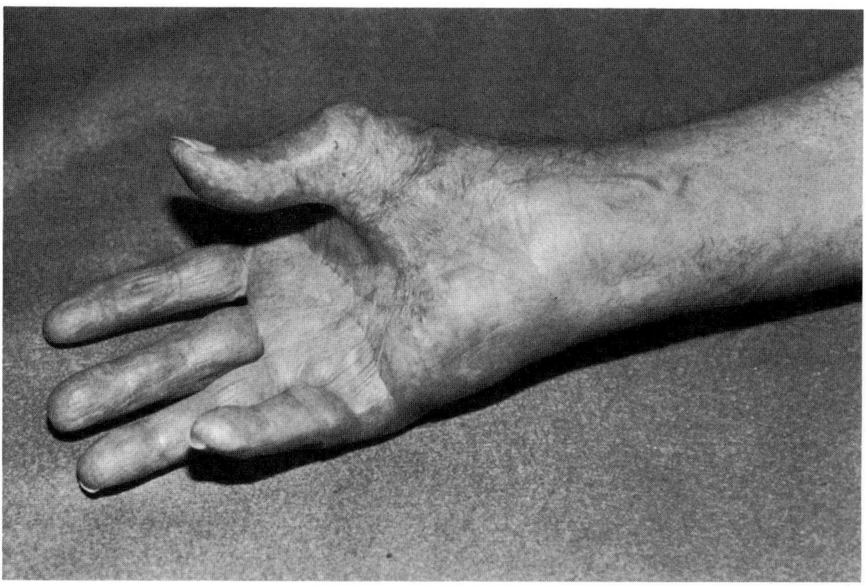

Fig 27-1. Adduction contracture of the thumb following partial-thickness burn injury to the first web.

joints can be blocked. Blocking is done with a finger or with a wood block. It should be started gently and is contraindicated in the early stages following tendon repair or transfer, lest it cause stretching or rupture of the tendon juncture. As time goes on and the repair becomes stronger, the proximal joints may be blocked in progressive degrees of extension or flexion for a flexor or extensor tendon repair, respectively.

Passive Motion

Passive motion is used to maintain or increase movement when active motion is insufficient or impossible, for example, as a result of tendon or nerve interruption. The patient must be able to distinguish between a sensation of pain and a sensation of stretch. The first must be avoided and the latter encouraged. Pain destroys the confidence of the patient and excites an inflammatory response which may cause further pain, stiffness, and scarring with subsequent loss of motion. Slow, gradual gains are safer than sudden, painful ones.

It should be noted that the tight conformity of the ligaments of the finger joints may impede gains in motion.[1] Distraction of the joint with a gentle axial pull, before therapy, stretches the joint capsule and collateral ligaments and may increase the range of motion subsequently obtained.

Passive motion can be increased with the aid of a splint, either static or dynamic (see "Dynamic and Static Splinting" below). A common static device for this purpose is the web strap. This is a simple strap which is tightened around the flexed finger, compressing the distal against the proximal phalanx. It increases motion at the extremes of the normal range.

Following a tendon repair in zone II, passive motion in the direction of the tendon pull is permitted in the immediate postoperative period. Passive motion in a direction opposite to the pull of the repaired tendon is the last activity to be allowed and is not permitted until the patient has been out of the splint for at least 4 weeks. If passive extension is indicated early, for example, because of incipient PIP joint contracture, it is applied to one joint at a time, keeping the adjacent joints flexed or extended so as to prevent tension on the repair. For example, the PIP joint can be extended after a flexor tendon repair, provided the MP joint and the wrist are fully flexed.

Dynamic and Static Splinting

The art of splint making has progressed from devices made of metal, cloth, or plaster, requiring great skill and time to fashion, to the present-day thermoplastics which can be molded accurately and adjusted quickly. In this way, hand splints have become readily available, disposable, and almost infinitely adjustable. Indeed, splint making is so deceptively easy that there is a danger of important mechanical principles being ignored[4] as well as simpler methods of treatment such as those already mentioned.

Static Splints

Static splinting may cause increased stiffness and should be interspersed with exercises and other measures to prevent stiffness and reduce swelling.

A common static splint is the wrist cock-up splint. It keeps the wrist in moderate dorsiflexion and by its tenodesis effect causes the MP joints and IP joints to flex, as well as the thumb to be abducted. Other factors that help maintain a functional posture in the wrist cock-up splint are activation of the intrinsic muscles and gravity.

Static splints may help to prevent deformity after burn injury. If indicated, the shoulder is splinted at 90° of abduction, the elbow in almost full extension, and the hand in the intrinsic plus position; the wrist is moderately dorsiflexed, the MP joints flexed 30° to 40°, the IP joints in almost full extension, and the thumb in palmar abduction parallel to the index metacarpal.

If the hand is not splinted, the wrist may fall into flexion and the hand may adopt a claw posture with hyperextension of the MP joints, flexion of the IP joints, loss of the transverse metacarpal arch, and contraction of the first web space (Fig 27-2).

All joints in the upper extremity may be deformed secondary to burn scar contracture, which usually occurs on the concave aspect of the joint. The exception is the MP joint, which contracts in a position of hyperextension. Timely static splinting interspersed with active and/or passive motion can prevent these deformities.

A splint designed to maintain elbow extension or shoulder abduction should not only immobilize the joint in this position (eg, an airplane splint for the

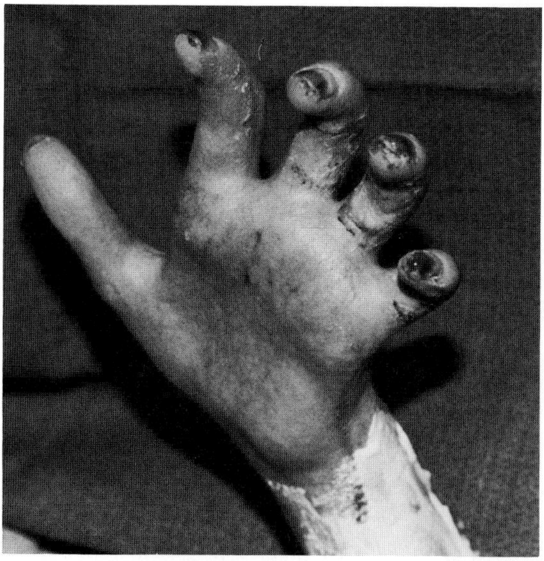

Fig 27-2. Claw hand posture following dorsal burns.

shoulder) but should also conform to the contours of the skin so as to apply constant pressure to the underlying scar tissue. This encourages the healed burn to mature in the stretched position. If the splint is not conforming, bands of contracted scar cut corners, obliterating flexion creases and recreating the deformity when splinting is discontinued. In the hand, wedges of foam or plastic spacers can be inserted into the web spaces with compression, to prevent burn syndactyly.

Static splints can substitute for loss of muscle action after nerve injury or disease. Following median nerve injury, a thumb abduction splint prevents contracture of the first web space and overstretching of the thenar muscles, which would prevent recovery of full strength after nerve regeneration.

Following an ulnar nerve injury, early application of a static splint maintains the MP joints in flexion, preventing a hyperextension deformity which might lead to a collateral ligament contracture as well as overstretching of the volar plate. The splint allows active extension of the IP joints by preventing hyperextension at the MP joint[5] (Fig. 27-3). When the patient tries to grip an object, the

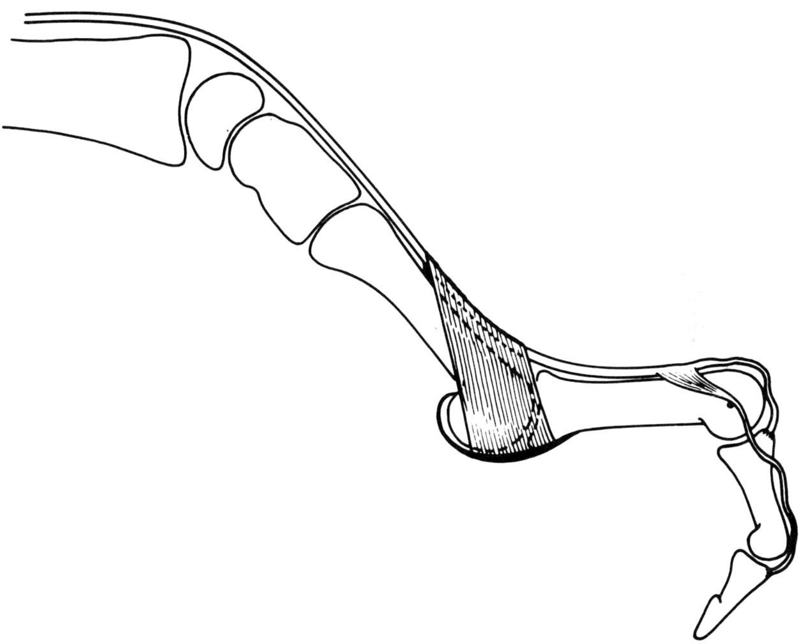

Fig 27-3. When the MP joint is hyperextended, the sagittal bands run progressively more transversely, finally blocking the extensor tendon. When thus blocked, the extensor tendon has less control over the IP joints, which then tend to fall into flexion. Source: Reprinted from "Intrinsic Muscles of the Fingers: Function, Dysfunction, and Surgical Reconstruction" by Smith RJ, *American Academy of Orthopaedic Surgeons Instructional Course Lectures* 24:203, with permission of CV Mosby Co, Copyright © 1975.

splint substitutes for intrinsic function by flexing the MP joints before the IP joints. Without the splint, digital balance is lost. The fingers will flex initially at the IP joints and then at the MP joints, without providing a wide enough grasp to enable the hand to pick up objects.

Following a radial nerve injury a static splint can be used to maintain the wrist in dorsiflexion with the thumb and fingers suspended in slings attached to rubber bands. This not only places the hand in a functional position for grasp but also permits resisted flexion exercises of the fingers and thumb against the dynamic traction and therefore helps to maintain power in the antagonistic muscles.

Dynamic Splints

Dynamic splints increase desirable movements, and static ones prevent undesirable movements (although static splints can also increase motion if used as serial splints, eg, finger casts for IP joint contractures).

Dynamic traction may be used early after tendon repair in zone II. Active extension is accompanied by synchronous relaxation of the finger flexors. Elastic bands flex the fingers passively, preventing active flexion. As a result of early motion, adhesions may be avoided or occur in such a manner as not to restrict tendon excursion.

In other conditions, dynamic traction may also be indicated, with or without static splints, if there is still significant stiffness after active and passive exercises.

Dynamic traction may be started when active motion plus a tolerance to mild stretch is present and as soon as the acute inflammatory response subsides (except following tendon repair, see above). The time to start therapy is assessed on an individual basis.

If therapy is begun too early or applied too vigorously, inflammation, new scarring, and increased stiffness will result. Other possible complications of dynamic traction are increased stiffness in other joints and injury due to failure to understand the mechanical forces involved.

Increased stiffness may be due to a bulky splint obstructing other joints as well as to lack of movement in the opposite direction from that in which traction is applied. Dynamic splinting may improve mobility in one plane at the expense of motion in the other planes. Hence, stiffness may occur in the other planes of motion. To prevent this, traction should be alternated with static or dynamic splinting in other planes or with active and passive exercises out of the splint.

Failure to appreciate the mechanical forces involved can cause skin ulceration or intra-articular damage. For example, when a dorsal splint is made to block MP extension and combined with dynamic traction of the IP joints, the fingers may pivot over the edge of the splint, causing necrosis of dorsal skin unless the splint applies pressure evenly and is designed so that the forces at the end of the finger are counteracted by opposing forces on the hand and dorsum of the proximal phalanx (Figs 27-4 and 27-5). If a joint is subluxed and the volar

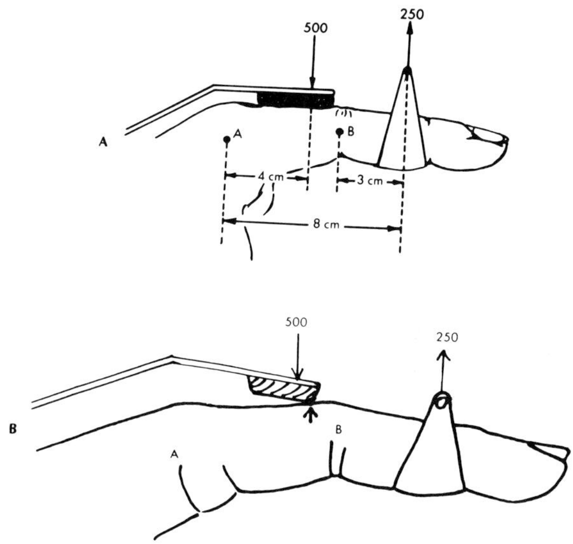

Fig 27-4. *a,* Diagram of finger subjected to force of 250 g through a sling 3 cm from the axis of the IP joint *(B).* The proximal segment of the finger is held in flexion by a felt pad, which is 4 cm from the axis of the MP joint *(A).* This pad receives a thrust of 500 g to balance the force on the sling (500 g × 4 cm = 250 g × 8 cm). *b,* Same finger as in *a,* but because the proximal part of the hand was not supported, the whole finger has tilted. Now only the edge of the felt pad presses on the finger, creating high pressure. Source: Reprinted from "The Forces of Dynamic Splinting: Ten Questions Before Applying a Dynamic Splint to the Hand" by Brand PW, in Hunter JM et al (eds): *Rehabilitation of the Hand,* ed 2, with permission of CV Mosby Co, Copyright © 1984.

plate and pericapsular structures are tight, as in the stiff type of rheumatoid arthritis, traction applied distally, instead of producing a gliding motion of the joint surfaces, may pivot the distal articular surface on the proximal. Pressure necrosis of the compressed articular surfaces may result. This is prevented by applying traction close to the joint so as to minimize the force applied and avoid angulation, thus encouraging a gliding motion of the joint surfaces.[4]

Dynamic splinting is monitored by measuring the volume of the hand and the skin temperature at affected joints. Frequent visual inspection for swelling, redness, and tenderness is essential. Increased volume of the whole or a part of the hand, as well as elevated temperature of a joint, are additional signs of inflammation. If any of these signs are present, traction should be discontinued until the process subsides.

A dynamic splint may constrict tissues, preventing venous return. Therefore splinting is used after the initial postoperative edema has settled but before intractable stiffness has occurred.

A hand that responds well to gentle passive stretch may receive no benefit from a dynamic splint. However, a joint that fails to respond to passive stretch

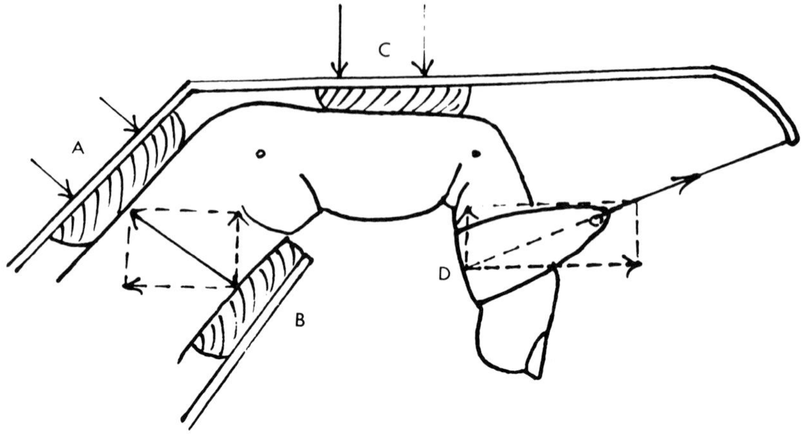

Fig 27-5. Vector diagram showing how both horizontal and vertical forces need to be balanced. Whereas in Fig 4*a* the sling was pulling dorsally, here it pulls obliquely because the IP joint is flexed. The horizontal vector at *D* is double the dorsal vector. Thus, the felt pad *(C)*, which balances the dorsal force, will not take much force. However, the felt pad in the palm *(B)* must be capable of considerable horizontal restraint. It also has a dorsal vector *(C)* which keeps the hand snug against the pad and prevents titling as shown in Fig 4*b*. Pad *A* has no force to exert or absorb. It is there to stabilize against B and prevent unexpected shifts of position of the hand as a whole. Source: Reprinted from "The Forces of Dynamic Splinting: Ten Questions Before Applying a Dynamic Splint to the Hand" by Brand PW, in Hunter JM et al (eds): *Rehabilitation of the Hand*, ed 2, with permission of CV Mosby Co, Copyright © 1984.

or that has an almost full range of motion, but shows significant stiffness at the end points, is likely to benefit from dynamic traction.

Dynamic splinting should allow gains in range of motion while avoiding injury and stimulation of edema production through excessive force. *A dynamic splint will increase the passive range of motion but will neither improve power nor greatly affect tendon glide of the involved muscle-tendon units. Active and active resisted exercises must be performed for improvement to occur, particularly in power and also in tendon glide.* However, a dynamic splint can be used for performing active resisted exercises by muscle contraction in a direction opposite to the pull of the elastic bands.

Tight joints and tight muscle-tendon units may be found in the same hand. A dynamic splint is used to increase the passive range of motion of stiff joints, and later it may be used to stretch tight muscle-tendon units.

The aim of dynamic traction should be to maintain gains in movement as well as to increase passive motion between active exercises. Tension must be gentle enough not to excite an inflammatory response. The aim is not to increase the force but to increase the duration in which the force is applied. Ultimately the patient should feel comfortable wearing the splint throughout the day and/or the night.

Splinting throughout the night lessens morning stiffness and makes it easier for the patient to start active motion of the involved part earlier in the morning. Extension splinting is less constrictive and is tolerated better than flexion splinting at night. Flexion splinting is tolerated better in the day when there are distractions to divert the patient's mind from a less-than-comfortable splint.

Dynamic splints are poorly tolerated at night, a static splint may be used with continuation of the dynamic splint during the day.

It is vital to make patients aware that the gains they achieve with splinting can be lost within hours or days if they neglect to apply their splints. Even with full cooperation it may be several months before the gains made are retained without the constant wearing of splints. The lag represents the time it takes for the collagen fibers to realign themselves and for the scar to mature. Explaining this at the time therapy begins will give the patient realistic expectations and prevent dissatisfaction and noncompliance.

Sensory Reeducation

Hypersensitivity is defined as the condition of extreme discomfort or irritability at or near the injury site in response to normally nonnoxious tactile stimulation. More diffuse pain syndromes are discussed under "Pain Reduction" below.

The theory of desensitization of hypersensitive areas is based on the premise that if painful or potentially painful neuromas are repeatedly percussed, their nerve fibers will gradually degenerate and be replaced by fibrous tissue.[6]

A bulky bandage, a sock, or a mitten enclosing an injured part, "protecting" it from noxious stimuli, prevents sensory input and may lower the patient's sensory threshold, leading to hypersensitivity. Such practices should be discouraged. At best, such a limb is only of use as a paperweight to stabilize objects for the opposite limb, and at worst it amounts to a physiological amputation of the part.

The patient will usually avoid hypersensitive areas, and this leads to abnormal patterns of use. The patient must be informed that it is actually beneficial to use and stimulate the injured and hypersensitive areas.

Various methods of desensitization may be used. They include application of ultrasound and vibrators, rubbing and tapping with materials of different textures attached to dowels, and immersing the part in containers of particles of various consistency. Vibration and the application of textures or particles can be graded according to level of stimulation so that a program of therapy can be planned that starts with mild stimuli and progresses to more noxious ones as tolerance increases. Local infiltration or regional nerve blocks may be required to initiate therapy.

Dowel textures range from felt or moleskin to Velcro hooks. These may be tapped or rubbed adjacent to or directly on the sensitive site. Contact particles range from cotton to buckshot. Vibration varies from 83 cycles near the sensitive site but without actual contact to 100 cycles continuous contact over the site itself. Exercises can be done at home. Rehabilitation should include simulated work activities as soon as the patient is able to cooperate. Using tools with which the patient is familiar may be more helpful than a formal desensitization program.

The end of treatment comes when the patient is able to return to work, not when he or she no longer has symptoms. With sufficient progress the patients cure themselves.

If these methods should fail, surgery may offer a solution, excising a neuroma in continuity and repairing the nerve or transposing an end-bulb neuroma into a well-padded location where it will be protected from noxious stimuli.

Compression

Intermittent and constant compression (including Ace bandage wrapping), elevation, string wrapping, retrograde massage, and active motion are all means of dispersing edema. Edema can be quantified by measuring the girth of a hand or a finger with a tape measure or by measuring its displacement of an equal volume of water according to Achimedes' law.

Constant compression (eg, Jobst compression garments) prevents edema and may prevent hypertrophic scarring. They are comfortable to wear and patients can become addicted to them. They should be examined often to be sure that they fit properly and should be replaced when loose. Because they take several weeks to be made, the patient should be measured before the wounds are healed. Small, unhealed wounds can be dressed and tolerated beneath a compression garment. Larger areas should be healed, or application and removal of the garments will traumatize the wound edges and retard epithelialization.

Retrograde Massage

Retrograde massage is a way of establishing the relationship between therapist and patient. It gives the patient positive feedback. As a therapeutic exercise, it helps to disperse edema and makes subsequent exercises easier to perform. Therefore, it is frequently used as a preliminary to an exercise session.

Elevation

The arm should be held in the "Statue of Liberty" position when the patient is standing upright and on two pillows when sitting and at night. A sling is not recommended. At best it keeps the hand over the heart. At worst, the hand is held immobile at waist level. A sling places the joints of the upper extremity in flexion, obstructing arterial inflow and venous return. Elevation should continue for as long as there is swelling or a tendency to swelling.

Biofeedback

The simplest form of biofeedback is the physician's or the therapist's tabulation of progress and advice about exercises as the patient recovers. Electrodes applied to the skin or placed within a muscle can record active contraction on a meter. This may be of use following tendon transfer when the patient is learning to use the transferred muscle-tendon unit. It is also indicated when co-contraction is a problem (see above). Other feedback aids are a grip dynamometer and a pinch meter with which the patient can record progress and attempt to exceed previous results.

Heat

Cold and inactive tissues have a low metabolic rate and are inelastic. Activity and heat increase the metabolic rate and increase tissue elasticity. Therefore, heat is a useful modality to increase tissue elasticity prior to an exercise program. Warm water soaks, whirlpool baths, and hot wax are all accepted methods of warming the limb. However, dependency in a whirlpool can aggravate edema, and we do not recommend this method.

Pain Reduction

Rehabilitation has two aims: to relieve pain and to improve function. The pain "threshold" is the least stimulus at which a patient perceives pain.[7] The pain "tolerance level" is the greatest stimulus intensity causing pain that a patient is prepared to tolerate.[7] A patient's readiness to communicate pain is a function of character and does not imply that the patient has a low pain threshold.

Personality traits can be measured by the Eysenck Personality Inventory (EPI) and the Minnesota Multiphasic Personality Inventory (MMPI). Patients with scores on the EPI, suggesting neuroticism, and with scores on the MMPI, suggesting depression, hypochondriasis, and hysteria, are those most likely to develop chronic pain syndromes.[8]

Passive exercises help to reduce pain and maintain mobility. However, active exercises build strength and dexterity, which are more important because they prepare patients for an independent existence and allow them to cure themselves.

Among the recognized causes of pain associated with upper extremity disease and injury are:

- peripheral painful stimulus
- reflex sympathetic dystrophy
- inflammatory pain of peripheral origin
- personality disorder
- cancer and other causes of intractable pain.

Peripheral Painful Stimulus

A peripheral painful stimulus is usually associated with a trigger point. A neuroma may be a terminal type or a neuroma in continuity. Terminal bulb neuroma is seen most commonly in amputation stumps.

Hypersensitivity or hyperpathia associated with a neuroma may be treated in several ways. Desensitization procedures are discussed above. Percutaneous injections of bupivacaine hydrochloride or triamcinolone acetonide combined with a short-acting local anesthetic may relieve symptoms.[9]

If these methods should fail, surgery may help, placing the neuroma in a new site where compression and traction are unlikely. A neuroma in continuity may be excised and the nerve repaired (end to end or with a graft).

This syndrome may be associated with tenderness of the respective nerve (median, ulnar, radial) proximally at the wrist, elbow, and in the supraclavicular fossa. If so, local treatment is less likely to help. A proximal 'neuritis' may respond to anti-convulsant medication such as Phenytoin (dilantin sodium) or Tegretol (carbamazepine). Consultation with a neurologist is recommended.

Reflex Sympathetic Dystrophy

"One must be alert to recognize early cases that will go on to edematous, immobile hands by recognizing signs of trophic disturbance and disposition on the part of the patient to hold his hand completely immobile."[1] Three conditions must be present for a dystrophy to develop. These are a persistent source of pain, a susceptibility on the patient's part, and an abnormal sympathetic reflex.

The cardinal signs are pain, swelling, stiffness, and vasomotor instability (temperature or color change). Pain is characteristically of a burning nature. The limb is usually warm. Hypersensitivity and cold intolerance are common. Technetium-99m-pertechnetate (^{99m}Tc04) and technetium-99m-distannous ethane-1-hydroxy-1-1-diphosphonate (^{99m}Tc-EHDP) scintigraphy may show localization of nuclide predominantly in the juxta-articular tissues. Radiographs may show osteoporosis in either a diffuse or a juxta-articular distribution, but this is not apparent for at least 6 weeks.[10]

Ultimately the extremity may become contracted, atrophic, stiff, pale, cool, sweaty, or dry. The syndrome is believed to be a prolongation of the normal sympathetic response to injury. The essential goal of treatment is interruption of the sympathetic reflex. The earlier this is done, the better the result.

Aggressive exercise programs at an early stage may prevent an incipient case from becoming established. The hand therapist should avoid any painful exercises as these may exacerbate the condition.

Median nerve compression at the wrist is associated with reflex sympathetic dystrophy. When present, decompression of the nerve is indicated. No subsequent surgery should be performed without cover of a sympathectomy or a stellate ganglion block.

Patients with Raynaud's phenomenon who have a positive cold stress test[11] and who do not show obstructive disease on arteriography may respond to medications that decrease peripheral sympathetic activity.

Drugs recommended for intra-arterial injection include α-receptor blockers such as tolazoline hydrochloride (Priscoline) and phenoxybenzamine hydrochloride as well as β-adrenergic blocking drugs such as propranolol hydrochloride and neuronal norepinephrine depletors such as reserpine, methyldopa, or guanethidine. Oral guanethidine, phenoxybenzamine, and propranolol have also been used.[11,12] Regional intravenous blocks with reserpine and guanethidine have been used effectively.[13–16]

A stellate ganglion block is a useful diagnostic test. A therapeutic response will usually confirm the value of a surgical sympathectomy, which may be indicated if a single or repeated blocks fail to relieve the pain for more than a brief duration. Surgery may relieve the burning pain of sympathetic overactivity. It will not affect pain secondary to a neuroma or arthritis.

If chemical or surgical sympathectomy fails, transcutaneous electrical nerve stimulation (TENS) may be considered. This is most effective when started within 3 months of the onset of pain.

The transcutaneous electrical nerve stimulator is an electric device that emits a pulsed current in the form of a biphasic, asymmetric wave form. The use of this device is based on the gate control theory proposed by Melzack and Wall[17] in 1965. Pain receptors (nocireceptors) transmit their impulses through A-delta and unmyelinated (C) fibers. When the impulses arrive in the posterior horn of the spinal cord, a gate mechanism controls the passage of signals to the spinothalamic tract and thence to the brain. Increased C fiber activity inhibits the gate, allowing transmission of more impulses. Increased large unmyelinated A fiber activity closes the gate, blocking pain. TENS is thought to stimulate the A fibers. The inhibitory agent released is an opioid peptide (endorphin).

"Conventional" TENS is usually administered at a frequency of 60 to 120 pulses per second (pps) with a low pulse width and a low amplitude, which is adjusted until the patient has a pleasant tingling sensation in the area that was previously painful. "Low-frequency" TENS has a frequency of 1 to 5 pps with a high pulse width and an amplitude adjusted until a visible muscle contraction occurs. Pain relief occurs 15 to 30 minutes after the start of conventional or low-frequency TENS and may last from 30 minutes to several hours after it is discontinued. "High-frequency" TENS has a frequency of 60 to 120 pps with a high pulse width and high amplitude adjusted until a strong muscle contraction occurs. This is in effect a form of counterstimulation. Pain relief is sudden and transient with variable carryover. This may be useful for brief procedures such as suture removal and wound débridement. Because an active muscle contraction occurs with low-frequency and high-frequency TENS, the patient must be cleared for active exercises. A muscle contraction does not occur with conventional TENS.

Therapy is usually initiated with conventional TENS, and converting to low frequency TENS if ineffective. For therapy to be evaluated properly, the patient should refrain from analgesics for 6 to 8 hours prior to TENS and should be experiencing pain when treated. Too often, TENS becomes a 'beacon' of the patient's disability labelling them as an impaired member of the community. Although TENS may relieve pain, it has not, in our experience, speeded recovery. Frequently, the patient becomes addicted to this expensive and complex form of treatment making discontinuation impossible. It is often prescribed too readily by both physician and therapist.

Inflammatory Pain

See the section titled "Drugs" below, for a discussion of nonsteroidal anti-inflammatory agents (NSAIA). Steroids are of use in certain conditions such as rheumatoid arthritis. We have no experience with intravenous blocks using prednisone and lidocaine.[18] Intra-articular steroids are particularly helpful in degenerative joint disease involving a single joint (eg, thumb basal joint arthritis). Flexor tenosynovitis may also respond to local injections of steroids. Half to one cc of Triamcinolone acetonide (Kenalog-40) combined with 0.5–1.0 cc of 1% lidocaine is the usual amount injected.

As pain subsides, massage and heat are combined with a program of exercises and NSAIA.

Personality Dysfunction

Medications for emotional instability and depression may be required. Phenytoin (Dilantin) and amitriptyline hydrochloride (Elavil) are commonly used drugs. These may be combined. Hypnosis may be helpful.

Cancer and Other Causes of Intractable Pain

When pain is intractable, invasive procedures such as spinal dorsal sensory root rhizotomy[19] may be of use in cases of unilateral pain involving the brachial plexus when the involved extremity is useless. Cordotomy is indicated for diffuse pain involving areas innervated by many nerve roots. Destructive lesions at higher levels (eg, cingulotomy) are of temporary benefit only.

Drugs

Infiltration with bupivacaine (Marcaine) at the end of an operation (with or without indwelling catheters) to provide continuous pain relief following tenolysis or capsulotomy, will enable the patient to begin early exercises.

Following trauma or disease, NSAIAs are the first-line medications after the acute stage, when narcotic analgesics can be used. Of the NSAIAs, phenylbutazone and indomethacin are not recommended for long-term therapy because of their gastric irritation. NSAIAs that we use regularly are ibuprofen (Motrin), naproxen (Naprosyn), diflunisal (Dolobid), piroxicam (Feldene), and meclofenamate sodium (Meclomen). In long-standing, active arthropathies, remitting agents such as penicillamine (Cuprimine) and aurothioglucose (Solganal) are of use in controlling the frequency of attacks.

Conclusion

The indications for rehabilitation are loss of function (ie, movement, strength, dexterity, and sensibility) as well as loss of parts. Pain and emotional disturbance may cause impairment of function. The best treatment, as always, is prevention; early motion prevents stiffness. The best therapist is the patient himself or herself. The best therapy is the patient's own work. A motivated patient will do well with a minimum of therapy.

Postoperatively, patients are instructed on the operating table at the termination of surgery and in the recovery room to exercise the shoulder and elbow as well as the unsplinted parts of the injured hand. Exercises are done every hour for 4 to 5 minutes and, after the acute stage, two to three times daily for 25 to 30 minutes.

In all cases, whether after injury or disease, patients are taught to distinguish between the sensation of stretch and the sensation of pain. The first is encouraged and the latter is not. The axiom, "It may hurt but it won't harm," is wrong. If it hurts it may harm, and it may excite an inflammatory reaction that leads to further cicatricization and stiffness. "The inevitability of gradualness" is to be stressed. Gentle exercises done with increasing frequency or duration will achieve more than sudden, impatient jerks performed on the unsuspecting patient.

Active motion is the safest and most effective exercise. It improves tendon glide and strength as well as range of motion. Active assistive and active resisted exercises are complementary. Active exercises are not possible after a recent tendon repair, however. Dynamic traction is used early after a flexor tendon repair in zone II.

Static splinting is used most frequently in the acute stage to prevent undesirable positions of rest. The wrist cock-up splint as well as the intrinsic plus splint are those in common use. The former places the hand in a "position of function." The wrist is in 20° to 30° of dorsiflexion, the MP joints in 20° to 30° of flexion, and the IP joints in 10° to 20° of flexion. The latter places the hand in the intrinsic plus position. The wrist is in the same position, but the MP joints are now flexed to 50° to 60° and the IP joints are in neutral. The thumb is held in 45° of palmar abduction and is opposite the index metacarpal.

Dynamic splinting may be started when active motion plus a tolerance to mild stretch is present. Dynamic splinting encourages motion in desirable planes.

Although splints are much easier to construct with thermoplastic materials, the mechanical principles involved in their construction are frequently misunderstood, and it behooves the physician to be cognizant of these principles and to be sure that splints are made and applied correctly. The price of misunderstanding is skin and joint injury. Splints should be reviewed by the physician at each office visit and adjusted as often as necessary. Frequently, one splint will not achieve all that is necessary, and then two or more splints should be used during the day or night to achieve the desired goals.

Other methods such as compression, massage, elevation, biofeedback, heat, and anti-inflammatory drugs may be used singly or in combination to decrease swelling, stiffness, and inflammation.

In the acute stage, elevation and static splinting are all that is indicated. As the inflammatory reaction subsides, gentle active and passive range-of-motion exercises are suitable. Gentle traction may also be of use at this time. As time progresses, active assistive and resistive exercises as well as more aggressive passive stretching, particularly in planes opposite to the plane of motion activated by the repaired tendon, are indicated. This sequence may be altered depending on the individual patient or the structure injured; for example, dynamic traction is used early following a tendon repair in zone II.

Pain may be localized to the site of a neuroma or may be diffuse as in reflex sympathetic dystrophy. A desensitization program is useful for a local cause of hypersensitivity. If the patient is encouraged to use the part normally from the beginning, the incidence of hypersensitivity is lessened considerably.[20]

Reflex sympathetic dystrophy can be prevented by "being alert to recognize early cases that will go on to edematous hands by recognizing signs of trophic disturbance and disposition on the part of the patient to hold his hand completely immobile."[1] An early, aggressive program of therapy may help. Other modalities of treatment have been discussed. Despite the best treatment, there will always remain a small percentage of patients who will do badly and develop chronic pain syndromes that are refractory to treatment. Personality dysfunction is frequent in this minority and may respond to treatment.

Inflammatory pain may respond to splinting and drugs, intractable pain such as that due to cancer may require surgery.

Early motion as well as functional activities prevent stiffness, swelling, and pain. An understanding of the purpose of each method of treatment and the correct timing for application of each will prevent injury and encourage rapid recovery of the hand to a level of maximum function consistent with the initial injury or the disease.

References

1. Bunnell S: *Surgery of the Hand,* ed 3. Philadelphia, JB Lippincott Co, 1948.
2. Peacock EE: Some biochemical and biophysical aspects of joint stiffness: Role of collagen synthesis as opposed to ultra molecular binding. *Ann Surg* 1966; 163:1–6.
3. Scott FA, Boswick JA: Palmar arthroplasty for the treatment of the stiff swan-neck deformity. *J Hand Surg* 1983; 8:267–272.
4. Brand PW: The forces of dynamic splinting: Ten questions before applying a dynamic splint to the hand, in Hunter JM, Schneider LH, Mackin EJ (eds): *Rehabilitation of the Hand.* St Louis, CV Mosby Co, 1984, pp 847–852.
5. Smith RJ: Intrinsic muscles of the fingers: Function, dysfunction and surgical reconstruction. *American Academy of Orthopaedic Surgeons Instructional Course Lectures* 1975; 24:200–220.

6. Russell WR, Spalding JMK: Treatment of painful amputation stumps. *Br Med J* 1950; 2:68–73.
7. Mersky H: Pain terms: A list with definitions and notes on usage (International Association for the Study of Pain [IASP] Subcommittee on Taxonomy). *Pain* 1979; 6:249–252.
8. Bond MR: *Pain: Its Nature, Analysis and Treatment.* Edinburgh, Churchill Livingstone, 1979.
9. Smith JR, Gomez NH: Local injection therapy of neuromata of the hand with triamcinolone acetonide: A preliminary study of twenty-two patients. *J Bone Joint Surg Am* 1970; 52A:71–83.
10. Kozin F, Genant HK, Bekerman C, et al.: The reflex sympathetic dystrophy syndrome II. Roentgenographic and scintigraphic evidence of bilaterality and of periarticular accentuation. *Am J Med* 1976; 60:332–338.
11. Porter JM, Snider RL, Bardana EJ, et al.: The diagnosis and treatment of Raynaud's phenomenon. *Surgery* 1975; 77:11–23.
12. Simson G: Propranolol for causalgia and Sudek atrophy. *JAMA* 1974; 227:327.
13. Chuinard RG, Dabezies JE, Gould JS, et al.: Intravenous reserpine for treatment of reflex sympathetic dystrophy. *J Hand Surg* 1980; 5:289.
14. Hannington-Kiff JG: Intravenous regional sympathetic block with guanethidine. *Lancet* 1974; 1:1019–1020.
15. Hannington-Kiff JG: Relief of Sudek's atrophy by regional intravenous guanethidine. *Lancet* 1977; 1:1132–1133.
16. Wynn Parry CB: Brachial plexus lesions, causalgia and Sudek's atrophy. *Am Soc Surg Hand Newsletter* 1981; 2.
17. Melzack R, Wall PD: Pain mechanisms: A new theory. *Science* 1965; 150:971–979.
18. Wiley AM, Poplawski ZB, Murray J: Post-traumatic dystrophy of the hand. *Orthop Rev* 1977; 6:59–61.
19. Leavens ME: Neurosurgical relief of pain in cancer patients. *Cancer Bull* 1981; 33:98–100.
20. Fisher GT, Boswick JA: Neuroma formation following digital amputations. *J Trauma* 1983; 23:136–142.
21. Omer GE: Management of pain syndromes in the upper extremity, in Hunter JM, Schneider LH, Mackin EJ (eds): *Rehabilitation of the Hand.* St Louis, CV Mosby Co, 1984, pp 503–508.

28

Work Evaluation: Returning the Hand-Injured Patient to Work

Pat McKenna and
Marilyn Meyers

A comprehensive study by the US Department of Labor showed that injury and severe illness resulted in a loss to the economy in 1981 of $62 billion. This figure is derived from the medical costs and compensation and disability benefits paid by industry and government for the care of injured workers. Another study has shown that for every $10,000 spent in rehabilitation of an injured worker, $35,000 is returned to the economy by that worker's returning to the work force.[1]

With dwindling resources to draw upon, it becomes apparent that the economy cannot continue to pay people disability or worker's compensation essentially forever, as has often been the case. It is also apparent that with all the new technology available, it should no longer be assumed that a person who is injured and has a residual handicap cannot be a profitable member of society. Indeed, with present resources, there are very few individuals who could not either resume their previous job, with some modifications in their manner of performing it, or be retrained into a new profession that is within the limits of their disability. However, in many cases, our regulations, social precedent, business and/or union policies, and motivation deter this from becoming a reality.

Insurance companies, industry, and government are becoming more and more attuned to the possibilities for rehabilitation, and the days of "permanent disability" are being reevaluated. In some states, it is becoming an accepted practice for injured workers to receive a comprehensive evaluation and program of rehabilitation, including job retraining, if necessary, before a settlement is determined. Colorado is moving very close to this approach with the worker's compensation regulations that were signed into effect in November 1983.[2] These regulations require that the insurance carrier provide for a vocational evaluation:

A. Immediately upon receipt of the first report of an injury in which liability is admitted and that involves any of the following:
   1. Mangling, crushing, or amputation of a major portion of an extremity
   2. Traumatic injury to the spinal cord that has caused or may cause paralysis
   3. Severe burns that require burn center care
   4. Serious head injury or loss of both eyes

B. Immediately upon knowledge that an injured employee is unlikely to be able to return to his or her usual and customary occupation on a permanent basis, as determined by competent medical evidence and opinion.

In the past, virtually the entire burden of determining a person's fitness to return to work has rested on the shoulders of the physician, who was expected to make this determination usually with very little objective data. In many cases, this placed the physician in an awkward situation. How could one say for certain that this person who was seen in the physician's office for a short time, and who could squeeze his or her hand or a dynamometer, could sustain this effort over time or in very different, even precarious situations? Coordination and fine manipulative ability were almost impossible to assess adequately.

If the patient were turned over to the vocational rehabilitation counselors because of doubt that the patient could work at his or her previous job, the counselors were not always trained in the real medical effects of the disability and its relationship to the job. Thus, persons who could actually return to their work with some modifications were sometimes unnecessarily retrained into new jobs. Vocational counselors also lacked the resources to observe a person's abilities over time, and so were forced to make subjective judgments as well.

If, however, we utilize all the skills of the resource people available, as a team, a competent approach is possible. If we are to work as a team it is helpful to understand who all the players are and what are their primary roles. Although there may be considerable overlap, depending on the situation, this may be helpful in delineating the basic roles.

The Vocational Rehabilitation Team

The vocational rehabilitation team includes the following personnel:

- physicians, physical therapists, and occupational therapists, whose primary role is in acute medical care and medical analysis;
- the occupational therapist, who analyzes the patient's job and abilities in relation to the medical conditions;
- the vocational evaluator, who analyzes the patient's achievements, aptitude, intelligence, and interests with relation to possible transferable skills;

- the vocational rehabilitation counselor, who performs an analysis of information collected from all of the above and develops a program for the patient's rehabilitation for submission to the insurance carrier, the employer, and so forth as appropriate;
- the insurance carrier, the employer, and the state department of vocational rehabilitation, whose role involves analysis and approval for funding of the rehabilitation plan;
- lawyers, social workers, and job market analysts, who are called on to meet the specific needs of the patient, as appropriate.

Work Evaluation

One important component that the occupational therapist can provide the team is the evaluation of the patient's medical condition in relation to his or her work. Occupational therapists have been doing this since before 1923, when hospitals were mandated by the Vocational Rehabilitation Act to provide these services to injured workers. In the past 5 years, partly as a result of the strong new demand, the following new descriptors of these services have been developed to help delineate more clearly which specific services may be most appropriate for a given patient:

- Work capacity evaluation: a comprehensive process that focuses upon the measurement of the patient's potential for work. It includes feasibility for employment and physical and emotional work capabilities.
- Work tolerance screening: the objective measurement of the patient's physical strength, coordination, range of movement, and/or endurance in performing particular tasks, with a focus on critical job demands, based on an analysis of the patient's job.
- Work simulation: the staging of a particular work task under simulated environmental conditions. Work simulation is used as a component of work capacity evaluation or work tolerance screening.

Components of the work capacity evaluation include[4]:

- physical capacity evaluation, including range of motion, strength, endurance, hand function, sensation, gross and fine motor coordination, ability to work under a load and over time, use of tools, visual-perceptual skills, body positioning, and cardiopulmonary response to work
- job analysis, including on-site job assessment when necessary and step-by-step breakdown of specific job tasks as needed in defining problem areas
- use of standardized tests, such as Valpar Work Samples, the Purdue Pegboard, the Jebsen Hand Function Test, and the Pennsylvania Bi-Manual Work Sample, in evaluating assets and limitations

- assessment of the patient's characteristics as a worker and his or her cognitive functioning, including problem-solving skills, motivation, adaptability, ability to follow instructions, and stress tolerance, while performing tasks.

Components of work tolerance screening include[5]:

- physical capacity evaluation, as noted above, which includes physical strength and range of movement while performing tasks
- analysis of work performance in a simulated setting, over time, which measures endurance in performance of specific skills in specific positions, based on critical job demands determined in job analysis
- assessment of strengths and weaknesses as well as modifications to be made in the method of performing the job, to allow the maximum amount of work to be performed by the patient with the least amount of physical or emotional stress
- analysis of modifications to the equipment or workplace that would permit the patient to perform the job more easily and/or more safely.

Components of work simulation include:

- job analysis
- evaluation and reevaluation using the BTE Work Simulator, a computerized device that simulates virtually every functional movement of the upper extremity and provides objective measurements of the ability to perform those movements
- structured, graded, and supervised simulation of a job task or tasks.

The work capacity evaluation begins when the hand-injured patient is referred to therapy. Often one of the first questions the patient asks is, "Will I be able to return to work?" and the next is often, *When* will I be able to return to work?"

It is difficult for the physician to assess a patient's ability to return to work. The physician sees the patient briefly in the office and does not see the injured hand after it has been exposed to a work situation.

There are many components to evaluate in a person's job. In one case, for example, a patient was referred to occupational therapy to increase the strength and range of motion in his left (nondominant) hand. His injury was a paint injection in the palm of his hand. He had a 10-pound grip and lacked 30° of extension in the metacarpophalangeal joints. The physician had released this patient to return to full duty, 5 days later, as a painter. The physician had reasoned that the patient had full use of his dominant hand and would therefore have no difficulties. The patient expressed concern to the therapist about returning to work. What the physician had not considered was that the patient

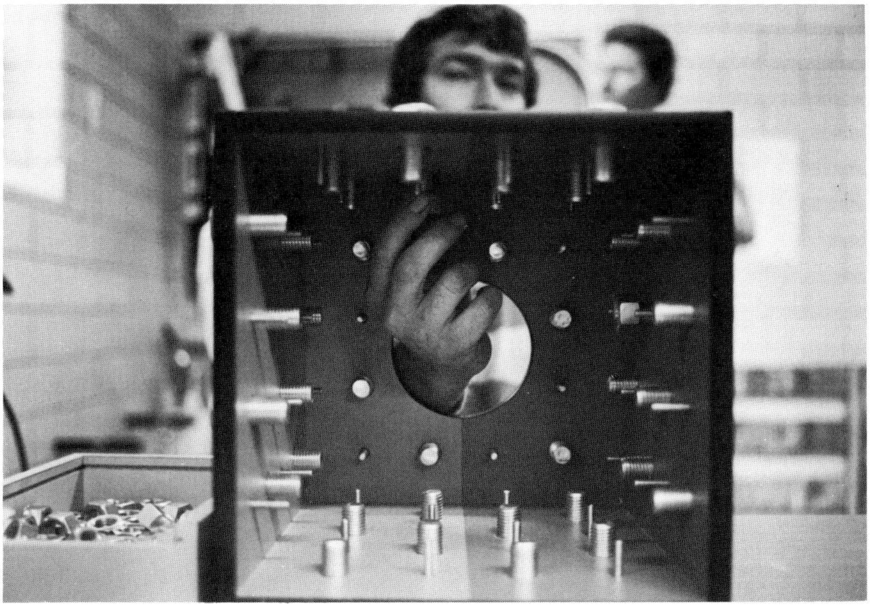

Fig 28-1. The Valpar Upper Extremity Work Sample is a standardized test that can assist in assessing the functional abilities of a patient's arms and hands.

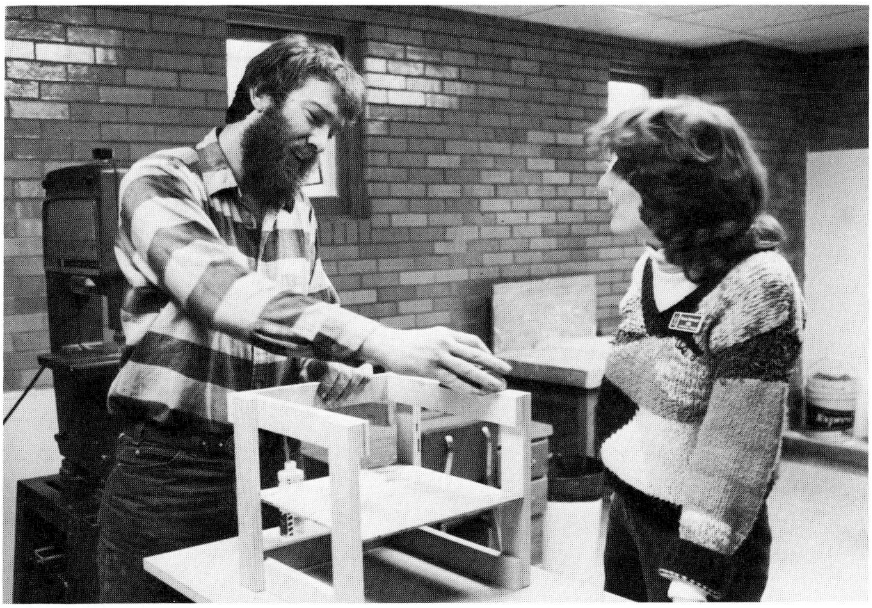

Fig 28-2. Woodworking encourages full upper extremity range of motion, coordinated hand function, and endurance as well as reintegration of carpentry skills to assist in returning to work.

needed to use his left hand to hold the can of paint, which he held at the bottom of the can with his wrist and fingers fully extended. He also painted from a ladder and needed his left hand to support himself.

The therapist took the patient to the paint shop in the hospital, and the patient was not able even to hold an empty paint can. The physician was called, and the patient's work release was delayed. The patient began a work simulation program and within 4 weeks was able to return to work, safely, and to full duty (Fig 28-2).

A work capacity evaluation is needed when the hand-injured patient has attained close to his or her full strength, range, and dexterity, and there is a question whether the patient can return to his or her previous job, or when it is determined that the patient will not be able to return to his or her previous job, but it is unknown what skills the patient has.

Several components are involved in a work capacity evaluation. First are physical measurements of range of motion, strength, endurance, sensation, and gross and fine motor coordination. Second is a job analysis. This is a step-by-step breakdown of specific job tasks. The information is obtained from the patient, the patient's employer, the *Dictionary of Occupational Titles,* and, if necessary, an on-site job assessment.

Several standardized tests to assess objectively the patient's abilities are available.

Valpar Whole Body Range of Motion[8]

The Valpar Whole Body Range of Motion test[3] measures the ability of a person's gross body movements of the trunk, arms, hands, legs, and fingers as they relate to the functional ability to perform job tasks. It provides insight into the relationship of gross body movements to finer manual dexterity found in many different work situations. For example, how well can a person grasp and manipulate objects while reaching overhead? Many dexterity tests have the patient sitting or standing comfortably, unlike actual work situations which require flexion or extension of the trunk and limbs, which often produces tension on the worker. The stress of physical demands can affect the dexterity of the client.

The Valpar evaluation is performed by having the client transfer forms to an overhead position, to a midbody position, to a kneeling position, and back up to standing. Each transfer is timed separately, and at the end of each the client is asked if he or she is experiencing any physical discomfort.

Valpar Upper Extremity Range of Motion

The Valpar Upper Extremity Range of Motion test[4] measures range of motion in the shoulder, upper arm, forearm, elbow, wrist, and hand. It provides information about factors such as neck and back fatigue, finger dexterity, and finger tactile sense (Fig 28-1).

The evaluation has two sections. In the assembly section, the client is required to pick up one nut at a time, reach through an opening in the front of a box, place the nut on a bolt, and screw the nut down snugly. Each hand is tested separately, and the client is timed on each panel.

The second section involves disassembly. The client removes the nuts one at a time using either the right or the left hand. The client has the option to change hands as often as needed. Again, after each section the client is asked to describe any pain or fatigue.

Lifting Evaluation

This evaluation is used to measure lifting capacity. A weight is placed in a box on a metal bar, which can be lifted from the floor to varying heights of between 13 and 78 inches. The evaluation is begun with 10 pounds, and with each trial a 5-pound weight is added until the patient reaches his or her maximum lifting capacity at each level.

This tool can also be used to evaluate carrying bilaterally and on each side by using the box and bar. The patient is instructed to carry the weighted box and bar 100 yards. Again, 5-pound increments are added progressively until the patient reaches his or her maximum level.

If it has been determined how much weight a person needs to lift or carry for a given job, and approximately how many times, this is a good tool to use to evaluate the client's ability to perform his or her job.

Purdue Pegboard

The Purdue Pegboard evaluation is one of many fine motor coordination tests that can be used. It is a timed test used to evaluate bilateral fine-motor coordination. It is a good assessment to utilize in evaluating someone in an assembly job. Other evaluations that could also be used are the Pennsylvania Bi-Manual Work Sample, the Nine-Hole Peg Test, and the Minnesota Rate of Manipulation Test.

Work Simulator

A work simulator is a computerized device that can simulate virtually every functional movement of the upper extremity and provides objective measurements of the patient's ability to perform those movements. Exercise machines assist a patient in strengthening specific muscles, but their limited, stylized movements do not permit the kind of therapy necessary to enable a patient to return to a previous occupation.

A work simulator can simulate a work environment by providing a rotatable shaft to which a variety of tools can be attached. These tools can reproduce the motions of the hand and upper extremity. The tools provide the patient with the "feel" to which he or she is accustomed (Fig 28-3).

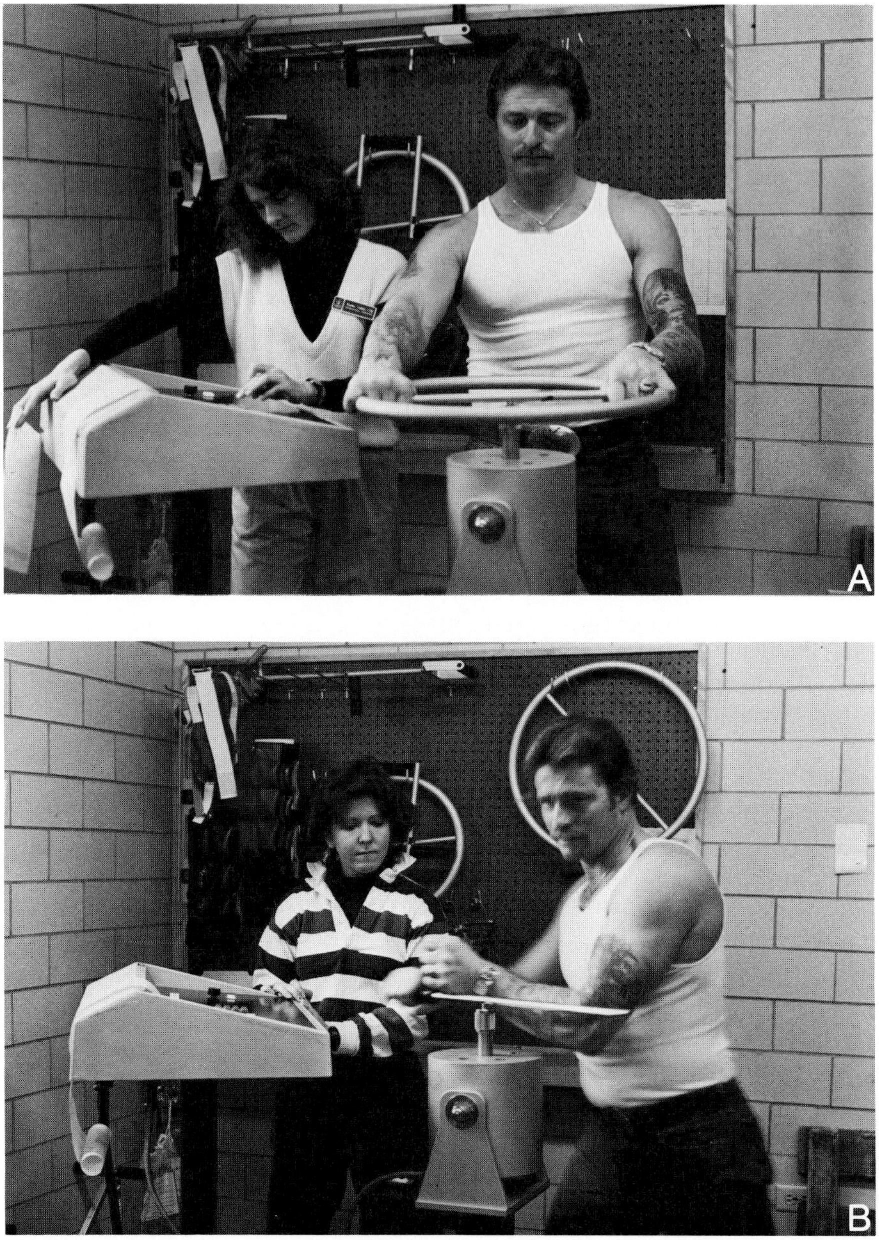

Fig 28-3. Tasks on the work simulator that replicate movements required in the patient's job. *A*, Truck driver simulating steering wheel, *B*, patient required to push heavy carts.

There are three major components of a work simulator:

1. An electrically controlled variable-resistance device, which adjusts in height to accommodate the individual and the requirements of the job and its tools;
2. A control console, which provides a printout of:
   a. degrees of rotation
   b. elapsed time in seconds
   c. amount of resistance
   d. work done and power achieved by the patient;
3. A variety of tools which attach to the resistance device.

When using the work simulator, the therapist needs to work with the patient to learn what tools the patient uses and what movements he or she performs on the job. Attachments are then chosen based on this information, and levels of repetitions and resistance are set.[5] A benefit of the work simulator is that the patient gets immediate feedback and can see the close relationship between treatment and what he or she does on the job.

Finally, if necessary, the work capacity evaluation includes simulation of the actual job. For example, a patient seen in therapy was injured at a meat-cutting plant. His injury was a stabbing wound to his right forearm, involving muscle and circulatory damage. His initial grip strength was 5 pounds. After 5 months his grip was 65 pounds, and the physician was asked if the patient could return to work. The problem was that after activities requiring a prolonged grasp, such as meat cutting would involve, his grip decreased to 40 pounds and his hand and forearm became edematous. With this information it was decided that it would be unsafe for him to return to work as a meat cutter as he might lose his grip on the knife.

The patient became involved in vocational rehabilitation, and his vocational evaluator asked the occupational therapist to do a work capacity evaluation to determine whether this patient could do janitorial work. Besides doing the standardized tests, a simulation of janitorial activities was also done. Activities that needed to be assessed were lifting trash bags, sweeping, mopping, operating a buffing machine, pushing a cart, and using spray cans, a sponge, and a dust broom. The results of this assessment demonstrated this to be a realistic option for the patient.

Work capacity evaluations are a new area of hand rehabilitation that is providing objective measurements and more reliable information to assist in determining whether the hand-injured patient can safely return to his or her occupation. This is an exceedingly important determination for the patient, his or her co-workers, the employer, and the physician.

References

1. Eckenhoff EA: Medical rehabilitation for disabled employees. *Business and Health* 1984;(May).

2. Rules of Procedures of Colorado: Rules and regulations pursuant to CRS 1973 §8-46-108 regarding benefits under the *Workman's Compensation Act of Colorado,* the *Colorado Medical Disaster Insurance Fund Act,* and the *Colorado Major Medical Insurance Fund Act.* part V, Nov 1983.
3. *Valpar Component Work Sample Series: Whole Body Range of Motion, No. 9.* Tucson, AZ, Valpar Corp, 1974.
4. *Valpar Component Work Sample Series: Upper Extremity Range of Motion, No. 4.* Tucson AZ, Valpar Corp, 1974.
5. Curtis RM, Clark GL, Snyder RA: *Work simulator. J Hand Surg* 1981; 6:499–501.
6. Matheson L: *Work Capacity Evaluation,* Trabuco Canyon CA, ERIC, 1984.
7. Spackman CS, Willard HS: *Occupational Therapy.* Philadelphia, JP Lippincott Co, 1947, pp 223–234.
8. Spackman CS, Willard HS: *Occupational Therapy,* Hopkins HL, Smith HD (eds). Philadelphia, JP Lippincott Co, 1978, pp 203–218.
9. US War Department: *Occupational Therapy.* Technical Manual 8-291. Government Printing Office, 1944.

29

Joint Protection in Rheumatic Disease

Debbie Post

Joint protection is essential in treating patients with rheumatic diseases and vital in the treatment regime. Joint protection is based on the knowledge of joint anatomy, the mechanics of the soft tissues surrounding the joint, and the kinesiology and pathology of the varieties of arthritis. A detailed look at the patient's daily activities along with the joint and body mechanics they use during these activities is necessary. This examination enables the therapist to become aware of those actions and movements that contribute to the exacerbation of the patient's disease, to decrease in function, and to possible production of joint changes.

One of the primary goals of the occupational therapist is to educate all arthritis health professionals, including physicians, in the area of joint protection and its importance. Physicians will not refer the patient for joint protection education until they are made aware of its purpose. To accomplish this goal, the therapist must be knowledgeable in the pathomechanics of normal and rheumatic joints in relation to daily activities.

To illustrate these principles, let us look at the hand, and specifically at the metacarpophalangeal (MP) joints. The asymmetry of the metacarpal heads and the inequality in length and attachment of the collateral ligaments account for a normal tendency toward ulnar deviation of the fingers. This action is further accentuated by the long flexor tendons, which move ulnarly and palmarly during pinch and grip activities.

In rheumatic disease with hand involvement, the ulnar and palmar forces generated by the flexor tendons in their sheaths may act adversely, actually stretching the accessory collateral ligaments. The intrinsic muscles, which help provide flexor forces across the MP joint, can also become a deforming element. Ligamentous instability at the carpometacarpal (CMC) joint contributes to a "widening" of the transverse arch in flexion. This increased width of the hand causes ulnar displacing forces to be applied to the extensor tendons.

When the extrinsic extensor tendons across the MP joint become displaced ulnarly, the balance of the intrinsic extensor tendons is lost. These intrinsic muscles then further increase the tendency toward volar subluxation of the MP joint.

Once ulnar deviation and volar subluxation have occurred, the mechanics of muscle pull and the normal forces developed in functional activities will accentuate any structural joint changes or deformities. The main purpose of joint protection education is to teach the patient techniques of redistributing the forces during these functional activities proportionately to the strength, vulnerability, and mechanics of the involved joint.

General Principles

In educating the patient in joint protection, certain general principles must be outlined. The therapist must consider the patient's personality, educational level, and rate of compliance and then individualize the principles to the patient's specific problems.

Respect for Pain

It is important for the patient to understand the source of joint pain and how to monitor activity appropriately. Fear of joint pain will allow the patient to become inactive, whereas total disregard for joint pain can lead to unnecessary joint damage and a possible flare-up of the disease. The patient must learn to distinguish between "usual" arthritic discomfort and the pain resulting from excessive stress to the joints. The patient needs to be taught that when pain occurs and lasts for more than 1 hour after finishing an activity, the time, energy, and effort spent on that activity should be reduced. The patient should also learn to carry out activities and exercises only up to the point of fatigue or discomfort, *before* any pain occurs.

Importance of Rest

Taking the time for rest periods is probably the hardest principle of joint protection for patients to learn to incorporate into their life-styles. It should be stressed to the patients, however, that rest is one of the most effective weapons they can use against the demands of their disease if it is used efficiently and appropriately. It is important that the patient learn to rest *before* becoming exhausted. Allowing for a 5- to 10-minute rest between activities can be difficult, but it can significantly increase the patient's overall endurance. Although it may lengthen the total time spent on activities such as household duties, it will allow more energy for enjoyable leisure activities.

The Four Ps of Joint Protection

The following points should be stressed with all patients in therapy for rheumatic disease.

Planning

Educate patients to plan out their activities for each day. Planning will help with organization and will decrease total energy spent.

Priorities

Teach patients to become more goal oriented. Each day the individual patient should plan which three to four goals are to be accomplished. Encourage patients to keep the goals within easy reach, varying from one specific household chore to that necessary coffee break at work.

Pacing

Patients should be taught to balance their activities with their rest periods. For example, they should plan to follow their shopping chores with a more restful activity such as paying the bills. Patients should also remember not to attempt any activity that cannot be stopped immediately.

Positioning

Any activity requiring static positions should be modified to provide frequent joint range of motion. Prolonged periods of sitting, holding a book, or writing cause an increase in stiffness. Patients need to learn to shift positions every 15 to 30 minutes, depending on the activity, to prevent stiffness from occurring.

Transferring Work to Stronger Joints

The principle of using larger, stronger joints to perform any given activity should become an unconscious habit with the patient. The larger joints, having more muscle bulk, often are not as involved in the disease and therefore are not as susceptible to structural joint changes as the smaller joints. A common example of this principle is the use of a strap to pull open a cabinet door, thus taking the stress off the finger joints and applying it to the forearm. The patient needs to be taught to rely on the strong leg and stomach muscles for lifting, pushing, and pulling activities rather than strain the back.

Avoiding Positions of Deformity

It is extremely important for the patient to remember to avoid positions of deformity, keeping in mind the deforming mechanical forces in a normal joint. Cordery demonstrates this principle with an excellent example of the normal hand using a hand-operated can opener. The left hand grips the levers of the can opener, forcing the MP joints into hard flexion. The collateral ligaments of the MP joints (which are tight in flexion) are under great strain, compounded by the large volar forces of the long flexor tendons. In the right hand, the tips of the fingers and the lateral tip of the thumb pinch against each other to twist the key of the opener. The flexor digitorum profundus flexes the distal interphalangeal joint (DIP). The intrinsics flex the MP joint and through the lateral bands extend the proximal interphalangeal (PIP) joint. The flexor digitorum sublimus cannot hold the PIP joint out of extension at this point, so the position of swan-neck deformity occurs. Also, during this strong grasp the extensor digitorum communis does not contract, allowing the hood of the extensor expansion to be stretched at its most distal point on the joint. This stretch allows the long extensor tendon to be displaced in an ulnar direction on the fingers with a lateral force being applied to the thumb.

This obvious example of stress to a normal joint during a simple activity underlines the need for education in joint protection in the rheumatoid hand, to aid in the minimization of pain, inflammation, and possible deformities while maintaining and increasing the patient's functional abilities.

Reducing the Force Applied to the Joint

Reduction of the amount of force applied to a joint may be accomplished in several different ways. One option is to change the method of carrying out the activity by redistributing the forces. The patient should be taught to hold items parallel to the MP joints rather than diagonally to reduce the stress on the radial side of the fingers, for example, when stirring food or using eating utensils. The use of special equipment is another example of reducing stress to the involved joint. The patient may use a raised toilet seat to aid the knee joints, a wrist brace to help support the wrist joint, or a reacher to decrease active movement in a painful shoulder. The method of last resort in reducing stress is elimination of the activity.

Patients need to be encouraged that joint protection education is something positive that can be done for their arthritis. By incorporating joint protection principles into their life-styles, patients will find they can reduce flare-ups and combat fatigue and pain, thus decreasing unnecessary stress to the involved joints. Each patient can then become the "director" of his or her own rehabilitation team, giving a sense of accomplishment and control in working with such a chronic disease.

Bibliography

Backhouse KM: Mechanics of normal digital control in the hand and an analysis of the ulnar drift of rheumatoid arthritis. Read before the Royal College of Surgeons of England, London, Jan 6, 1966.

Cordery JC: Joint protection—A responsibility of the occupational therapist. *Am J Occup Ther* 1965;19:285–294.

Hakstian RW: Ulnar deviation of the fingers. *J Bone Joint Surg Am* 1967; 49A:299–316.

Melvin JL: Joint protection training and energy conservation, in *Rheumatic Disease: Occupational Therapy and Rehabilitation.* Philadelphia, FA Davis Co., 1977, pp 191–206.

Smith EM, Juvinall RC, Bender LF, et al: Role of the finger flexors in rheumatoid deformities of the metacarpophalangeal joints. *Arthritis Rheum* 1964;7:467–479.

Smith RJ: Balance and kinetics of the fingers under normal and pathological conditions. *Clin Orthop Rel Res* 1974;104:92–110.

Smith RJ, Kaplan EB: Rheumatoid deformities at the metacarpophalangeal joints of the fingers. *J Bone Joint Surg Am* 1967;49A:31–46.

Swanson A: Pathomechanics of deformities in hand and wrist, in Hunter JM, Schneider LH, Mackin EJ, et al (eds): *Rehabilitation of the Hand.* St. Louis, CV Mosby Co, 1984, pp 638–650.

Index

H

I

J

K

L

M

T